MEDICAL RADIOLOGY

Diagnostic Imaging

P. Lefere · S. Gryspeerdt (Eds.)

Virtual Colonoscopy

A Practical Guide

2nd Edition

With Contributions by

Y. Arai · D. Bielen · F. Booya · D. Burling · F. Cerri · A. H. Dachman · A. H. de Vries
H. Fenlon · J. G. Fletcher · S. Gryspeerdt · L. S. Guimaraes · S. Halligan · G. Iinuma
A. Laghi · P. Lefere · A. Maier · T. Mang · B. G. McFarland · R. Mendelson · M. Miyake
N. Moriyama · K. J. Mortelé · Y. Muramatsu · D. Murphy · E. Neri · P. R. Obara
A. S. Odulate · M. Raquel Oliva · P. Pokieser · W. Schima · J. Stoker · S. A. Taylor · F. Turini
K. Uchida · J. Yee · H. Yoshida · M. E. Zalis

Foreword by

A. L. Baert

With 198 Figures in 355 Separate Illustrations, 146 in Color and 16 Tables

Springer

Philippe Lefere, MD
Stedelijk Ziekenhuis Roeselare
Department of Radiology
Bruggesteenweg 90
8800 Roeselare
Belgium

Stefaan Gryspeerdt, MD
Stedelijk Ziekenhuis Roeselare
Department of Radiology
Bruggesteenweg 90
8800 Roeselare
Belgium

Medical Radiology · Diagnostic Imaging and Radiation Oncology
Series Editors:
A. L. Baert · L. W. Brady · H.-P. Heilmann · M. Knauth · M. Molls · C. Nieder

Continuation of Handbuch der medizinischen Radiologie
Encyclopedia of Medical Radiology

ISBN: 978-3-540-79879-8 e-ISBN: 978-3-540-79886-6

DOI: 10.1007/978-3-540-79886-6

Springer Heidelberg Dordrecht London New York

Medical Radiology · Diagnostic Imaging and Radiation Oncology ISSN 0942-5373

Library of Congress Control Number: 2009931697

Cover design: Publishing Services Teichmann, 69256 Mauer, Germany

Printed on acid-free paper

9 8 7 6 5 4 3 2 1

Springer is part of Springer Science+Business Media (www.springer.com)

Foreword

Rapid progress in the technique and practice of virtual colonoscopy as well as the continuing clinical high interest for this radiodiagnostic procedure made this second edition, only 3 years after the publication of the first edition of this successful volume, necessary.

This new edition includes the latest study results and technical developments of this exciting noninvasive diagnostic modality for the evaluation of the colon. The technical presentation and lay out of the text and of the many new illustrations are impeccable.

The editors were again able to ensure the collaboration of many international leaders in the field and the book offers a very comprehensive overview of all aspects and issues of CT colonography with a focus on how to perform practically this examination, which requires meticulous technique starting from rigorous preparation, then the conduct of the study itself, and finally the interpretation of the results.

I am very much indebted to the editors and the collaborating authors for preparing this outstanding volume in a record short time period, which enabled them to include the latest technical advances in this rapidly evolving important radiological method. It is highly recommended to general and gastrointestinal radiologists as well as gastroeneterologists as a most welcome update of their knowledge and as a practical guide in their daily practice. I am convinced that this second edition will meet the same success with our readership as the first one.

Leuven, Belgium

Albert L. Baert
Series Editor

Preface to the Second Edition

The publication of this second revised edition of the practical guide on virtual colonoscopy less than 4 years after the publication of the first edition underscores the big interest for CT colonography. In the past 4 years, the promising expectations of the technique were confirmed by several large multicenter studies obtaining very good results for colorectal neoplasia detection. This was possible by establishing a state-of-the-art technique of CT colonography (CTC) in combination with image interpretation performed by experienced teams. This updated edition confirms the efforts of the international CTC community to promote this technique as a widely accepted imaging technique for exploring the colon for colorectal neoplasia. In the past 4 years, these efforts have been focused on the development and fine tuning of the state-of-the-art application of CTC in order to allow widespread implementation of a high-quality total colonic examination. All different aspects of the CTC technique are widely covered in this edition. In the past years, it also became obvious that a structured education is mandatory in obtaining sufficient expertise in CTC before starting the technique in a clinical practice. This expertise will prove invaluable for CTC to become a robust technique performed on a high scientific level by a large community of radiologists. Once this goal is achieved, it will be possible considering reimbursement of CTC and its use as tool for population-based screening for colorectal cancer.

We are very grateful to all authors of the first and second edition, who made both issues a very rich resource of information on CT colonography and to the series editor of this book, Professor Dr. A.L. Baert, who enabled this second revised edition.

Roeselare, Belgium

Philippe Lefere
Stefaan Gryspeerdt

Preface to the First Edition

Virtual colonoscopy or computed tomographic (CT) colonography is a recent radiological technique enabling detection of tumoral lesions in the colon. As in the past two decades its radiological predecessor, double-contrast barium enema (DCBE), has lost most of its adherents, CT colonography constitutes a real opportunity for gastrointestinal radiologists to play a preponderant role in the diagnosis and treatment of colorectal cancer and the adenoma. Since its introduction by David Vining in 1994, CT colonography has very rapidly shown its virtues as a possible substitute for DCBE. The first important study on CT colonography by Helen Fenlon from the Boston Medical Center, published in 1999 in the *New England Journal of Medicine,* reporting very good lesion detection, underscored this aspiration. Since then, CT colonography has markedly evolved by the refinement of existing techniques and the introduction of new ones: fecal tagging with the option of reducing the cathartic or laxative part of the preparation, the use of carbon dioxide to inflate the colon, the introduction of multidetector CT scanners producing spectacular images with isotropic resolution and reducing the examination time for the patient, the use of ultra-low-dose scan protocols reducing the radiation burden, improvement of the image postprocessing with fast three-dimensional functions, and computer-aided diagnosis (CAD). These technical improvements help both the radiologist and the patient. For the former, there is an improvement of the reading conditions, possibly improving diagnostic accuracy; for the latter, the preparation and examination are more comfortable.

Despite these improvements in technique, however, CT colonography has not yet been able to break through as an acceptable tool for colorectal cancer screening. This is because of the disappointing results in some recent large multicenter trials. Most probably suboptimal technique in preparation, colonic distension, scanning parameters, and image postprocessing was the main cause of this failure. In fact, each of these stages needs rigorous attention if one is to achieve optimal results like those obtained in another momentous study, performed by Perry Pickhardt and published in the *New England Journal of Medicine* in 2003. Based upon a meticulous technique of preparation with fecal tagging, colonic inflation, scanning parameters, and reading conditions, CT colonography obtained better scores than optical colonoscopy in this study. Furthermore, the examinations were interpreted by a team of radiologists experienced in CT colonography. This brings us to another important aspect of CT colonography. As was the case with DCBE, the degree of experience needed to adequately read and interpret CT colonography should not be underestimated.

In experienced hands, CT colonography seems to be ripe for prime-time colorectal cancer screening. However, it is not yet ready for widespread application of screening for the aforementioned reasons. CT colonography is now at an important crossroad, and serious efforts should be undertaken to take it to the level of being a widely accepted screening method for colorectal cancer. To fulfill this goal, tremendous efforts are being undertaken in both Europe and the United States to educate radiologists with workshops, data banks, and numerous scientific publications.

With contributions from several leaders in the field, this book, entirely dedicated to this exciting technique, sets out to be a guide for both the beginner and the experienced CT colonographer. It provides the reader with a wealth of information on all the prerequisites to perform state-of-the-art CT colonography.

We want to express our sincere gratitude and appreciation to all the renowned radiologists experienced in CT colonography who have contributed to this volume. We also thank Professor Albert L. Baert, who gave us the unique opportunity to edit this book and to bring it to a successful conclusion.

We hope that the reader will enjoy this work and will find it a help when performing CT colonography.

Roeselare, Belgium

Philippe Lefere
Stefaan Gryspeerdt

Contents

Why We Do CTC: Screening for Colorectal Cancer

Richard M. Mendelson

CONTENTS

Richard M. Mendelson, MD
Department of Diagnostic and Interventional Radiology, Royal Perth Hospital, Wellington Street, Perth, Western Australia 6001, Australia

1.1 Introduction: What Is Screening?

Screening is a method of secondary prevention by testing to detect a target disease in individuals with no symptoms of that disease to identify those at increased risk and/or to detect the disease or its precursor with the purpose of reducing the risk of dying from the disease. The aim of population screening is to reduce the mortality rate from the disease in the community. Screening is not necessarily equivalent to diagnosis but it identifies those with an increased chance of having the disease. In most situations further diagnostic tests are required for those individuals testing positive at screening. However, in the case of colorectal neoplasm (CRN) screening, if colonoscopy is the chosen method, diagnosis (by biopsy of any abnormality) can be performed at the same time as screening.

It is important to note that any screening program should identify and redirect those with significant symptoms or those with increased risk factors towards more appropriate investigations.

1.2 Types of Screening: Some Definitions

All three of the screening strategies outlined below are applicable to colorectal cancer (CRC):

- *Mass population screening*: This is a strategy aimed at risk reduction from the disease in large populations containing groups at variable risk. Asymptomatic people are screened for the target disease in order to classify them as likely or unlikely to have the disease and to reduce the mortality rate from the disease in *the population.* In the case of screening tests with only moderate sensitivity, such as fecal occult blood testing for colorectal neoplasia, this concept may be difficult for the *individual* to comprehend and accept the need for serial testing over time.
- *Selective (or targeted) screening:* Individuals or groups of people at higher than average risk of disease are screened.
- *Case-finding:* This occurs in a clinical setting and may be opportunistic, the physician initiating the test in patients consulting him/her for unrelated problems, or it may be initiated by the patient himself/herself. In the context of CRC, the individual asymptomatic person aged 50 years or over who is concerned about the possible presence of CRC may be directed by their physician to appropriate testing depending on their risk factors, such as family history (see Sect. 1.5.1).

1.3 Why Screen for Colorectal Neoplasm?

CRC is a disease ideally suited to screening, in that it satisfies all of the WHO Principles of Screening: (Wilson and Jungner 1968)

- *The target disease should be an important and/or common one with high morbidity and/or mortality:* CRC is in the top two or three most common noncutaneous cancers in the developed world and is the second most common cause of cancer death in the USA. A 50-year-old woman or man at average risk for CRC has a 5.25–5.37% lifetime

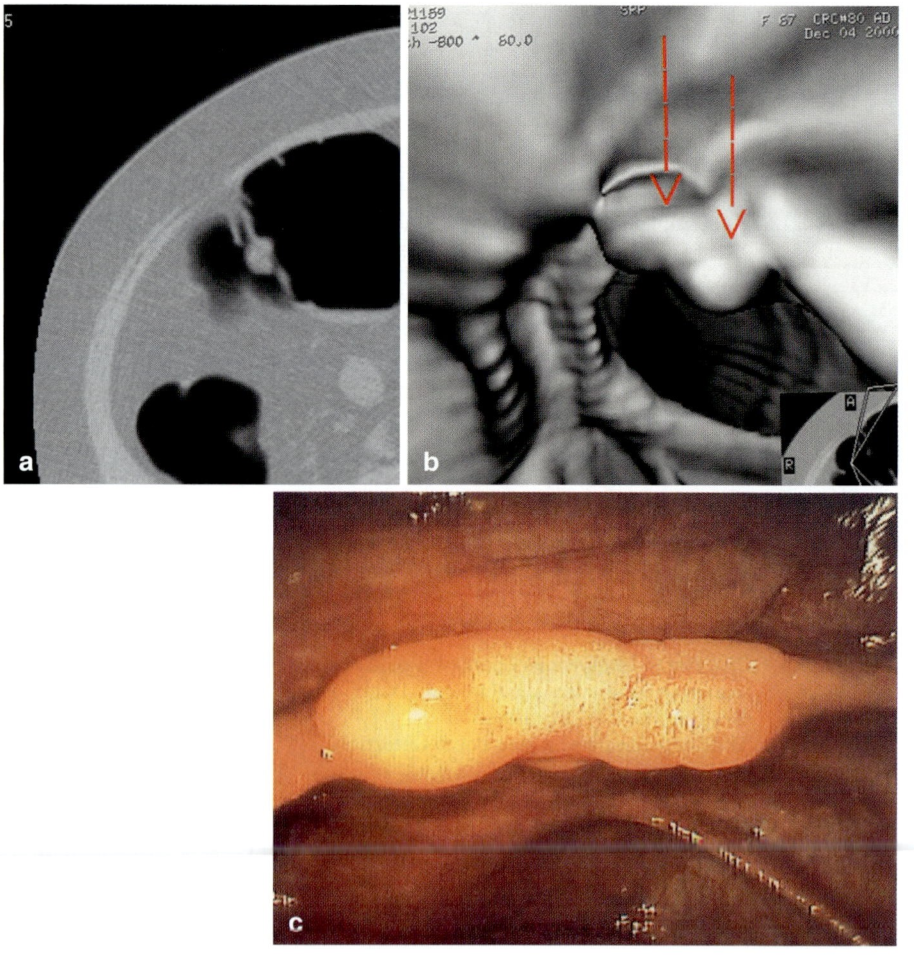

Fig. 1.1. Twelve millimeter polyp in ascending colon demonstrated in 67-year-old asymptomatic woman undergoing screening CTC (**a**) axial image (**b**) 3D endoluminal view (**c**) endoscopic image. Polypectomy performed. Histology showed adenoma with high grade dysplasia

chance, respectively, of developing CRC and a 2–3% chance of dying from it (EDDY 1990).

- *The natural history of the disease should be understood*: It is widely recognized that most CRCs develop from preexisting adenomas – the adenoma–carcinoma sequence (MORSON 1974). The risk of cancer being harbored within a polyp is related to its size. A 10 mm polyp has about 1% chance of being malignant. The chance of malignancy developing within a polyp is increased if it is an "*advanced adenoma*" – that is, one measuring 10 mm or more and/or having villous components and/or showing dysplasia (Fig. 1.1). About 6–9% of average-risk asymptomatic individuals over 50 years of age have advanced adenomas at screening colonoscopy (LIEBERMAN et al. 2000). There is evidence that a polyp 10 mm or larger in size has a cumulative risk of about 8% of developing into cancer at 10 years (STRYKER et al. 1987). Diminutive polyps (5 mm or less) are as likely to be hyperplastic as adenomatous; those that are adenomas are highly unlikely to have advanced features and the chance of malignancy within the lesion at diagnosis is negligible. The 10-year risk for CRC is estimated to be 0.08% in diminutive polyps and 0.7% for intermediate-size polyps (6–9 mm). Furthermore, there is evidence that these intermediate-size polyps are indolent or may even regress. Lastly, in the recent years it has become apparent that there is an intermediate type of polyp – the serrated polyp – that occupies a position on the spectrum between classical adenomas and hyperplastic polyps that is intermediate and has a propensity for malignant change (see later).
- *There should be a recognizable latent or early symptomatic phase*: the colorectal adenoma is a premalignant lesion which is usually asymptomatic, and although only a small minority of adenomas, perhaps one in twenty, become malignant, a subset – the advanced adenomas (see above) – are known to have a greater malignant potential than adenomas without these features. The prevalence of such polyps is up to approximately 9% in asymptomatic average-risk individuals over 50 years of age. Some screening tests (such as optical colonoscopy and CT colonography) can detect adenomas, while others (such as fecal occult blood tests [FOBT]) predominantly detect CRC.
- *There should be an effective and acceptable treatment available for those with the disease*: Adenomas can be reasonably safely removed by colonoscopic polypectomy. Early invasive carcinomas can also be removed at surgery with acceptably small attendant morbidity and mortality.
- *Treatment should be more effective if started early in the natural history of the disease*: Polypectomy effectively prevents development of cancer in that lesion. In addition, in a cohort of patients undergoing polypectomy there is a lower than expected incidence of CRC. Dukes Stage D cancers carry a 5-year survival of about 5% whereas following surgery for early invasive cancer there is a 5-year survival of about 95%.
- Test procedures should be:
  - Acceptable to the general population
  - Repeatable
  - Quick and easy to interpret
  - Safe
  - Have high specificity and high sensitivity
- *Cost of screening and treatment should be cost-effective and economical in relation to expenditure on health as a whole.* Cost-benefit analysis may be computed in several ways but essentially balances the various financial and other costs including, time off work, costs of follow-up diagnostic tests and treatment, as well as the burden of false-positive results and complications, compared to the benefit of reducing loss of net earnings from premature death and other desired outcomes. Measurement of cost-effectiveness is usually expressed in terms of cost per life-year saved. The financial and emotional costs of a screening test may be set too high if the test has poor specificity, leading to expensive and possibly hazardous investigation of false-positive results. In this situation specificity of the screening test should be optimized, even at the sacrifice of a small reduction in sensitivity (COLE and MORRISON1980; MILLER 2008). This issue is pertinent with regard to fecal occult blood testing (see later).
- *Case-finding should be a continuous process.* There is no convincing evidence that one-off screening for CRN is effective in reducing lifetime risk of CRC. Particularly for tests of relatively low sensitivity such as fecal occult blood testing it is important that subjects are part of a program that involves serial testing.

1.4 Screening Tests

1.4.1 The "Ideal" Screening Test

In the setting of population screening, the test attributes of feasibility, acceptability and participation rates, safety and cost-effectiveness are vital.

Effectiveness measures the outcome in the screened population against the outcome in an equivalent unscreened population and determines if the testing does more good than harm. As healthy people are the subjects, any test must have a minimal potential for harm and the screening method must have been shown to offer benefit at a population level.

Any effective screening test must reduce the overall mortality from the target disease. *Cost-effectiveness* measures the cost (in financial terms) or the relative value of the test – usually in terms of cost per year of life gained in the target population.

For most target diseases and most screening tests, serial testing is required – the interval determined by the natural history of the disease, the sensitivity of the test, and the risk profile of the individual or group. Ideally a screening test will detect all the prevalent cases in the target population at the first screening event (that is, the disease existing in that population at the time of initiation of screening) and detect the incident cases (that is, new or interval cases) at subsequent screening events.

All individuals testing positive on screening should progress to a diagnostic test. Ideally a screening test should have *high sensitivity* – that is, it should be able to detect most of the disease with few false negatives – but also have a *low false-positive* rate. False-positives expose the screened individual to harm without benefit, including financial cost, anxiety, and the risks associated with any subsequent diagnostic test or intervention. *False negative* results may lead to a false belief by the screened individual that the disease has been entirely excluded.

Of the tools that are available for CRN screening, none is perfect. It is important to recognize that some tests, such as FOBT, are used essentially for CRC screening, whereas others such as optical colonoscopy and CT colonography are methods of CRN screening in that they detect neoplastic precursors of CRC (polyps) with the aim of preventing CRC, as well as detecting CRC itself.

1.4.2 Problems with Screening

These are manifold:

- *Test related.* A suitable screening test has high sensitivity and satisfactory specificity. Many screening tests, such as FOBT may be "set" at a level to provide maximum sensitivity, but usually at the trade-off of reduced specificity. In this scenario, false positives are increased and lead to unnecessary further tests (colonoscopy) with attendant costs and risks, as well as engendering misguided anxiety in the subjects. Semiquantitative tests may therefore be set to maximize specificity (see Sect. 1.5.2).
- *Preparation.* Many tests require preparation of the patient. In the case of CRN screening, this may constitute dietary manipulation and/or cathartic use, which many individuals find problematic or uncomfortable.
- *Psychological.* Many people prefer not to know whether they have cancer or a precursor of cancer and anticipate problems dealing with a positive result. Others find it difficult to accept, due to lack of knowledge or psychological factors, that they can be well and still harbor a disease that could be potentially fatal.
- *Costs.* Even though population screening programs should have to be shown to be effective before adoption, it is only the rich countries that can afford to run them. If the health system requires the subject to contribute financially to the cost of the test, this will inevitably reduce uptake and compliance.
- General acceptability
  - *Preparation.* It has been consistently demonstrated that patients find bowel preparation the worst part of large bowel imaging. Compliance would undoubtedly be increased if a preparation-free method of examining the colon could be reliably achieved.
  - *Procedure.* All the methods for CRN screening involve some potential unpleasantness for the subject. Some individuals find the need for preparing their stool for FOBT unacceptable, others do not like the idea of sedation for colonoscopy, and still others find the discomfort of bowel distension without sedation for CT Colonography unacceptable. This emphasizes the desirability of offering a menu of options to the would-be screened.

- *Likelihood of repeating.* Current recommendations require repeated testing at regular intervals for all the recognized modalities. Whether "once-off" negative colonoscopy or CTC will prove to have lifelong protection remains to be proven.

1.5 Screening Tests for Colorectal Neoplasm

1.5.1 Risk Stratification for CRN

Symptomatic patients require diagnostic testing and are not the subject of this chapter.

Asymptomatic individuals may be stratified largely by their family history into (1) average or slightly above average risk, (2) moderately increased risk, and (3) high risk.

About 98% of the population is at average or slightly above average risk, usually defined as people with no personal history of colorectal neoplasia or inflammatory bowel disease, and up to one first- or second-degree relatives diagnosed with cancer at the age of 55 or over.

Those individuals at moderate and high risk are normally advised to undergo colonoscopy. These will not be further discussed here.

For individuals at average or slightly increased risk it is generally agreed that screening should start at the age of 50 years and there are several options available for screening. Recommendations will vary from country to country. In the UK and Australia only stool testing for occult blood is sanctioned, being the only method that has been shown to be effective at a population level at the highest level of evidence. In the USA several methods are recommended, the main thrust of advice being that a range of options be made available (Davila et al. 2006; Levin et al. 2008). The recently revised guidelines, published jointly by the American Cancer Society, the US Multisociety Taskforce on CRC and the American College of Radiology, indicate that screening aimed at prevention of CRC – that is, strategies for detection of adenomas – is the preferred primary goal of screening (Levin et al. 2008). This would tend to militate against fecal occult blood testing (see below).

1.5.2 Fecal Occult Blood Testing

The first study to show reduced mortality from population screening by FOBT (Mandel et al. 1993) in a randomized controlled trial (RCT) was followed by other RCTs showing similar results (Hardcastle et al. 1996; Kronborg et al. 1996). FOBT is the only screening test which has been shown at this highest level of evidence to reduce mortality from CRC in a screened population (Hewitson et al. 2007). These trials used chemical (guaiac) tests but fecal immunochemical testing (FIT) is now available which has greater specificity for human hemoglobin and is not affected by diet or medications. However, RCTs comparing guaiac and FIT have not been carried out. FOBT is safe and reasonably acceptable, but with variable compliance. In the Nottingham and Danish population-based studies (which used guaiac tests) (Hardcastle et al. 1996; Kronborg et al. 1996) the compliance rate was 60% or more for those completing at least one screening round. However, some studies have shown considerable reduction in compliance for subsequent rounds of screening. The Australian FOBT pilot study employed FIT and resulted in a compliance rate of 45% (Australian Bowel Cancer Screening Pilot Program 2005). Guaiac FOBT has variable sensitivity for cancer; various commercially available tests can be grouped into those of high and low sensitivity, but high sensitivity is traded for some reduction in specificity. FIT is more sensitive and specific than guaiac tests (Allison et al. 2007) since only human hemoglobin is detected, and is associated with greater compliance as dietary restriction is unnecessary (Federici et al. 2005; Young and Cole 2007; Mandel 2008). While being successful in risk-reduction within the population tested, guaiac tests will only detect 40–60% of asymptomatic CRC, that is, at least 40% of CRCs will be missed. The sensitivity of FIT for cancer is on the order of 80%, but only a minority of advanced adenomas is detected. Sensitivity for polyps >10 mm is about 45–50% (Nakama et al. 2000).

In addition, the level of sensitivity of FITs can be adjusted (Smith et al. 2004). Quantitative FIT involves an inverse relationship between levels of sensitivity and specificity.

In the Australian Bowel Cancer Screening Pilot Program which employed two varieties of FIT, there was a 9% positivity rate. The PPV was 19.2% – that is, in those FIT-positive individuals progressing to colonoscopy, there was almost a one-in-five chance of having an advanced adenoma or cancer.

In view of the intermittent nature of bleeding from cancers and advanced adenomas, multiple fecal samples need to be tested. Relatively low sensitivity for CRN also means that individuals need to be in a screening program. Annual or biennial testing is advised for this test to achieve its full potential. Because of its variable and often only moderate PPV and NPV at an individual level, many people choose to undergo examinations with higher predictive values, such as colonoscopy or virtual colonoscopy.

In view of its unique place in being proven to be effective in RCTs, several countries including the United Kingdom and Australia, Australian Government National Bowel Cancer Screening Program, 2008 rely on FOBT for CRC screening of average-risk individuals and it is on the menu of options in the USA guidelines. Additional 5-yearly flexible sigmoidoscopy is recommended by several authorities.

1.5.3 Flexible Sigmoidoscopy

Flexible sigmoidoscopy (FS) has some advantages over colonoscopy in that less bowel preparation is required than for whole-colon examinations, it can be undertaken without sedation, and primary care physicians and paramedical staff can be trained to perform it. However, by definition it only examines the rectum and sigmoid colon and, at best, the descending colon.

The principles behind the use of FS for CRC screening are that 50–60% of cancers and advanced polyps are within detectable reach of the instrument (Imperiale et al. 2000; Lieberman and Weiss 2001) and that distal polyps are markers for increased risk of proximal neoplasms (Imperiale et al. 2000). Therefore, individuals with distal lesions should undergo a full colon examination.

However, between one third and one half of subjects (and probably more in older individuals and women) with advanced proximal neoplasms do not have a distal adenoma, and therefore would have a negative FS (Imperiale et al. 2000; Lieberman and Weiss 2001).

No RCTs of FS for population screening have been completed (but are currently ongoing), but high-quality case-control studies have shown a decrease in mortality in those individuals screened. (Davila et al. 2006; Levin et al. 2008)

Some authorities recommend 5 yearly FS in combination with yearly FOBT although the added benefit of FS appears to be minimal (Davila et al. 2006).

1.5.4 Colonoscopy

Optical colonoscopy (OC) alone, among the potential tools for CRN screening, additionally provides diagnostic and therapeutic options. All other screening strategies require the subject with a positive test to proceed to colonoscopy. Although, on balance, it is the most accurate of the modalities with the best predictive values (with the proviso that some studies have shown CT colonography to rival OC – see later), there are issues related to compliance, cost and complications. OC has not been the subject of RCTs for population screening for CRN and, therefore, in many health systems, it is not officially sanctioned. Nevertheless, several authorities do recommend OC as a primary screening procedure in average-risk subjects (Pox et al. 2007) and, even in constituencies where it is not, screening "by stealth" occurs on a moderately large scale (best described as case-finding) when patients within the appropriate age group, with minimal or questionable bowel symptoms are referred for colonoscopy. In Australia, more than 10% of the community have undergone OC or barium enema in the preceding 5 years.

A meta-analysis of screening colonoscopy publications found ten prospective cohort studies with a total of over 68,000 participants (mixed low and increased-risk subjects) in whom colonoscopy was completed in 97%, CRC was diagnosed in 0.78% (77% of which were Stage I or II), advanced adenomas were found in 5% and complications occurred in 0.06% (Niv et al. 2008). In the USA National Polyp Study, patients who underwent colonoscopy and clearing polypectomy had a 76% reduction in CRC incidence compared to the general population (Winawer et al. 1993). The data support the contention that detection and clearing of polyps at colonoscopy has a long-term impact on CRC incidence and mortality, but the reduction within the first 10 years was almost entirely due to the baseline colonoscopy. However, there are no published studies showing reduction in CRC mortality due to screening colonoscopy and some studies have documented greater rates of incident cancer after clearing colonoscopy than that demonstrated in the National Polyp Study (Rex and Eid 2008) – see Sect. 1.6.1.1.

The disadvantages of colonoscopy for population screening of average-risk individuals include the need for bowel preparation, risks and inconvenience of sedation, time off-work for the subject, risks of perforation and cost. There is also a dependency on the skill of the operator and studies have shown considerable variance in performance. There are also doubts as to whether there is capacity in the health system to perform the increased numbers of colonoscopies required for a screening program. However, modeling studies have shown that screening colonoscopy can be cost-effective (Lieberman 1995; Sonnenberg et al. 2000; Bolin et al. 2001; Pignone et al. 2002; Provenzale 2002).

Compliance with regard to population screening has important implications on cost-effectiveness (Lieberman 1995) and participation rates have been poor to moderate in most published series (Lieberman et al. 2000; Scott et al. 2004; Macs 2006; Pox et al. 2007).

Those authorities recommending colonoscopy as an option for screening suggest examination every 10 years for average-risk subjects with a normal baseline OC (Levin et al. 2008). This has the potential advantage of increasing cost-effectiveness and compliance rates over the need for more frequent FOBT (Sonnenberg et al. 2000).

1.5.5 Barium Enema

Although double contrast barium enema (DCBE) examination remains one of the options approved in the United States (Levin et al. 2008), it is being largely superseded by OC and CTC. Among trainee and recently qualified radiologists there are diminishing numbers who have sufficient expertise to provide an adequate service. In the screening context (and, indeed, for symptomatic patients) DCBE has little to offer over CTC. CTC is quicker, more accurate (Rockey et al. 2005), more comfortable for the patient (Taylor et al. 2003), and safe.

1.6 CT Colonography as a Screening Test for CRN

Recent large trials of CTC in screening asymptomatic subjects for CRN have led to guidelines jointly drawn up by the American Cancer Society, the U.S. Multisociety Task Force on Colorectal Cancer, and the American College of Radiology to recommend 5-yearly CT Colonography as an option for screening for average-risk individuals (Levin et al. 2008)

Considering the necessary criteria for a good screening test for CRN, how does CTC perform?

1.6.1 Accuracy (Table 1.1)

Like OC, CTC examines the whole of the large bowel and is aimed at detecting both CRC and its precursor, the advanced polyp.

There have been several meta-analyses of CTC accuracy (Sosna et al. 2003; Halligan et al. 2005; Mulhall et al. 2005; Rosman and Korsten 2007) which have analyzed studies which included low-prevalence subjects and increased prevalence subjects or symptomatic patients. These meta-analyses showed 85–93% sensitivity on a per patient basis for larger polyps and specificity of 95% or greater. There has certainly been variability of accuracy among

Table 1.1. Per patient accuracy of CTC for lesions 10 mm or larger: meta-analyses and studies in low-prevalence cohorts

	Sosna et al. 2003	Mulhall et al. 2005	Halligan et al. 2005	Rosman and Korsten 2007	Pickhardt et al. 2003	Johnson et al. 2008
Study type	Meta-analysis	Meta-analysis	Meta-analysis	Meta-analysis	Single center	Multicentre
Prevalence within study population	Mixed	Mixed	Mixed	Mixed	Low	Low
Sensitivity ≥10 mm	0.88 (CI 0.84–0.93)	0.85 (CI 0.79–0.91)	0.93 (CI 0.73–0.98)	0.82 (CI 0.76–0.88)	0.94	0.90
Specificity ≥10 mm	0.95 (CI 0.94–0.97)	0.97 (CI 0.96–0.97)	0.97 (CI 0.95–0.98)	0.96 (CI 0.94–0.98)	0.96	0.86

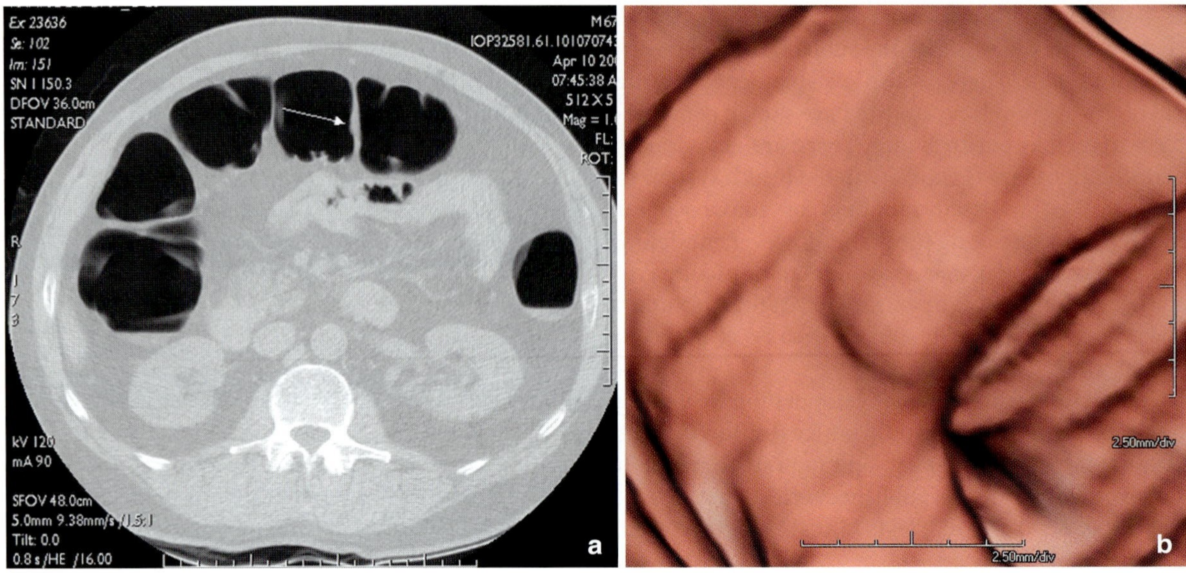

Fig. 1.2. Flat polyp in transverse colon. (**a**) Axial image showing height approximately one quarter of its width. (**b**) 3D endoluminal view. Endoscopic biopsy showed hyperplasia only

several individual studies. Two studies that have been widely quoted (Cotton et al. 2004; Rockey et al. 2005), in patients with clinical indications for investigation, cast doubts on the accuracy of CTC, reporting poor per patient sensitivity, even for lesions greater than 10 mm in size. The methodology of both of these studies has been criticized, particularly, with regard to the Cotton trial, the lack of experience of reporting radiologists. However, other studies have gone a long way towards abating criticism over the variability of accuracy of previous reports. A landmark study, employing meticulous methodology, and one of the few large studies of CTC in asymptomatic average-risk individuals, published by Pickhardt et al. (2003), reported excellent accuracy for CTC, equal or better than OC. This group's results have been attributed to state of the art scanning and software, using 3D as the primary read, and fecal tagging. Similarly, the recently published American College of Radiology Imaging Network (ACRIN) multicentre trial (Johnson et al. 2008a, b) reported excellent sensitivity for large adenomas and cancers. A further study compared the diagnostic yield from parallel OC and CTC screening programs and found similar detection rates of advanced neoplasia in the two groups (Kim et al. 2007).

What remains uncertain is the performance of CTC for so-called "flat" lesions and more importantly their significance, both numerically and pathologically (See Sect. 1.6.1.1). These lesions, however, are difficult to detect by any means, including conventional colonoscopic examination.

1.6.1.1 The Problem of Flat, Depressed and Serrated Lesions (Fig. 1.2)

Reports from Japan in the 1980s and 1990s documented that flat or depressed CRNs were common and frequently contained carcinoma. Flat polyps are defined as lesions whose height is less than half their greatest diameter. Despite initial skepticism in the West, it is now apparent that these Nonpolypoid Colorectal Neoplasms (NP-CRNs) (a name preferable to the oxymoronic "flat and depressed polyps") are not uncommon in non-Asian populations. Soetikno et al. (2008), using chromoendosocopy techniques, were able to document NP-CRNs in 9.3% of male veterans. These lesions harbored in situ or submucosal carcinoma at a rate five times higher than polypoid lesions of the same size. NP-CRNs are difficult to detect at conventional colonoscopy (spray dye techniques are necessary) and CTC. Less than 50% of flat lesions could be detected at CTC in one study (Park et al. 2006). It is highly likely that the failure to detect NP-CRNs accounts for a high proportion of interval cancers after apparent polyp clearance at baseline colonoscopy.

Most colorectal carcinomas develop through the "classic" pathway of the adenoma–carcinoma sequence.

Conventional teaching has also held that hyperplastic polyps (HPs) have no malignant potential. However, in recent years it has become apparent that there is an alternative pathway for colorectal carcinogenesis – the serrated pathway (East et al. 2008). Approximately 15% of sporadic CRCs are thought to arise de novo. These lesions are associated with high level microsatellite instability (MSI-H). MSI-H also occurs in a variant form of hyperplastic polyp which is intermediate between typical HPs and adenomas – the *serrated adenoma*. Some of these serrated adenomas (about 11%) show severe dysplasia or intramucosal carcinoma. In turn there are two types of serrated adenoma, the "traditional" serrated adenoma (TSA) and the sessile serrated adenoma (SSA). TSAs tend to be more pedunculated, villous and tubulovillous and situated distally in the colon. SSAs have a predilection for the proximal colon and, being sessile, account for some of the flat lesions missed at conventional colonoscopy and CTC and alluded to above. It is of interest that interval cancers after polyp "clearance" at colonoscopy are three times more likely to occur in the proximal colon than the left side and nearly four times more likely to be MSI-H lesions. It remains to be seen whether this alternative pathway for carcinogenesis proves to be a problem for screening programs that employ serial conventional colonoscopy or CT colonography examinations and whether the emerging technology of screening stool for DNA mutations, with or without a total colon examination, will address this issue. The issue of the flat lesion will extensively be discussed by Iinuma in Chap. 12.

1.6.2 Acceptability and Participation Rates

CTC is well tolerated, although comparisons of acceptability with optical colonoscopy show variable results – possibly due to the variable levels of sedation used for OC (Forbes and Mendelson 2000; Akerkar et al. 2001; Svensson et al. 2002; Gluecker et al. 2003). As for OC and barium enema, the bowel preparation is regarded by subjects as the least acceptable part of the examination.

Reduced preparation techniques accompanied by fecal tagging and electronic subtraction of feces have shown some success but have not yet been tested in large studies of asymptomatic subjects.

A completely preparation-free CTC examination is as yet an unfulfilled promise but would undoubtedly increase participation, compliance and acceptability.

Participation and compliance rates are critical to the success of any population screening program (Lieberman 1995), having a marked effect on risk-benefit and cost-benefit ratios. The participation rate in a study in Western Australia based on mail-out invitation only was 28.4% (Edwards et al. 2004). Further Australian studies showed no significant difference in participation rates between OC and CTC (Scott et al. 2004) and offering a choice of test made little difference (Macs 2006). It is apparent that any population-based program requires adequate publicity, "marketing" and education of doctors and patients (Zubarik et al. 2000).

1.6.3 Availability of CTC

The availability of CTC is dependent on the provision of a multidetector CT scanner, and technician and reader expertise. The pool of radiologists available to perform CTC is continually growing. One of the advantages of CTC over OC is the ability to read CTC remotely after images are transferred electronically over any distance. The question of whether enough radiologists can be provided to service a mass population screening program by CTC can only be addressed at a country by country level. In this, CTC has similar specialist staffing drawbacks to OC.

1.6.4 Cost-Effectiveness of CTC Screening

Attempts to model the cost-effectiveness of CTC are exercises in trying to hit a moving target. Results are self-evidently dependent on the sensitivity and specificity values and the unit cost of CTC used for the modeling, but also on other variables such as compliance rates. One such study, using the accuracy figures from the meta-analysis performed by Mulhall et al. (2005), found 3D CTC to be less effective and more expensive than optical colonoscopy but noted that 5-yearly 3D CTC could be a dominant strategy if colonoscopy costs were 1.6 times more than CTC and if sensitivity of CTC is greater than 83% for 10 mm adenomas (Vijan et al. 2007). Given the improved performance of CTC as shown in the ACRIN trial (Johnson et al. 2008a, b) it may be time to undertake another modeling exercise. See also Sect. 1.6.6

1.6.5
Risks and Side-Effects of CTC

1.6.5.1
Risks of Preparation (See Chap. 5)

1.6.5.2
Radiation Exposure

See Chap. 8

1.6.5.3
Colorectal Perforation

See Chap. 7

1.6.6
CTC as Triage in FOBT Positive Subjects

Because of the relatively high false positive rates in FOBT screening programs, concerns have been raised regarding access and availability of colonoscopy services to investigate subjects with a positive FOBT. To reduce the number of unnecessary colonoscopies the possibility has been mooted of using CTC as a triage tool for selection of these subjects for colonoscopy. One Australian study has modeled this strategy and found it not to be cost-effective (Walleser et al. 2007). However, this study used for calculation a pooled CTC sensitivity of only 63% for lesions of 10 mm or larger. A further study, published in abstract form (Liedenbaum et al. 2008) did not report cost-effectiveness, but reported that CTC can reduce the number of colonoscopies required, although the number is, as expected, influenced by the FOBT true positive rate. Further studies are required on this issue. However, there is likely to be an increased demand for CT colonography in those subjects having an incomplete follow-up optical colonoscopy subsequent to a positive FOBT. See also Sect. 1.6.4

1.7
CT Colonography Screening: Technique

1.7.1
Preparation

Currently, colon preparation is essential for accurate CTC. Residual fecal material can mimic polypoid lesions and obscure polyps. Preparation consists of three elements: diet, purgation and fecal and/or fluid tagging. The issue of preparation is further addressed by Yee in Chap. 5 and by Lefere in Chap. 6.

1.7.1.1
Diet

Most centers institute a low-residue and/or clear-fluid diet for 24–48 h prior to the examination.

1.7.1.2
Purgation

Bowel cleansing can be divided into "wet" and "dry" preparations. Wet preparations utilize colonic lavage solutions – usually polyethylene glycol (PEG) – up to 4 L in volume. This is the same preparation that is used by many colonoscopists. It has the disadvantage over "dry" preparations of being less well-tolerated and resulting in more residual fluid in the colon (Ginnerup Pedersen et al. 2002). The author uses a combination of 1 L of PEG followed by two sachets of sodium picosulphate on the day prior to the examination (Forbes et al. 2005).

1.7.1.3
Fecal and Fluid Tagging

The use of oral contrast agents, for fecal tagging and for tagging of residual fluid, is optional but the European Society of Gastrointestinal and Abdominal Radiology (ESGAR) consensus statement notes that it "should be considered" for screening CTC (Taylor et al. 2007). It should also be noted that the major trials of CTC screening that have shown the best results also employed both fecal and fluid tagging (Pickhardt et al. 2003; Johnson et al. 2008a, b).

1.7.2
Colonic Distension

Adequate colonic distension is imperative for a good quality CTC examination. The variables that determine the degree of distension include the method of insufflation (manual or automatic insufflator), the use of spasmolytics, the rate and volume of inflation and the end point for obtaining CT images. The latter is largely determined by patient tolerance (Dachman 2006). Colonic distension is extensively described in Chap. 7 by Burling.

An answer will be given on the following issues:

- Carbon dioxide vs. room air?
- Automated insufflation vs. manual insufflation?
- Which rectal catheter?
- The use of spasmolytics

1.7.3 The Use of Intravenous Contrast Agents

Within the context of CRN screening, there is no indication for the routine use of intravenous iodinated contrast agents. However, there may be an argument for performing the low-radiation dose, noncontrast prone scan before the supine scan and, if there is an obvious cancer on fast review of these images, undertaking a standard-dose supine scan with intravenous contrast material.

1.7.4 Scanning Parameters and Radiation Dose

Low-dose CTC has been shown to be effective in demonstrating CRN (Kim et al. 2007; Johnson et al. 2008a, b) and should be employed in screening of average-risk asymptomatic individuals in the interest of reducing the risk–benefit ratio of the examination. The aim should be to keep the total effective dose of the complete procedure (supine and prone scans combined) below 5 mSv. This issue will be discussed by Laghi in Chap. 8.

Table 1.2. Recommendations for reporting of colorectal lesions

CTC finding	Recommendation
Cancer likely	Urgent colonoscopy or surgical referral[a, b]
Polyp(s) ≥10 mm	Colonoscopy with view to polypectomy[a, b]
Polyp 6–9 mm (less than 3 in number)	Surveillance after 3 years[a] or refer for colonoscopy[a]
Polyps 6–9 mm (≥3 in number)	Colonoscopy[a]
Polyp(s) ≤5 mm	Not necessary to report, continue routine surveillance (5-yearly)[a, b] (alternative: report but add qualifying comments[c])
Polyps ≤5 mm (≥3 in number)	Consider follow-up at 3 years[c]

[a]Recommendation endorsed by Working Group on Virtual Colonoscopy (Zalis et al. 2005)
[b]Recommendation endorsed by ESGAR (Taylor et al. 2007)
[c]Author's discretionary practice

1.7.5 Reading the CTC Examination

Utilizing the above protocols, a complete two-position examination will usually yield between 1,000 and 1,200 images. Despite the use of CTC for over a decade, the technology for reading examinations continues to evolve.

Major CT scanner manufacturers and third-party vendors provide dedicated software packages for reading CTC examinations. Adequate interpretation requires a combination of 2D (axial images and multiplanar reformats) and 3D (endoluminal) views. Some readers use 2D images for primary interpretation and 3D for problem-solving, while others use the converse approach. The issue of image interpretation is covered by McFarland, Gryspeerdt, De Vries, Mang, and Fletcher in Chaps. 9–11, 16, and 17, respectively.

1.7.6 Effect of Computer Aided Polyp Detection on Screening CTC

Computer aided polyp detection (CAPD) software is a potentially valuable tool for training personnel to read CTC examinations. In the context of a mass screening program using CTC for CRN detection, CAPD is likely to prove useful in increasing the speed of reading examinations. Whether CAPD should be used as a primary, secondary or parallel reader remains uncertain. This subject is dealt with more fully by Yoshida in Chap. 14.

1.7.7 CT Colonography Reporting

In attempts at standardization, both the Working Group on Virtual Colonoscopy (Zalis et al. 2005) and the European Society of Gastrointestinal and Abdominal Radiology (Taylor et al. 2007) have published consensus on reporting of CTC.

The Working Group presents a practical guide – the CT Colonography Reporting and Data System (or "C-RADS") – which deals with lesion description and size and extra-colonic findings.

1.7.7.1 Reporting of Polyps at CTC (Table 1.2)

The natural history of colorectal polyps is described earlier in this chapter. In summary, size is an important determinant of risk of cancer development and is essentially the only parameter that can be assessed at CTC. In view of the increased risk associated with polyps 10 mm or larger, the consensus is that subjects with one or more of these found at screening CTC should be referred for colonoscopy and polypectomy. With regard to diminutive polyps of 5 mm or less, about half of these are hyperplastic and have no malignant potential (but see Sect. 1.6.1.1). Diminutive polyps that are adenomas are of almost negligible risk of malignancy at the time of detection and have a low risk of progression to cancer (see Sect. 1.3, above). Moreover, the estimated dwell time for conversion from adenoma to cancer for a polyp of less than 10 mm is estimated to be in the order of 10 years. Therefore if the subject is in a screening program, it can be anticipated that those diminutive polyps that do progress will be detected at the next screening event.

However, it is the author's discretionary practice depending on the referring doctor and the patient's clinical situation (1) to report polyps ≤5 mm but with a qualifying comment to the effect that "this is of negligible significance" or "risk" and (2) to report polyps ≤5 mm if they are greater than 3 in number and suggest follow-up in 3 years. The latter policy is in line with the opinion that the presence of three or more diminutive polyps increases the risk of developing CRC (Rex 2005).

Moreover, there can be little doubt that reporting of diminutive polyps at CTC leads to an increased false-positive rate and unnecessary colonoscopies with associated costs and risks. In one series the false-positive rate (by patient) fell from 12% when all suspected polyps were reported to 4.2% when a 5 mm threshold for reporting was applied, without loss of sensitivity for larger polyps (Edwards et al. 2004).

For these reasons, consensus guidelines from ESGAR (Taylor et al. 2007) and the Working Group on Virtual Colonoscopy (Zalis et al. 2005) recommend that polyps of 5 mm or less in size are not reported. Decision analysis modeling has recently shown that colonoscopic referral for diminutive polyps is not cost-effective given the low likelihood of advanced neoplasia and the high costs of colonoscopic polypectomy, and that for polyps of 6–9 mm, CTC surveillance may be a reasonable management option (Pickhardt et al. 2008).

The issue of what to do with intermediate sized polyps (6–9 mm) is a more difficult one. Intermediate sized polyps (6–9 mm) should be reported, but the question of how to proceed remains, to some extent, controversial. The risk of cancer at diagnosis is very small and the risk of development of cancer over 10 years is also small. It has also been shown that some 6–9 mm polyps can regress (Hofstad et al. 1996). The options are to recommend colonoscopic polypectomy (Rex 2005) or periodic surveillance (Zalis et al. 2005). Some advocate an individualized, informed choice by the patient rather than a physician-driven decision. Revised colorectal screening guidelines resulting from the joint effort of the American Cancer Society, US Multisociety Task Force on Colorectal Cancer and the American College of Radiology, recommend that subjects with three or more polyps of 6 mm or larger should be referred for colonoscopy (McFarland et al. 2008) on the assumption that these are adenomas and that subjects with three or more adenomas are at increased risk of advanced neoplasia. However, there is a lack of consensus on what to do for subjects with one or two 6–9 mm polyps. These guidelines arrive at a current expert consensus that recommendation should be made for colonoscopy. However, others suggest (as stated above) that surveillance may be a reasonable option (Pickhardt et al. 2008). For extensive explanation of CTC reporting see Chap. 15 by Dachman and Zalis.

1.7.7.2 Extracolonic Pathology

Among the CRN screening methods, CTC allows detection of extra-colonic abnormalities. This presents an opportunity to prevent or anticipate later morbidity (and mortality) but, conversely, poses a potential threat to the cost-effectiveness of CTC as a screening tool. Clinically important abnormalities, such as aortic aneurysms and extra-colonic malignancies, such as renal cancers, can be detected even at low-dose imaging. However, responsible reporting is essential to prevent unnecessary anxiety, inconvenience and cost to the patient in investigating lesions which are almost never clinically important – including liver lesions in subjects with no risk factors for significant focal liver pathology, and renal cystic disease. An Australian study (Chin et al. 2005) detected clinically relevant abnormalities in 7.4% of subjects; a potential clinical benefit from further investigation and treatment was estimated in 2.1%, with an incremental cost of CTC, spread over the entire cohort of 14.2%. The authors also state that limiting reporting to aortic aneurysms and renal masses would have reduced the need for follow-up imaging to 3.2% and the incremental cost to 4.7%.

The extracolonic findings are described by Neri in Chap. 13.

1.8 Future Developments

The future of CTC as a clinical tool in symptomatic patients is probably secure. Its role in screening is less certain. It is likely that compliance will only improve significantly if a reliable, truly preparation-free method is developed. In the interim, CTC remains one of several options that can be offered to asymptomatic average-risk individuals seeking CRN screening.

Other emerging technologies include capsule endoscopy of the colon (Adler et al. 2008), fecal DNA tests (Young and Cole 2007), and innovate endoscopic techniques, such as confocal microendoscopy (Anandasabapathy 2008). The role of these techniques in CRN screening remains to be assessed.

References

Adler DG, Chand B, Conway JD et al (2008) Capsule endoscopy of the colon. Gastrointest Endosc 68:621–623

Anandasabapathy S (2008) Endoscopic imaging: emerging optical techniques for the detection of colorectal neoplasia. Curr Opin Gastroenterol 24:64–69

Australian Bowel Cancer Screening Pilot and Beyond (2005) Final evaluation report. Screening monograph no 6. Commonwealth of Australia, Canberra

Australian Government: Department of Health and Ageing (2008) National Bowel Cancer Screening Program, 2008. http://www.cancerscreening.gov.au/internet/screening/publishing.nsf/Content/bowel-1lp. Accessed September 2008

Akerkar GA, Yee J, Hung R et al (2001) Patient experience and preferences toward colon cancer screening: a comparison of virtual colonoscopy and conventional colonoscopy. Gastrointest Endosc 54:310–315

Allison JE, Sakoda LC, Levin TR et al (2007) Screening for colorectal neoplasms with new fecal occult blood tests: update on performance characteristics. J Natl Cancer Inst 99: 1462–1470

Bolin TD, Lapsley HN, MGl K (2001) Screening for colorectal cancer: what is the most cost-effective approach? Med J Aust 174:298–301

Chin M, Mendelson R, Edwards J et al (2005) Computed tomographic colonography: prevalence, nature, and clinical significance of extracolonic findings in a community screening program. Am J Gastroenterol 100:2771–2776

Cole P, Morrison AS (1980) Basic issues in population screening for cancer. J Natl Cancer Inst 64:1263–1272

Cotton PB, Durkalski VL, Pineau BC et al (2004) Computed tomographic colonography (virtual colonoscopy): a multicenter comparison with standard colonoscopy for detection of colorectal neoplasia. JAMA 291:1713–1719

Dachman AH (2006) Advice for optimizing colonic distention and minimizing risk of perforation during CT colonography. Radiology 239:317–321

Davila RE, Rajan E, Baron TH et al (2006) ASGE guideline: colorectal cancer screening and surveillance. Gastrointest Endosc 63:546–557

Eddy D (1990) Screening for colorectal cancer. Annals Intern Med 113:373–384

Edwards JT, Mendelson RM, Fritschi L et al (2004) Colorectal neoplasia screening with CT colonography in average-risk asymptomatic subjects: community-based study. Radiology 230:459–464

East JE, Saunders BP, Jass JR (2008) Sporadic and syndromic hyperplastic polyps and serrated adenomas of the colon: classification, molecular genetics, natural history and clinical management. Gastoenterol Clin N Am 37:25–46

Federici A, Rossi P, Borgia P et al (2005) The immunochemical faecal occult blood test leads to higher compliance than the guaiac for colorectal cancer screening programmes: a cluster randomized controlled trial. J Med Screen 12: 83–88

Forbes GM, Edwards JT, Foster NM et al (2005) Randomized single blind trial of two low-volume bowel preparations for screening computed tomographic colonography. Abdom Imaging 30:48–52

Forbes GM, Mendelson RM (2000) Patient acceptance of virtual colonoscopy. Endoscopy 32:274–275

Ginnerup Pedersen B, Moller Christiansen TE, Viborg Mortensen F et al (2002) Bowel cleansing methods prior to CT colonography. Acta Radiol 43:306–311

Gluecker TM, Johnson CD, Harmsen WS et al (2003) Colorectal cancer screening with CT colonography, colonoscopy, and double-contrast barium enema examination: prospective assessment of patient perceptions and preferences. Radiology 227:378–384

Halligan S, Altman DG, Taylor SA et al (2005) CT colonography in the detection of colorectal polyps and cancer: systematic review, meta-analysis, and proposed minimum data set for study level reporting. Radiology 237:893–904

Hardcastle JD, Chamberlain JO, Robinson MH et al (1996) Randomised controlled trial of faecal-occult-blood screening for colorectal cancer. Lancet 348:1472–1477

Hewitson P, Glasziou P, Irwig L et al (2007) Screening for colorectal cancer using the faecal occult blood test, hemoccult (review). Cochrane Database Syst Rev (1):CD001216

Hofstad B, Vatn MH, Andersen S et al (1996) Growth of colorectal polyps: redetection and evaluation of unresected polyps for a period of three years. Gut 39:449–456

Imperiale TF, Wagner DR, Lin CY et al (2000) Risk of advanced proximal neoplasms in asymptomatic adults according to the distal colorectal findings. N Engl J Med 343:169–174

Johnson CD, Chen M-H, Toledano AY et al (2008a) Accuracy of CT colonography for detection of large adenomas and cancers. N Engl J Med 359:1207–1217

Johnson CD, Manduca A, Fletcher JG et al (2008b) Noncathartic CT colonography with stool tagging: performance with and without electronic stool subtraction. AJR Am J Roentgenol 190:361–366

Kim DH, Pickhardt PJ, Taylor AJ et al (2007) CT colonography versus colonoscopy for the detection of advanced neoplasia. N Engl J Med 357:1403–1412

Kronborg O, Fenger C, Olsen J et al (1996) Randomised study of screening for colorectal cancer with faecal-occult-blood test. Lancet 348:1467–1471

Levin B, Lieberman DA, McFarland B et al (2008) Screening and surveillance for the early detection of colorectal cancer and adenomatous polyps, 2008: a joint guideline from the American Cancer Society, the US Multi-Society Task Force on Colorectal Cancer, and the American College of Radiology. Gastroenterology 134:1570–1595

Lieberman D (1995) Cost-effectiveness model for colon cancer screening. Gastroenterology 109:1781–1790

Lieberman DA, Weiss DG (2001) One-time screening for colorectal cancer with combined fecal occult-blood testing and examination of the distal colon. N Engl J Med 345: 555–560

Lieberman DA, Weiss DG, Bond JH et al (2000) Use of colonoscopy to screen asymptomatic adults for colorectal cancer. Veterans Affairs Cooperative Study Group 380. N Engl J Med 343:162–168

Liedenbaum MH, van Rijn AF, de Vries AH et al (2008) CT colonography with limited bowel preparation: diagnostic performance in a FOBT positive screening population. Eur Radiol 18(Suppl.1):B471

The Multicentre Australian Colorectal Neoplasia Screening Group (MACS) (2006) A comparison of colorectal neoplasia screening tests: a multicentre community-based study of the impact of consumer choice. Med J Aust 184:546–550

Mandel JS (2008) Screening for colorectal cancer. Gastroenterol Clin North Am 37:97–115

Mandel JS, Bond J, Church J et al (1993) Reducing mortality from colorectal cancer by screening for fecal occult blood. N Engl J Med 328:1365–1371

McFarland EG, Levin B, Lieberman DA et al (2008) Revised colorectal screening guidelines: joint effort of the American Cancer Society, U.S. Multisociety Task Force on Colorectal Cancer, and American College of Radiology. Radiology 248:717–720

Miller AB (2008) Implementation of colon cancer screening: techniques, costs, and barriers. Gastroenterol Clin North Am 37:83–95

Morson BC (1974) The polyp-cancer sequence in the large bowel. Proc Roy Soc Med 67:451–457

Mulhall BP, Veerappan GR, Jackson JL et al (2005) Meta-analysis: computed tomographic colonography. Ann Intern Med 142:635–650

Nakama H, Fattah A, Zhang B et al (2000) A comparative study of immunochemical fecal tests for detection of colorectal adenomatous polyps. Hepatogastroenterology 47: 386–389

Niv Y, Hazazi R, Levi Z et al (2008) Screening colonoscopy for colorectal cancer in asymptomatic people: a meta-analysis. Dig Dis Sci 53:3049–3054

Park SH, Ha HK, Kim AY et al (2006) Flat polyps of the colon: detection with 16-MDCT colonography – preliminary results. AJR Am J Roentgenol 186:1611–1617

Pickhardt PJ, Choi JR, Hwang I et al (2003) Computed tomographic virtual colonoscopy to screen for colorectal neoplasia in asymptomatic adults. N Engl J Med 349: 2191–2200

Pickhardt PJ, Hassan C, Laghi A et al (2008) Small and diminutive polyps detected at screening CT colonography: a decision analysis for referral to colonoscopy. AJR Am J Roentgenol 190:136–144

Pignone M, Saha S, Hoerger T et al (2002) Cost-effectiveness analyses of colorectal cancer screening: a systematic review for the U.S. Preventive Services Task Force. Ann Intern Med 137:96–104

Pox C, Schmiegel W, Classen M (2007) Current status of screening colonoscopy in Europe and in the United States. Endoscopy 39:168–173

Provenzale D (2002) Cost-effectiveness of screening the average-risk population for colorectal cancer. Gastrointest Endosc Clin N Am 12:93–109

Rex D, Eid E (2008) Considerations regarding the present and future roles of colonoscopy in colorectal cancer prevention. Clinical Gastroenterology and Hepatology 6:506–514

Rex DK (2005) PRO: patients with polyps smaller than 1 cm on computed tomographic colonography should be offered colonoscopy and polypectomy. Am J Gastroenterol 100: 1903–1905

Rockey DC, Paulson E, Niedzwiecki D et al (2005) Analysis of air contrast barium enema, computed tomographic colonography, and colonoscopy: prospective comparison. Lancet 365:305–311

Rosman AS, Korsten MA (2007) Meta-analysis comparing CT colonography, air contrast barium enema, and colonoscopy. Am J Med 120:203.e4–210.e4

Scott RG, Edwards JT, Fritschi L et al (2004) Community-based screening by colonoscopy or computed tomographic colonography in asymptomatic average-risk subjects. Am J Gastroenterol 99:1145–1151

Smith A, Young GP, Cole P et al (2004) A quantifiable fecal immunochemical test (FIT) for hemoglobin facilitates balancing sensitivity with specificity when screening for colorectal cancer. Gastroenterology 126:A-199

Soetikno RM, Kaltenbach T, Rouse RV et al (2008) Prevalence of nonpolypoid (flat and depressed) colorectal neoplasms in asymptomatic and symptomatic adults. JAMA 299: 1027–1035

Sonnenberg A, Delco F, Inadomi JM (2000) Cost-effectiveness of colonoscopy in screening for colorectal cancer. Ann Intern Med 133:573–584

Sosna J, Morrin MM, Kruskal JB et al (2003) CT colonography of colorectal polyps: a metaanalysis. AJR Am J Roentgenol 181:1593–1598

Stryker S, Wolff B, Culp C et al (1987) Natural history of untreated colonic polyps. Gastroenterology 93:1009–1013

Svensson MH, Svensson E, Lasson A et al (2002) Patient acceptance of CT colonography and conventional colonoscopy: prospective comparative study in patients with or suspected of having colorectal disease. Radiology 222:337–345

Taylor SA, Halligan S, Saunders BP et al (2003).Acceptance by patients of multidetector CT colonography compared with barium enema examinations, flexible sigmoidoscopy, and colonoscopy. AJR Am J Roentgenol 181:913–921

Taylor SA, Laghi A, Lefere P et al (2007) European Society of Gastrointestinal and Abdominal Radiology (ESGAR):

Consensus statement on CT colonography. Eur Radiol 17: 575–579

Vijan S, Hwang I, Inadomi J et al (2007) The cost-effectiveness of CT colonography in screening for colorectal neoplasia. Am J Gastroenterol 102:380–390

Walleser S, Griffiths A, Lord SJ et al (2007) What is the value of computed tomography colonography in patients screening positive for fecal occult blood? A systematic review and economic evaluation. Clin Gastroenterol Hepatol 5: 1439–1446

Wilson JMG, Jungner J (1968) Principles and practice of screening for disease. from http://whqlibdoc.who.int/php/WHO_PHP_34.pdf. Accessed September 2008

Winawer SJ, Zauber AG, Ho MN et al (1993) Prevention of colorectal cancer by colonoscopic polypectomy. The National Polyp Study Workgroup. N Engl J Med 329:1977–1981

Young GP, Cole S (2007) New stool screening tests for colorectal cancer. Digestion 76:26–33

Zalis ME, Barish MA, Choi JR et al (2005) CT colonography reporting and data system: a consensus proposal. Radiology 236:3–9

Zubarik R, Eisen G, Zubarik J et al (2000) Education improves colorectal cancer screening by flexible sigmoidoscopy in an inner city population. Am J Gastroenterol 95:509–512

The Performance of CTC

DIDIER BIELEN

CONTENTS

DIDIER BIELEN, MD
UZ Gasthuisberg, Herestraat, 3000 Leuven, Belgium

2.1 Introduction

In Western Europe and the United States, colorectal carcinoma (CRC) remains the second leading cause of cancer-related death (JEMAL et al. 2005; FERLAY et al. 2007). In Belgium, each year 7,700 new colorectal cancers are diagnosed (DE LAET et al. 2006). Fortunately, the majority of these cancers originate from pre-existing benign lesions from the mucosal lining of the bowel wall. These "adenomatous polyps" have the potential to progress into a malignant lesion, a carcinoma, over a period of 10 years, the dwelling time (STRYKER et al. 1987). Identification and subsequent removal of these adenomas by way of endoscopy determines a significant decrease in the incidence of CRC (WINAWER et al. 1993). Once a cancer has been diagnosed, the 5-year survival declines significantly. This justifies a population-based screening for the early detection of the disease. Such screening tests should be sufficiently accurate, i.e. be able to detect polyps ≥10 mm, be acceptable to "patients", be feasible in clinical practice, and be neither harmful nor too expensive. The test should be cost-effective where the potential benefits must outweigh the costs.

Depending on genetic and environmental factors, the risk for cancer transformation is variable and associated with the histological characteristics of a polyp, in particular the villous component of a lesion or the flat aspect of a lesion. But since these histological characteristics can only be determined after the removal of a lesion, it would be more convenient to determine this risk prior to removal. Unfortunately, most of these characteristics can be evaluated only after polyp resection, either surgically or after an endoscopy. Further, endoscopic polyp resection has both an inherent procedural risk and an additional risk because of the need for pharmacological sedation (BOWLES et al. 2004).

The clinically important polyp seems to be a lesion measuring at least 6 mm. The rationale behind this is the fact that the majority of polyps ≤5 mm are hyperplastic and harbour a risk of malignancy of less than 1%, while larger polyps ≥10 mm harbour a risk of 10%, which further increases with size (Nusko et al. 1997). Additional risk factors are the histological characteristics, with a risk of nearly 30% for tubulovillous and villous lesions vs. 3.9% for tubulous polyps, and lesion location, with a risk of 6.4% for right-sided lesions, 8.0% for left-sided lesions and 23.0% for lesions in the rectum (Nusko et al. 1997). Considering small (<5 mm) and intermediate (6–9 mm) lesions, follow-up studies showed that there is a tendency to grow for polyps <5 mm, and a tendency to regress for those >5 mm (Hofstad et al. 1994). In this series, only one lesion showed an increase in diameter >10 mm.

For practical reasons, the main determinant of the risk for CRC is believed to be the polyp's size (Winawer et al. 1997). While small adenomas (<10 mm) have a negligible potential for short-term degeneration, the so-called advanced adenomas, i.e. those with a diameter ≥10 mm, and/or ≥20% villous component and/or high-grade dysplasia, carry a significantly increased risk of cancer (Shinya and Wolff 1979).

The prevalence of such adenomas in 20–40% of the population aged ≥60 years (Imperiale et al. 2000) offers opportunities for secondary prevention or screening for risk stratification and subsequent patient management based on the polyp size.

Such screening tests should be sufficiently accurate for detecting polyps ≥10 mm, be acceptable to the otherwise healthy persons to be screened, be feasible in clinical practice, and be neither harmful nor too expensive. The test should be cost-effective where the potential benefits must outweigh the costs.

Multiple screening options are available because no single test offers an unequivocal superiority (Winawer et al. 2003). Until today conventional colonoscopy (CC) is the most accurate technique, because it offers a high sensitivity for polyp detection. Although the CC has the possibility for polyp removal, this might not be taken into account in a screening setting since polyp removal will only be performed in the second therapeutic session. Further, the majority of lesions are not advanced adenomas and can be left in place if not detected.

On the other hand, optical colonoscopy has some disadvantages, especially the laxative bowel preparation which is experienced as an unpleasant procedure since it causes a lot of patient discomfort, and the rather high cost. Although there is a risk of bowel perforation, in particular in case of polyp removal, this might not be taken into account in case of a screening programme, since polyp removal will only be performed in the second therapeutic session.

In addition, the participation rate for CRC screening programmes is rather low, be it ±30% for flexible sigmoidoscopy and ±57% for FOBT (Seeff et al. 2004). In general, the majority of US population remains unscreened. Information regarding this topic is lacking for Belgium, since there are no organized screening programmes yet. A pilot project on CRC screening supported by the Flemish Community will start soon.

This low prevalence may be due to the lack of awareness, an inadequate provider counselling, the fact that patients had to make an appointment by themselves (Golder et al. 2007), and seems to be related to the number of primary care office visits (Zimmerman et al. 2006). Although the degree of participation remains higher in men (Meissner et al. 2006), women with up-to-date mammography and cervical cancer screening were more likely to be up to date concerning CRC screening (Carlos et al. 2005). A positive family history of CRC (Hlavaty et al. 2005), the knowledge of a sibling's illness (Gili et al. 2006), a tailored telephone outreach (Basch et al. 2006), or a patient navigator system (Jandorf et al. 2005) are likely to increase the participation rate.

2.2 CT Colonography

Since its introduction in 1994 (Vining and Gelfand 1994) many papers on CTC technique and its reliability have been published in both radiology and gastroenterology-related journals. CTC did just recently become an accepted screening tool according to the guidelines of the American Cancer Society (Levin et al. 2008a, b).

Besides the detection and characterisation of polyps, one of the advantages of CTC is that the technique is also able to measure polyps. This allows risk stratification of patients according to polyp size, since the main determinant of the risk for CRC is believed to be polyp size. The success of the patient's risk stratification by CTC can be judged using the criteria as proposed by the Working Group on Virtual Colonoscopy (Zalis et al. 2005a).

Further, CTC offers the possibility to evaluate not only the colonic lumen and mucosal surface, but also the colonic wall and the extracolonic structures, allowing, for example, the staging of disease in case of a colonic malignant tumour in one session.

To become acceptable and be able to compete with the CC, CTC should be sufficiently accurate, i.e. be able to detect at least significant polyps. Although there is no consensus on what should be the targets, guidelines recommend to target on the advanced adenomas, whereas the importance of lesions 6–9 mm remains controversial (Winawer et al. 2003). This topic, especially, gives rise to a lot of controversy. One study, examining a large patient population resembling the target population for a screening programme, proved that CTC with the use of a 3D approach is an accurate screening method in an average risk population and compared favourably with optical colonoscopy, with a sensitivity for lesions >10 mm that was >90% (Pickhardt et al. 2003). Another study stated that the sensitivity for lesions >10 mm was only 55% and that the accuracy varied considerably between centres, leading to the conclusion that CTC by these methods is not yet ready for widespread use, and that techniques and training need to be improved (Cotton et al. 2004; Rockey et al. 2005).

Two recent publications (Kim et al. 2007; Johnson et al. 2008) are more optimistic, indicating that primary screening strategies with CTC and CC resulted in similar detection rates for advanced neoplasias.

An explanation for these different conclusions might be found in the fact that the above mentioned Pickhardt-study was performed under optimal conditions with a standardized CTC technique and reading conditions, whereas the other studies grouped different centres, different CTC techniques and readers' experiences, very close to what might be found in daily practice.

Today, the CTC examination promises to be sufficiently sensitive and specific for the detection of large and medium sized polyps and symptomatic cancers (Halligan et al. 2005). It shows a similar detection rate for advanced neoplasias, i.e. adenocarcinoma and advanced adenoma, as that of CC (Kim et al. 2007), and is a valuable tool for tumour staging and detecting polyps and cancers in case of suspicion of colorectal cancer (Chung et al. 2005). Since the sensitivity and negative predictive value for 8 mm lesions is as high as 94 and 99% using four or eight channel multidetector CT scanners and double dose oral colon cleansing, CTC should even replace the double contrast barium enema for screening purposes.

2.3 Our Experience

The basic principles of the CTC technique have been described in detail in many publications. These include the necessary bowel preparation with laxatives and tagging, the bowel relaxation, the bowel distension with room air or carbon dioxide, the image acquisition in both supine and prone patient positions, the use of high resolution CT scan protocols, and the evaluation of the images in 2D as well as in 3D endoscopic view in both a colon window (e.g. 1,700/−500 HU) and soft tissue window (e.g. 450/50 HU).

All these different steps can be subject to personal interpretation and implementation by the radiologist, making the technique prone to variations and subsequently variable results.

2.3.1 Patient Acceptance

While the feasibility of reduced preparation with faecal tagging and/or rigorous dietary restrictions (Zalis et al. 2000; Callstrom et al. 2001; Gryspeerdt et al., 2002; Lefere et al. 2002; Thomeer et al. 2002; Bielen et al. 2003) has been described, our own study evaluated the effect of different preparation regimens on patient acceptance (Bielen 2008). The bowel preparation regimens contained a decreasing proportion of laxatives, with the intention to reduce patient discomfort i.e. diarrhoea. We evaluated the combination of moderate dietary restrictions, laxatives and faecal tagging preparation vs. a tagging-only preparation, i.e. without the use of any laxatives.

All participants were invited to complete a questionnaire on their pre-test expectation, their assessment of the two different CTC preparation regimens, their post-test experience, i.e. immediately and after 24–48 h, and their future preference in case a new colonic exam would be necessary: CTC, CC or no difference.

According to the pre-test expectation questionnaire, in which patients had to answer the question as to whether they expected CTC or CC to be least pleasant, more patients expected CC to be least comfortable compared to CTC. These findings were not related to the preparation regimen or a previous CC.

The rating of the CTC preparation, the CTC and the CC exams was scored using a visual assessment scale, with 0/9 being uncomfortable and 10/9 being highly comfortable.

The mean score for the preparation with the combination of laxatives and tagging was 5,4 whereas the mean score for the tagging-only preparation was 6, 7, indicating that the patients preferred the preparation without laxatives to the preparation with laxatives and this difference was statistically significant. Although even the use of the water-soluble iodinated contrast medium for tagging purposes might induce some laxation, only one patient mentioned a mild diarrhoea, which might be due to the tagging.

The mean score for the CTC exam was 6,7 whereas the mean score for the CC exam was 5,8, indicating that the CTC exams were preferred to the CC. This was the case for both preparation regimens. The mean score for the CC exam was significantly higher in case of a previous CC while this was not the case for the mean CTC score.

The CTC exams were experienced as least comfortable by a minority of patients, whereas this was the case in half of the CC exams, after completion of both exams and after 24–48 h. The same outcome is reflected in the future preference in case a new colonic exam would be necessary. More than 50% would prefer CTC compared to 15% who would choose CC. Neither post-test experience nor future choice was influenced by preparation regimen or previous CC.

Given the fact that reduced preparation for CTC seems to improve patient acceptance for undergoing a colonic exam, that a minority experiences CTC as least comfortable, and that a majority would prefer a CTC in case a new colonic exam would be necessary, CTC might become a more acceptable alternative for, or complement to, the CC in screening programmes, considering that the polyp detection would not be hampered by the use of a tagging-only preparation. Concerning the answers given after completion of the CC, it has been reported that these answers could be affected by the sedation used for the CC, especially for reasons of the retrograde amnesiac characteristics of midazolam (Svensson et al. 2002). However, the above does not impair the results of our survey, since the CTC procedure was chosen over the CC exam, irrespective of the side effects of sedation. Other parameters that might influence the results of such a questionnaire are the phrasing of the questions, the age and the education of the patients.

2.3.2 Polyp Detection

In our own study we evaluated the feasibility of polyp detection using three different preparation regimens with a decreasing proportion of laxatives, in order to reduce patient's discomfort. The goal was the correct referral to CC, based on the referral criteria of the Working Group on Virtual Colonoscopy (Zalis et al. 2005a). Therefore, we evaluated the accuracy of the CTC using both manual lesion size measurements as well as the use of an automated measurement tool delivering on the patient's risk stratification.

All patients underwent, besides dietary restrictions, one of three different bowel preparation regimens for which they received recommendations. Preparations contained a decreasing proportion of laxatives, with the intention to reduce patient discomfort, i.e. diarrhoea.

To evaluate the effect of a standard laxative bowel preparation, patients in "*Group 1*", the laxative-only group had to drink 4–5 L electrolyte solution on the morning of the colonoscopy (Na^+ 141 mEq, K^+ 10 mEq, Cl^- 121 mEq, HCO_3^- 30 mEq/L water).

To evaluate the effect of tagging, patients in "*Group 2*", the laxative-and-tagging group, had to drink a low volume laxative preparation with two doses (45 mL each) sodium phosphate (Fleet Phospho Soda®, Wolfs, Belgium) on the afternoon and evening prior to the colonoscopy.

For tagging purposes, patients had to drink 100 mL of a water-soluble iodinated contrast medium (meglmine ioxitalamate 3% – Telebrix Gastro® Guerbet/Codali Belgium): 10 mL diluted in a standard glass of water (250 mL) together with the three principal meals (breakfast, lunch, dinner) the day prior to the exam, 25 mL diluted in a standard glass of water together with each dose of the laxative and 20 mL diluted in a standard glass of water on the morning of the exam. The use of the contrast material is intended to enhance the density of possible residual stool ("faecal tagging") (Bielen et al. 2003) allowing discrimination between non-contrast containing polyps and contrast containing stool.

To evaluate the effects of a minimal preparation, patients in "*Group 3*", the tagging-only group, received a minimal preparation of "faecal tagging" only. The same tagging scheme as used in Group 2 was applied, but patients had to drink 25 mL of contrast medium diluted in a standard glass of water (250 mL) in the afternoon and in the evening, i.e. without the laxatives.

Considering the lesions 6–9, ≥10 mm and tumours (Figs. 2.1–2.4), the per patient sensitivity and negative predictive value were 62.5 and 96.7% respectively for Group 1 using the laxative only preparation, 90.0 and 99.1% respectively for Group 2 using the laxative with tagging preparation, and 100.0 and 100.0%

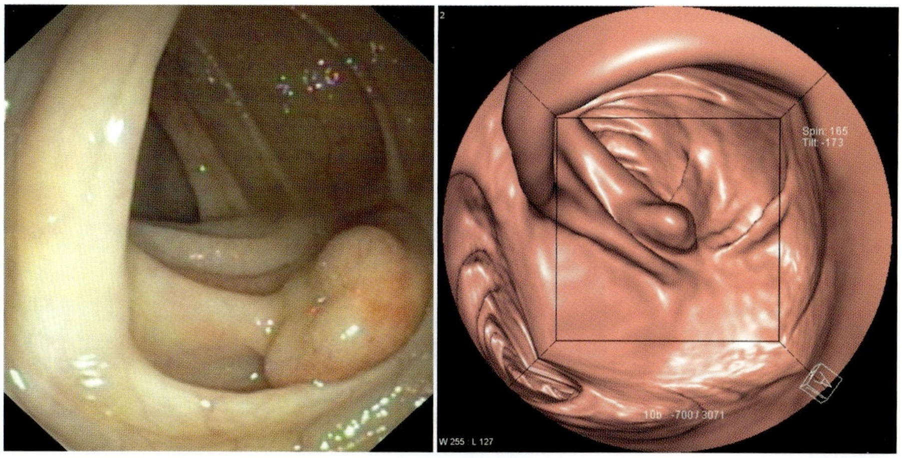

Fig. 2.1. Polyp 6–9 mm in endoscopic and CTC endo view

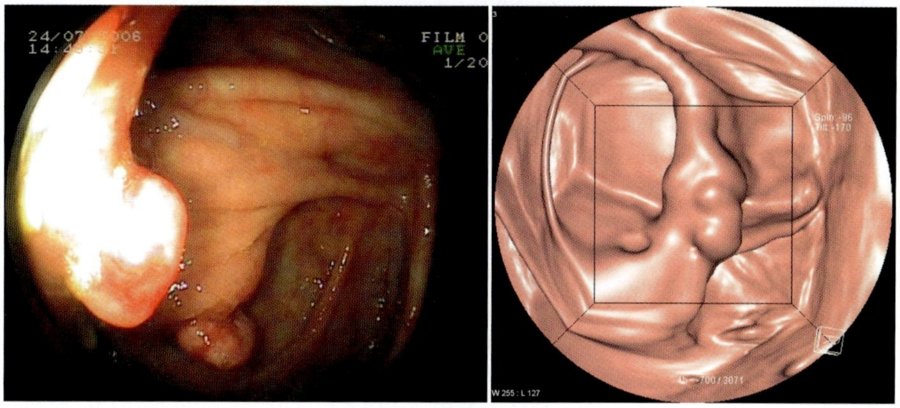

Fig. 2.2. ≥3 Polyps 6–9 mm in endoscopic and CTC endo view

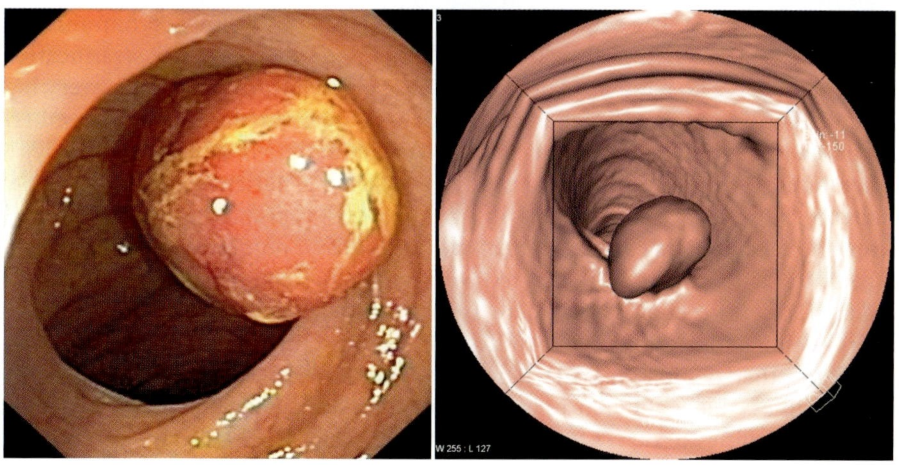

Fig. 2.3. Polyp ≥10 mm in endoscopic and CTC endo view

respectively for Group 3 using the tagging-only preparation. For the three groups together, the per patient sensitivity and negative predictive value were 81.8 and 98.53% respectively. These results are in line with recently presented studies (Johnson et al. 2008).

Considering the diminutive lesions, i.e. lesions measuring ≤5 mm, the results are far less beneficial. The same is true for the flat lesions, which remain eaily overlooked, both on CTC and CC. According to literature, less than 50% of flat lesions could be visualized, unless they were 2 mm or greater in height, 7 mm or larger in diameter. Contrast enhancement, location on a haustral fold, and abnormal 2D and 3D morphology contributed to lesion conspicuity (Park et al. 2006).

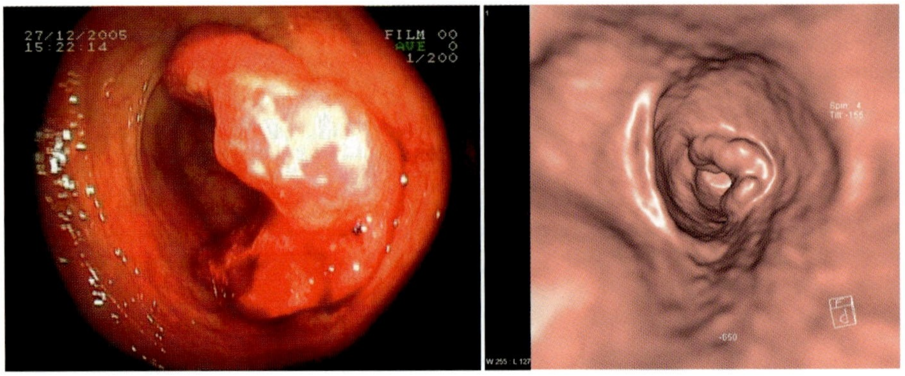

Fig. 2.4. Tumour in endoscopic and CTC endo view

This is remarkable since current CT scanners offer high spatial resolution that should make the detection of these lesions feasible. On the other hand, these lesions might be obscured due to the uncontrollable stretching or overstretching of the bowel wall as a consequence of the insufflation, whereas insufflation in CC can be controlled easily. The 3D evaluation software we used for problem solving did not present the lesions in a colour different to the surrounding normal bowel wall lining and so discrimination of lesions was not always clear, not even in 3D.

These shortcomings of the CTC technique will certainly be the subject of debate with the gastroenterology community, since especially the flat lesions constitute nearly 25% of colorectal polyps and harbour an increased malignant potential (Parra-Blanco et al. 2006). The prevalence of flat lesions in our own study was significantly lower, i.e. only three flat lesions in 296 patients. Further, the National Polyp Study did not show a higher risk for high-grade dysplasia in flat lesions (O'Brien et al. 2004). On the other hand, a recently published study revealed a rather high prevalence of flat lesions in a group of veteran patients, and that these lesions had a greater association with carcinoma compared with polypoid lesions (Soetikno et al. 2008). There are differences in prevalence of flat lesions in our study patients compared to other populations, but it remains unclear whether this is due to differences in the population or in the possibilities to detect these lesions by CC and CTC. These findings might lead to the discussion on the necessity for the search of these lesions.

Even on CC using white light, these flat lesions are overlooked easily. More advanced techniques, e.g. magnification chromo-colonoscopy, autofluorescence endoscopy and narrow-band imaging approve detection of adenoma, but necessitate a longer endoscopic procedure (Helbig 2006; Lapalus et al. 2006).

2.3.3 Referral to Optical Colonoscopy

Although there is evidence for the use of the referral criteria from the Working Group on Virtual Colonoscopy (Zalis et al. 2005a), other thresholds and referral criteria might be considered.

Selection criteria using a simple 8 mm threshold for referral to CC by CTC led to a per patient sensitivity and negative predictive value of 60.0 and 95.6% respectively for Group 1, 71.4 and 96.2% respectively for Group 2 and 83.3 and 98.5% respectively for Group 3. For the three groups together, the per patient sensitivity and negative predictive value were 70.0 and 96.6%, respectively.

Compared to the standard referral criteria, the use of a simple 8 mm threshold for polyp detection and patient's risk stratification resulted overall in slightly worse results for every individual group as well as for the three groups together.

It is clear that polyp detection and accordingly patient's risk stratification by CTC using a laxative preparation without tagging resulted in a significant number of failed referrals, using either the standard referral criteria or the simple 8 mm threshold. The main reason for this could be the amount of residual fluid and the lack of contrast difference between the low-density residual fluid covering the polyps of which the density is in the same range.

Sensitivity and NPV were clearly higher in both Group 2 and Group 3, which solely might be related to the use of tagging, since one preparation regimen was with, and the other without, the use of laxatives. In these groups, the polyp detection is enhanced, resulting in an improved patient's risk stratification compared to the preparation without tagging. This improvement is true for both sensitivity and NPV. However, most remarkable is the fact that the best results were found in Group 3, i.e. the group with the tagging-only preparation, findings which one would not expect in these setting, given this minimal preparation without any laxatives.

On the other hand, one should ask the question whether the improvement of these results are related to the preparation regimen only or are influenced by the improvement of the reader's skill as a consequence of a learning curve, since the three groups were examined in consecutive order.

For these reasons, a data sample of 60 patients, composed of patients from the three study groups with a mix of lesion types, was evaluated by three other readers: one with no CTC experience, one with limited CTC experience and one experienced reader. The purpose was to try to eliminate the possible effect of a learning curve by analyzing a new randomly composed study group.

As was the case with the initial reader, the sensitivity and NPV improved by adding tagging to the laxative preparation in Group 2 for the reader with no experience, the reader with limited experience as well as for the experienced reader.

There was no further improvement of the results in Group 3 for the reader with no CTC experience or for the reader with limited CTC experience. For the initial reader, who evaluated Group 3 at the end of the study, i.e. after having read at least 200 CTC examinations with endoscopic feedback, as well as for the experienced external reader, there was a further improvement of the results.

Besides improvement of the results as a consequence of more experience, one can expect that the reading time for an experienced reader might be far less than that for a non experienced reader, with consequences on the final cost of the CTC procedure.

Given these results, we can recommend CTC with a laxative and tagging preparation in case the reader has no or limited experience, allowing adequate polyp detection. In case the reader is experienced in reading CTC, the patient's bowel preparation can be simplified i.e. using a tagging-only preparation without laxatives, resulting in less patients' discomfort, without compromising the CTC results.

2.3.4 Interpretation

It remains unclear whether to use a primary 2D or 3D approach for evaluation of the CTC data. Some studies recommend the primary 3D approach for the detection of polyps, with 2D views used chiefly for correlation (Pickhardt et al. 2003). Other advocate using 2D axial images only, since this approach results in a very low rate of unnecessary referral for colonoscopy (Bruzzi et al. 2004), or since 2D and 3D show similar diagnostic performance (McFarland et al. 2001; van Gelder et al. 2007) (Fig. 2.5).

More important than this controversy on the 2D or 3D approach is the level of competency needed for CTC interpretation. Where on the one hand competence cannot be assumed even after directed training via 50 cases (Taylor et al. 2004), others recommend a specific training during hands-on courses with 40–50 cases under supervision or during mini fellowships (Soto et al. 2005). Reader errors are most of the time due to failure of detection rather than failure of lesion characterisation (Slater et al. 2006). Untrained reader performance is generally poor, so basic training should focus on lesion detection. Also the interpretation time depends on the reader's experience: the more the experience, the lesser the time needed for the image evaluation (Burling et al. 2006a). Less interpretation time is needed for normal cases. Compared to radiologists, technologists read CTC exams more slowly but more accurately.

It is clear from our study that a 2D approach is feasible, but a minimal level of experience is needed (Bielen 2008). Since we strive to a limited bowel preparation in the frame work of a screening programme, we should recommend that, in case such a low preparation CTC examination would be implemented, reading of these examinations should be done only by an experienced radiologist. In case the radiologist has little or no experience in reading CTC examinations, we should recommend doing the CTC examinations with a laxative and tagging preparation, favourable only in a clinical diagnostic setting, where a less stringent preparation can be used.

2.3.5 CAD

Another aspect regarding CTC is that it is unclear whether CTC might benefit from the use of computer aided detection (CAD). In the area of medical imaging, first CAD experiments involved the identification and classification of micro calcifications in mammography (Freer and Ulissey 2001). Positive results encouraged the development of algorithms to identify lung nodules on chest radiographs (Giger et al. 1988) and helical CT images (Kaneko et al.

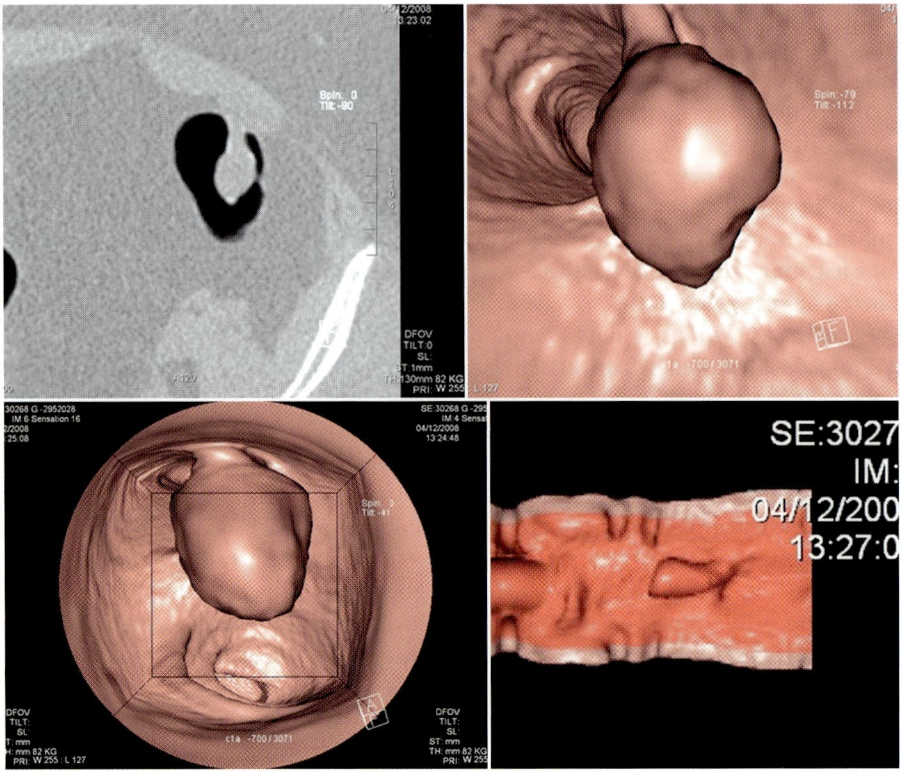

Fig. 2.5. Sessile polyp in axial 2D, endoscopic, wide-angle endoscopic and dissection view

1996). Whereas the idea behind CAD in CTC is quite simple – "Look for polyps and present them to the radiologist" – CAD is a multi step procedure typically consisting of (1) segmentation of the colonic wall, (2) generation of intermediate polyp candidates, (3) classification for detection of final candidates and (4) presentation of the polyp candidates.

In our study, we evaluated the added value of an experimental homemade CAD programme as a second reader for the three different bowel preparation regimens (Bielen 2008). The detection of polyps in this CAD software was based on sphere fitting and surface normals (Kiss et al. 2006). To judge the accuracy of our CAD technique, the same criteria for patient's risk stratification, as proposed by the Working Group on Virtual Colonoscopy (Zalis et al. 2005a) based on the size of the largest lesion detected, were used.

To evaluate the added value of the CAD on patient referral, the results from the radiologist and the CAD were combined: failed CTC referral became a correct referral in case of a correct CAD referral, unnecessary CTC referral was eliminated in case CAD decided a lesion not eligible for referral.

Based on the referral criteria of the Working Group on Virtual Colonoscopy (Zalis et al. 2005a), per patient sensitivity and negative predictive value were 87.5 and 98.9% respectively for Group 1 using the laxative only preparation, 90.0 and 99.1% respectively for Group 2 using the laxative with tagging preparation, and 100.0 and 100.0% respectively for Group 3 using the tagging-only preparation. For the three groups together, the per patient sensitivity and negative predictive value were 90.9 and 99.3% respectively.

By changing the selection criteria using a simple 8 mm threshold referral per patient sensitivity and negative predictive value were 80 and 97.8% respectively for Group 1, 71.4 and 96.4% respectively for Group 2 and 83.3 and 98.5% respectively for Group 3. For the three groups together, the per patient sensitivity and negative predictive value were 76.7 and 97.4% respectively.

The use of CAD alone shows only a slightly higher per patient sensitivity and NPV than CTC in Group 1 when using the referral criteria of the Working Group on Virtual Colonoscopy as well as the simple 8 mm threshold. The combined use of the CTC and CAD findings resulted in an improved risk stratification in Group 1 and for all three groups together, for the standard referral criteria of the Working Group on Virtual Colonoscopy as well as the simple 8 mm threshold. In the latter case, only the NPV in both Group 2 and Group 3 was slightly improved.

2.3.6 Polyp Measurements

Besides the detection of polyps, CTC has the inherent advantage to measure polyps. The measurements are performed with a calliper, either in the native transversal CT images, or in the multiplanar reformatted images (MPR), and in a coronal, sagittal or manually adjusted MPR plane along the longest axes of the polyp (BURLING et al. 2006c). Alternatively, the measurements may be carried out manually in 3D view or by using semi- or fully automated tools allowing either linear or volume measurements (BURLING et al. 2003, 2005; PICKHARDT et al. 2005, 2006). It is recommended for routine CTC examinations that polyps should be measured on 2D axial or MPR images using lung window settings (e.g. WW 1,500 HU and WL between −200 and −600 HU) or using dedicated 3D visualization software (YOUNG et al. 2007).

While CTC measurements in one study underestimated all polyps (BURLING et al. 2006b) and manual measurement techniques in another study either over- or underestimated polyp size, there is a wide variety among the observers, with CTC diameters less than the endoscopic reference measurements (BURLING et al. 2006b). The variations in the measurements of polyp diameters are related to the reader's experience and the viewing display used. Although the 3D display is commonly used for the detection of polyps, its use should not be recommended for polyp measurement (BURLING et al. 2006); this recommendation is not supported by other publications mentioning that linear polyp measurements in 3D are more accurate than measurements in 2D (PICKHARDT et al. 2005) and correlate better with the CC measurements (YESHWANT et al. 2006). The use of volume measurements instead of linear measurements allows better detection of small incremental polyp size changes in CTC (PICKHARDT et al. 2006).

Automated size measurements are technically feasible, resulting in an increased inter and intra reader agreement (BURLING et al. 2005). The automated size measurements are more precise than manual measurements, but the reader has to control the automated measurements, especially in case of small and flat polyps and lesions located on folds (FLETCHER et al. 2007). For lesions <10 mm, the measurement differences are within expected ranges of inter- and intra reader agreement for the manual 2D, the manual 3D and the automated measurement technique (TAYLOR et al. 2007).

In our own study (BIELEN 2008) some polyps were also over- or underestimated, with consequences of risk stratification. It remains unclear whether this distribution is related to the use of different WW/WL settings in the referred studies.

This distribution can also be explained by the use of the open biopsy forceps technique in all studies for the measurements, although this is the least accurate technique (GOPALSWAMY et al. 1997). The use of a linear probe measurement immediately after resection agrees best with polyp size. Alternatively, measurements can be done after polyp fixation or by the pathologist (SCHOEN et al. 1997). These uncertainties and the fact that endoscopic measurements may be operator dependent pose the question whether or not endoscopy is the gold standard for reference size estimation (FENNERTY et al. 1993; WAYE 1993).

The automated tool for polyp size measurement used in our study determined the longest dimension of polyps with high accuracy and reproducibility in the phantom study, even for low mAs values and irrespective of WW/WL settings. This also seems to be the case for the patient study, since differences between manual, endoscopic and automated measurements were not statistically significant, as long as we carried out the manual measurements using WW/WL setting of 1,700/−300 HU. The automated measurement tool provides an advantage over manual measuring since only one click on a lesion was necessary to measure it, avoiding timecosuming reconstruction, tilt and spin of MPRs along the axes of the polyp. Although the automated size measurement categorized the patients to the correct size groups without any significant difference to the radiologist, it slightly improved patient risk stratification by reducing failed and unnecessary colonoscopy referral using the referral criteria as described by the Working Group on Virtual Colonoscopy (ZALIS et al. 2005a) as well as the simple 8 mm threshold. However, it is not clear why fewer polyps were assigned to the correct size group by reader 2.

Further, it should be evaluated whether maximum linear dimension or polyp volume is the best indicator for cancer risk in polyps, and the best parameter to determine if patients are eligible for future surveillance or routine screening. In addition, the combined use of the automated tool with computer-assisted detection of polyps might be subject to future investigation.

2.3.7 The Issue of Radiation

There is an increased awareness of the possible adverse effects of the ionizing radiation of CTC, even at low dose. Although the dose used in CTC is lower than the dose in a diagnostic abdominal CT, we have to strive to use a CTC technique with a dose as low as reasonably achievable, according to the ALARA principle, with respect to both image quality and accuracy (van Gelder et al. 2002, 2004).

The effective dose (E) is currently believed to be the best available dose descriptor for quantifying risks in diagnostic radiology (McCollough and Schueler 2000; Huda and Vance 2007). In an attempt to estimate E, we recorded in our own study (Bielen 2008) for all acquisitions the effective mAs, and the for CT exams specifically DLP in mGy.cm and the CTDIvol in mGy. *E* reflects the equivalent whole-body dose that results in a stochastic risk, equivalent to the stochastic risk from the absorbed dose to those tissues irradiated in a non-uniform irradiation as CTC exams (International Commission on Radiological Protection 1991; McCollough and Schueler 2000; Bushberg et al. 2001).

Per individual, the calculated E ranged from 0.80 mSv for the prone acquisition with 140 kV, 15 mAs and CARE dose4D to 5.30 mSv for the supine acquisition with 120 kV, 55 mAs and CARE dose4D. These measured E is far below the calculated theoretical E for a routine abdominal CT examination acquisition with 120 kV, 200 mAs and CARE dose4D, or for CTC examinations in a diagnostic setting, this dose would be around 11 mSv for a man and 15 mSv for a woman (Liedenbaum et al. 2008).

To estimate the risk of an additional fatal cancer, we used the risk for a working population, of which the age is close to the age of the screening target group, i.e. 50–70 years.

We studied the assessment of image quality and the feasibility of polyp detection using the original data sets and simulated low dose data sets in a sample of 30 patients.

The calculated E for this study sample ranged from 0.40 mSv for the prone acquisition with 100 kV, 15 mAs and CARE dose to 3.0 mSv for the supine acquisition with 120 kV, 55 mAs and CARE dose. Related to the natural background radiation dose in Belgium, this would result in a multiplication factor of 0.002 for the prone acquisition with 100 kV, 15 mAs and CARE dose and up to 1.15 for the supine acquisition with 120 kV, 55 mAs and CARE dose. The theoretical risk of the induction of a fatal cancer would be 1/50,000 for the prone acquisition with 100 kV, 15 mAs and CARE dose and 1/6,667 for the supine acquisition with 120 kV, 55 mAs and CARE dose.

Besides having sufficient image quality for interpretation, the feasibility of polyp detection in the low dose scans should be as accurate as in high dose settings. All five radiologists detected the tumour, the lesions ≥10 mm and the two lesions 6–9 mm in all patients in both the high and the low dose series. This resulted in correct referral to CC in all four patients by all five readers. These findings corresponded to a per patient sensitivity and negative predictive value of 100%. Unfortunately, one reader erroneously detected three lesions 6–9 mm in the low dose series leading to unnecessary referral. Another reader erroneously referred two patients to CC in both the high and the low dose series, and a third reader erroneously referred one patient to CC in both the high and the low dose series, and two different patients in either the high or the low dose series. These three readers had knowledge in reading CTC examinations but were not experienced. While these findings had no influence on the per-patient sensitivity and negative predictive value, it led to a lower specificity.

2.4 Conclusion

In conclusion, polyp detection by means of CTC is feasible. Besides the implementation of CTC in a screening programme, the radiologists should offer this examination in a clinical diagnostic setting in case a CC is not possible, or in case patients are not able or willing to undergo a CC.

References

Basch CE, Wolf RL, Brouse CH et al (2006) Telephone outreach to increase colorectal cancer screening in an urban minority population. Am J Public Health 96:2246–2253

Bielen D (2008) Screening for colorectal cancer with CT colonography: facing the challenges. Leuven University Press, Leuven

Bielen D, Thomeer M, Vanbeckevoort D et al (2003) Dry preparation for virtual CT colonography with fecal tagging using water-soluble contrast medium: initial results. Eur Radiol 13:453–458

Bowles CJ, Leicester R, Romaya C et al (2004) A prospective study of colonoscopy practice in the UK today: are we adequately prepared for national colorectal cancer screening tomorrow? Gut 53:277–283

Burling D, Halligan S, Taylor S et al (2006) Polyp measurement using CT colonography: agreement with colonoscopy and

effect of viewing conditions on interobserver and intraobserver agreement. AJR Am J Roentgenol 186:1597–1604
Bushberg J, Seibert J, Leidholdt E et al (2001) The essential physics of medical imaging. Lippincott Williams & Wilkins, Philadelphia, PA
Carlos RC, Fendrick AM, Patterson SK et al (2005) Associations in breast and colon cancer screening behavior in women. Acad Radiol 12:451–458
Chung DJ, Huh KC, Choi WJ et al (2005) CT colonography using 16-MDCT in the evaluation of colorectal cancer. AJR Am J Roentgenol 184:98–103
Cotton PB, Durkalski VL, Pineau BC et al (2004) Computed tomographic colonography (virtual colonoscopy): a multicenter comparison with standard colonoscopy for detection of colorectal neoplasia. JAMA 291:1713–1719
De Laet C, Neyt M, Vinck I et al (2006) Health Technology Assessment Colorectale Kankerscreening: wetenschappelijke stand van zaken en budgetimpact voor België. In: KCE reports, vol 45A
Fennerty MB, Davidson J, Emerson SS et al (1993) Are endoscopic measurements of colonic polyps reliable? Am J Gastroenterol 88:496–500
Ferlay J, Autier P, Boniol M et al (2007) Estimates of the cancer incidence and mortality in Europe in 2006. Ann Oncol 18:581–592
Freer TW, Ulissey MJ (2001) Screening mammography with computer-aided detection: prospective study of 12,860 patients in a community breast center. Radiology 220: 781–786
Giger ML, Doi K, MacMahon H (1988) Image feature analysis and computer-aided diagnosis in digital radiography. 3. Automated detection of nodules in peripheral lung fields. Med Phys 15:158–166
Gili M, Roca M, Ferrer V et al (2006) Psychosocial factors associated with the adherence to a colorectal cancer screening program. Cancer Detect Prev 30:354–360
Golder S, Vogt W, Lichti H et al (2007) Acceptance of flexible sigmoidoscopy as a screening examination for colorectal cancer in an outpatient clinic. Int J Colorectal Dis 22:387–394
Gopalswamy N, Shenoy VN, Choudhry U et al (1997) Is in vivo measurement of size of polyps during colonoscopy accurate? Gastrointest Endosc 46:497–502
Gryspeerdt S, Lefere P, Dewyspelaere J et al (2002) Optimisation of colon cleansing prior to computed tomographic colonography. JBR-BTR 85:289–296
Halligan S, Altman DG, Taylor SA et al (2005) CT colonography in the detection of colorectal polyps and cancer: systematic review, meta-analysis, and proposed minimum data set for study level reporting. Radiology 237: 893–904
Helbig C (2006) Chromoendoscopy and its alternatives for colonoscopy: useful in the United States? Rev Gastroenterol Disord 6:209–220
Hlavaty T, Lukac L, Huorka M et al (2005) Positive family history promotes participation in colorectal cancer screening. Bratisl Lek Listy 106:318–323
Huda W, Vance A (2007) Patient radiation doses from adult and pediatric CT. AJR Am J Roentgenol 188:540–546
Imperiale TF, Wagner DR, Lin CY et al (2000) Risk of advanced proximal neoplasms in asymptomatic adults according to the distal colorectal findings. N Engl J Med 343:169–174
International Commission on Radiological Protection (2007) The 2007 recommendations of the International Commission on Radiological Protection. ICRP publication 103
Jandorf L, Gutierrez Y, Lopez J et al (2005) Use of a patient navigator to increase colorectal cancer screening in an urban neighborhood health clinic. J Urban Health 82:216–224
Jemal A, Murray T, Ward E et al (2005) Cancer statistics, 2005. CA Cancer J Clin 55:10–30
Johnson CD (2007) Results of the ACRIN Colonography Trial. In: RSNA annual meeting, Chicago, pp VG21-14
Kaneko M, Eguchi K, Ohmatsu H et al (1996) Peripheral lung cancer: screening and detection with low-dose spiral CT versus radiography. Radiology 201:798–802
Kim DH, Pickhardt PJ, Taylor AJ et al (2007) CT colonography versus colonoscopy for the detection of advanced neoplasia. N Engl J Med 357:1403–1412
Kiss G, Drisis S, Bielen D et al (2006) Computer-aided detection of colonic polyps using low-dose CT acquisitions. Acad Radiol 13:1062–1071
Lapalus MG, Helbert T, Napoleon B et al (2006) Does chromoendoscopy with structure enhancement improve the colonoscopic adenoma detection rate? Endoscopy 38:444–448
Lefere P, Gryspeerdt S, Marrannes J et al (2005) CT colonography after fecal tagging with a reduced cathartic cleansing and a reduced volume of barium. AJR Am J Roentgenol 184:1836–1842
Lefere PA, Gryspeerdt SS, Dewyspelaere J et al (2002) Dietary fecal tagging as a cleansing method before CT colonography: initial results polyp detection and patient acceptance. Radiology 224:393–403
Leung WK, Lam WW, Wu JC et al (2004) Magnetic resonance colonography in the detection of colonic neoplasm in high-risk and average-risk individuals. Am J Gastroenterol 99: 102–108
Levin B, Lieberman DA, McFarland B et al (2008a) Screening and surveillance for the early detection of colorectal cancer and adenomatous polyps, 2008: a joint guideline from the American Cancer Society, the US Multi-Society Task Force on Colorectal Cancer, and the American College of Radiology. Gastroenterology 134:1570–1595
Levin B, Lieberman DA, McFarland B et al (2008b) Screening and surveillance for the early detection of colorectal cancer and adenomatous polyps, 2008: a joint guideline from the American Cancer Society, the US Multi-Society Task Force on Colorectal Cancer, and the American College of Radiology. CA Cancer J Clin 58:130–160
Liedenbaum MH, Venema HW, Stoker J (2008) Radiation dose in CT colonography-trends in time and differences between daily practice and screening protocols. Eur Radiol 18: 2222–2230
Mang T, Graser A, Schima W et al (2007) CT colonography: techniques, indications, findings. Eur J Radiol 61:388–399
Mang TG, Schaefer-Prokop C, Maier A et al (2005) Detectability of small and flat polyps in MDCT colonography using 2D and 3D imaging tools: results from a phantom study. AJR Am J Roentgenol 185:1582–1589
McCollough CH, Schueler BA (2000) Calculation of effective dose. Med Phys 27:828–837
Meissner HI, Breen N, Klabunde CN et al (2006) Patterns of colorectal cancer screening uptake among men and women in the United States. Cancer Epidemiol Biomarkers Prev 15: 389–394

Morrin MM, Farrell RJ, Keogan MT et al (2002) CT colonography: colonic distention improved by dual positioning but not intravenous glucagon. Eur Radiol 12:525–530

Morrin MM, Hochman MG, Farrell RJ et al (2001) MR colonography using colonic distention with air as the contrast material: work in progress. AJR Am J Roentgenol 176:144–146

Nusko G, Mansmann U, Altendorf-Hofmann A et al (1997) Risk of invasive carcinoma in colorectal adenomas assessed by size and site. Int J Colorectal Dis 12:267–271

O'Brien MJ, Winawer SJ, Zauber AG et al (2004) Flat adenomas in the National Polyp Study: is there increased risk for high-grade dysplasia initially or during surveillance? Clin Gastroenterol Hepatol 2:905–911

O'Connor SD, Summers RM, Yao J et al (2006) CT colonography with computer-aided polyp detection: volume and attenuation thresholds to reduce false-positive findings owing to the ileocecal valve. Radiology 241:426–432

Park SH, Ha HK, Kim AY et al (2006) Flat polyps of the colon: detection with 16-MDCT colonography–preliminary results. AJR Am J Roentgenol 186:1611–1617

Parra-Blanco A, Gimeno-Garcia AZ, Nicolas-Perez D et al (2006) Risk for high-grade dysplasia or invasive carcinoma in colorectal flat adenomas in a Spanish population. Gastroenterol Hepatol 29:602–609

Pickhardt PJ (2004) Differential diagnosis of polypoid lesions seen at CT colonography (virtual colonoscopy). Radiographics 24:1535–1556; discussion 1557–1539

Pickhardt PJ, Choi JR, Hwang I et al (2003) Computed tomographic virtual colonoscopy to screen for colorectal neoplasia in asymptomatic adults. N Engl J Med 349:2191–2200

Rockey DC, Paulson E, Niedzwiecki D et al (2005) Analysis of air contrast barium enema, computed tomographic colonography, and colonoscopy: prospective comparison. Lancet 365: 305–311

Schoen RE, Gerber LD, Margulies C (1997) The pathologic measurement of polyp size is preferable to the endoscopic estimate. Gastrointest Endosc 46:492–496

Seeff LC, Nadel MR, Klabunde CN et al (2004) Patterns and predictors of colorectal cancer test use in the adult U.S. population. Cancer 100:2093–2103

Shinya H, Wolff WI (1979) Morphology, anatomic distribution and cancer potential of colonic polyps. Ann Surg 190: 679–683

Slater A, Taylor SA, Tam E et al (2006) Reader error during CT colonography: causes and implications for training. Eur Radiol 16:2275–2283

Soetikno RM, Kaltenbach T, Rouse RV et al (2008) Prevalence of nonpolypoid (flat and depressed) colorectal neoplasms in asymptomatic and symptomatic adults. JAMA 299:1027–1035

Sosna J, Kruskal JB, Bar-Ziv J et al (2005) Extracolonic findings at CT colonography. Abdom Imaging 30:709–713

Soto JA, Barish MA, Yee J (2005) Reader training in CT colonography: how much is enough? Radiology 237:26–27

Stryker SJ, Wolff BG, Culp CE et al (1987) Natural history of untreated colonic polyps. Gastroenterology 93:1009–1013

Svensson M, Svensson E, Lasson A, et al (2002) CT Colonography versus colonoscopy: comparing apples and oranges: reply to Forbes GM, Edwards JT, Mendelson RM (letters to the editor). Radiology 225:308–309

Taylor SA, Halligan S, Burling D et al (2004) CT colonography: effect of experience and training on reader performance. Eur Radiol 14:1025–1033

Taylor SA, Laghi A, Lefere P et al (2007) European Society of Gastrointestinal and Abdominal Radiology (ESGAR): consensus statement on CT colonography. Eur Radiol 17:575–579

Taylor SA, Slater A, Burling DN et al (2008) CT colonography: optimisation, diagnostic performance and patient acceptability of reduced-laxative regimens using barium-based faecal tagging. Eur Radiol 18:32–42

Vining D, Gelfand D (1994) Noninvasive colonoscopy using helical CT scanning, 3D reconstruction, and virtual reality. In: 23rd Annual Meeting and Postgraduate Course of the Society of Gastrointestinal Radiologists, Maui, Hawaii

Waye JD (1993) The accuracy of endoscopic estimates: what is large? What is small? Am J Gastroenterol 88:483–484

Winawer S, Fletcher R, Rex D et al (2003) Colorectal cancer screening and surveillance: clinical guidelines and rationale-update based on new evidence. Gastroenterology 124:544–560

Winawer SJ, Fletcher RH, Miller L et al (1997) Colorectal cancer screening: clinical guidelines and rationale. Gastroenterology 112:594–642

Winawer SJ, Zauber AG, Ho MN et al (1993) Prevention of colorectal cancer by colonoscopic polypectomy. The National Polyp Study Workgroup. N Engl J Med 329:1977–1981

Yeshwant SC, Summers RM, Yao J et al (2006) Polyps: linear and volumetric measurement at CT colonography. Radiology 241:802–811

Young BM, Fletcher JG, Paulsen SR et al (2007) Polyp measurement with CT colonography: multiple-reader, multiple-workstation comparison. AJR Am J Roentgenol 188: 122–129

Zalis ME, Barish MA, Choi JR et al (2005a) CT colonography reporting and data system: a consensus proposal. Radiology 236:3–9

Zalis ME, Perumpillichira JJ, Kim JY et al (2005b) Polyp size at CT colonography after electronic subtraction cleansing in an anthropomorphic colon phantom. Radiology 236: 118–124

Zimmerman RK, Nowalk MP, Tabbarah M et al (2006) Predictors of colorectal cancer screening in diverse primary care practices. BMC Health Serv Res 6:116

Starting CT Colonography in Your Department

Darra Murphy, Alan O'Hare, and Helen Fenlon

CONTENTS

3.1 Introduction

CT colonography (virtual colonoscopy) has rapidly evolved since its initial description in 1994. It has gradually moved from being a research tool that was largely confined to academic teaching hospitals to a clinical test that is now widely available in many community-based hospitals. Now that it has become accepted as a viable alternative to optical colonoscopy and a credible tool for colon cancer screening (Levin et al. 2008a, b; Kim et al. 2007), many radiologists are interested in establishing CT colonography in their departments. Physicians are requesting the test more frequently and patients are demanding it increasingly. This chapter examines the essential components, minimum requirements and potential hurdles in establishing an effective CT colonography service in a busy diagnostic radiology department.

3.2 Technical Requirements

Progress made in the clinical implementation of CT colonography would not have been possible without significant advances that have been made in CT imaging technology over the past 10 years. Availability and ease of access to this technology is crucial for any CT colonography service to allow rapid acquisition, processing and reading of CT colonography datasets.

Technologically, there are three basic components to a CT colonography examination: (1) multislice CT hardware for image acquisition, (2) software and associated platforms for post processing and reading of data sets, and (3) adequate transfer networks between the hardware and software components with appropriate image data storage facilities.

Darra Murphy, MD
Alan O'Hare MD
Helen Fenlon, MD
Department of Radiology, Mater Misericordiae University Hospital, Eccles Street, Dublin, 7, Ireland

While techniques for image post processing and rendering have a major impact on how the final image is viewed, the spatial quality of the dataset will fundamentally be determined by the initial CT acquisition parameters. Although much of the early work on CT colonography was performed on single row helical scanners (Fenlon et al. 1999), multidetector CT (MDCT) is now the accepted standard for CT colonography research protocols and for performing clinical examinations in everyday practice. MDCT allows acquisition of a single breath-hold thin section CT examination of the entire colon in very short scan times. A typical acquisition takes 6–8 s using a 64-slice MDCT with a decrease in both respiratory artifacts and improved colonic distension compared with single-slice acquisition (Fenlon et al. 1999). Image artifacts and misregistration secondary to motion and breathing at single-slice CT scanning have been shown to increase both diagnostic errors and evaluation times (Shinners et al. 2006). These artifacts are virtually eliminated using MDCT acquisition. With the development of dual-source CT, 320-detector-row CT and a new generation of scintillator materials, image acquisition times are steadily reducing and image quality improving, with careful consideration to dose reduction.

Once the CT data are acquired, images should be reconstructed according to a standard protocol and automatically transferred to a reading workstation for review. There are numerous options available with regard to CT colonography workstations. Appropriate software is available from both the leading CT manufacturers and specific CT colonography software vendors. Such workstations allow datasets to be read in a variety of formats, most commonly 2D images with multiplanar reconstructions (MPR) and 3D endoluminal views for problem solving. Furthermore, software programs are now capable of generating automated 3D reconstructions of the colonic mucosa from the acquired datasets with an average time for reconstruction in the order of seconds for a complete 3D flythrough. The relative merits of each method will be discussed in the subsequent chapter.

Consideration must also be given as to how CTC datasets will be archived and how datasets may be retrieved to facilitate comparison with previous CT colonography studies. The volume of data generated for each CT colonography examination precludes hardcopy printing of all acquired images. Using a 16-slice MDCT with 3 mm slice acquisition and 1.5 mm slice overlap, a standard study with 40 cm of *Z*-axis coverage in both supine and prone positions will typically comprise over 600 slices. At the standard 512 × 512 pixels per slice image each study will require over 500 MB of memory for storage. A single patient's examination will therefore occupy almost an entire conventional compact disc (CD), which has a memory capacity of 700 MB. This may be substantially greater with 64-slice and dual-source CT with use of thinner slice acquisition. An alternative to CD for archiving is DVD. While relatively inexpensive, use of DVD requires purchase of a DVD reader as most commercially available workstations come with only an integrated CD reader. Now that the formatting war between Blu-Ray and HD DVD has ended, we can expect to see 25 GB single-layer and 50 GB dual layer Blu-Ray discs being increasingly used. That said, physical disc media is giving way to storage on hard drives at a local level and PACS archives at a network level. The actual hard drive memory capacities of workstations vary (100 GB in our department) and alone can accommodate only a limited number of cases, especially when large studies containing over 1,000 images are being acquired and stored. In reality, these workstations are also used for 3D reconstruction of other studies including vascular and orthopedic examinations, resulting in a real need for robust image archiving.

Without an integrated PACS system, effective high volume CT colonography that allows rapid image retrieval and comparison with previous studies is extremely difficult. Many issues relating to memory storage and networking infrastructure are simply resolved with the implementation of PACS. PACS offers numerous potential advantages including the viewing of studies in remote locations, near elimination of lost datasets, and large image storage capacity. A major benefit is the facilitation of rapid retrieval of previous studies with reports, a significant advantage in the setting of a busy department or a screening program. Until recent years many CT workstations did not have a PACS compatible interface. Furthermore many radiology departments do not yet have PACS. When choosing a workstation for CT colonography interpretation, careful consideration should be given to its PACS compatibility.

The network interface between the CT workstations and reading workstations must be seamless, transfer of datasets must be fast and automatic, and datasets must be available for reading without any loss of diagnostic information. Transferring datasets of this size places a considerable demand on any network whether it involves transmission from CT workstations to reading workstations or from the primary reading stations to remote reader locations.

The connecting network cable must be at least category 5 UTP with switches producing network speeds up to 100 Mb/s, and increasingly Gigabit Ethernet. Speed of transfer should not be compromised if the network is of sufficient capacity, even if high volumes of data are being transferred simultaneously.

3.3 CT Colonography Protocols

Specific CT colonography protocols should be established at a local level and should be based on the currently available published evidence. Protocols should address the method of bowel preparation (clean colon vs. fluid or fecal tagging), use or not of intravenous contrast, use or not of spasmolytics, method of colon distension, scanning parameters and methods of interpretation. The specifics of many of these options are discussed in subsequent chapters.

The basic equipment required for the CT colonography examination is little more than a rubber catheter with a hand held insufflation bulb similar to that used for barium enema examinations. There are a variety of rectal catheters available in different sizes, typically 5–15 mm in diameter. Although we routinely use a balloon-tipped enema catheter, many researchers now avoid balloon insufflation. Traditionally room air has been the agent of choice for colonic insufflation at CT colonography due to its availability and lack of additional expense. However, there is a growing body of evidence advocating the use of carbon dioxide (CO_2) which is associated with less abdominal cramping and is more rapidly reabsorbed (Shinners et al. 2006). CO_2 is supplied from a refillable cylinder via a disposable administration set that allows constant gas pressure influx with the facility to record both gas pressures and the volume of CO_2 administered.

In our practice, the radiologist is responsible for the practicalities of rectal tube insertion and subsequent colonic insufflation. Depending on departmental time constraints, radiology staffing and volume of CT colonography examinations, consideration may be given to training a dedicated CT colonography technician or nurse and this has been successfully established in some institutions. Furthermore some centers allow patients to "self-inflate" in order to improve patient acceptance of the technique. Overall, it is well documented that there is a low risk of procedure-related complications (Pickhardt 2006; Burling et al. 2006a).

Much research has been published from both in vivo and phantom studies on the effect of different scan parameters (particularly slice collimation, pitch and mAs) on the quality of CT colonography studies, the associated artifacts and patient radiation doses. As with any radiologic study there will be a trade off between image quality (the diagnostic value of the study) and radiation dose. Typical parameters for CT colonography will be specifically discussed in a later chapter. In establishing a CT colonography service it is important to agree on a standard scan protocol so that patients are imaged and data set acquired in a consistent and reproducible manner. This creates a uniformity among studies, which facilitates interpretation and comparison with previous studies. Published literature advocates that all patients be scanned in both supine and prone positions as dual positioning allows redistribution of air, stool and fluid and is associated with an increased sensitivity for polyp detection. In one particular study, the reported sensitivity of CT colonography for detection of polyps greater than 10 mm in size was 92.7% for dual positioning compared with 58.5 and 51% for supine and prone scanning alone (Yee et al. 2003). If patients are unable to lie prone, it is acceptable to lay them in the lateral decubitus position in addition to the supine position.

3.4 Reading and Training

After image acquisition and transfer of datasets, studies should be read and reported in a timely fashion. The following discussion will address aspects of image interpretation including who should read the datasets, how much training is required, how many readers are required and when and where studies should be read.

The primary aim of CT colonography is accurate identification of significant colorectal polyps and cancers in a minimally invasive manner. For CT colonography to be a safe, accurate and attractive alternative to colonoscopy, radiologists reading these studies must confidently recognize polyps and cancers, identify pitfalls and therefore reduce the number of false positive findings, and report significant extracolonic findings in a consistent and reliable manner. It is increasingly clear that to achieve this, radiologists must have specific CT colonography training. The effect of training and experience on reader performance has been the subject of a number of studies to date and has been a topic of intense discussion at many scientific meetings including the annual International Symposia on Virtual Colonoscopy in Boston, now in its ninth year. Training and its relationship to an individual's ability to accurately report CT colonography studies is a complex issue and much has been published in both the radiology (European Society of Gastrointestinal and Abdominal Radiology CT Colonography Group Investigator 2007) and gastroenterology (Rockey et al. 2007) literature. It appears that radiologists with a specific interest in CT colonography who have read many, many hundreds of cases perform better than abdominal radiologists who have been trained on a limited number of cases alone, who in turn perform better than those with little or no specific CT colonography training. As one might expect, there is a difference in performance between experts, experienced or "trained" readers and novices. It is, however, not clear just how steep the learning curve is and when, or if, one reaches a plateau in reader performance.

Current recommendations are that radiologists should be specifically trained in a supervised manner on cases that have either endoscopic verification or have been read by an "expert" reader. The datasets should include an appropriate mix of normal studies, cancers of various morphology, polyps (pedunculated and flat), and extracolonic findings, as well as studies limited by under-distension and poor bowel preparation. Emphasis should also be placed on familiarity with CT colonography software applications and recognition of the various pathologies in both 2D and 3D formats. While supervised training on 50 proven cases has been regarded as a minimum initial requirement (Soto et al. 2005), it would be wrong to assume that this is adequate for every radiologist or that it provides a level of "expertise" as performance clearly improves with increasing experience.

Differences in reader experience have been identified as one of the factors contributing to the wide range of reported accuracies of CT colonography. In earlier studies, the reported sensitivities for detection of polyps >1 cm varied from 52 to 92% (Johnson et al. 2003; Cotton et al. 2004; Pickhardt et al. 2003). In another study, the performance of novice readers was recorded after every 25 patients for almost 100 CT colonography examinations. They found that the sensitivity achieved by readers for polyps of all sizes increased from 32% after the first 25 cases to 92% for the final 25 cases (Spinzi et al. 2001).

Although there were some differences in the study populations and the methods used for bowel preparation, image acquisition, and interpretation, it is widely believed that differences in performance were due, at least in part, to variability in reader experience. Comparisons between the performance of novice observers who had undergone directed training and radiologists experienced in CT colonography have been performed (European Society of Gastrointestinal and Abdominal Radiology CT Colonography Group Investigator 2007), with colonoscopy as the gold standard. This found that the interpretation of experienced observers was significantly better than novices trained with 50 studies. Although no difference was observed between trained radiologists and trained technologists, individual performances were variable and some trainees outperformed some experienced observers. Recent data from the ACRIN 6664 trial provides further supporting evidence that in experienced hands the per-patient sensitivity for detecting polyps 10 mm and larger is 90% or greater (Johnson et al. 2008). Adequate and widespread access to reader training will be required now that studies such as these and others (Levin et al. 2008a, b; McFarland et al. 2008) enhance the acceptance of CT colonography as a screening tool.

A comparison has previously been made between a colonic screening program and the template that already exists for mammographic screening (Ferrucci 2000). In it, Ferrucci correctly predicts that in the setting of a colon screening program there will be a demand by certain third parties such as insurance companies or the American college of Radiologists that radiologists reporting CT colonography studies reach certain levels of competence and maintain those standards. The impact of such a step is to be welcomed, as it would establish pre-requisites that every reporting radiologist should meet in terms of their training and level of experience.

Even with suitable training, errors of judgment will continue to be made by even the most experienced of radiologists. Potential "pitfalls" leading to both false positive and negative results must be highlighted. These pitfalls typically relate to retained stool, complex fold and polyp morphology, and the relationship of polyps to folds and flexures. A number of publications have addressed these pitfalls (Fenlon 2002; Mang et al. 2007a; Dachman et al. 2007), and training courses should include examples. Training courses should also include formal lectures on image acquisition parameters, non-interpretive matters and a review of the data supporting virtual colonoscopy for screening. European Society of Gastrointestinal and Abdominal Imaging (ESGAR) offers both hands-on workshops and doctor-to-doctor training several times a year in various locations around Europe. Similar workshops are also available in the USA and around the world. These courses are typically held over a 2- to 3-day period. In addition, the ESGAR released a consensus statement in 2007, which offers excellent guidelines regarding training (Taylor et al. 2007).

3.5 Reading Conditions

Reading conditions also impact on reader performance. CT colonography studies should ideally be batch-read in a quiet environment with each batch consisting of no more than five or six cases. This helps to reduce the impact of reader fatigue, which adversely affects reader concentration and performance in terms of polyp detection. Although an experienced radiologist may take as little as 5 min to read a study in 2D format, interpretation requires a high level of concentration to maintain ones focus on the lumen while scrolling back and forth through the colon. In the setting of a busy department with many conflicting demands on radiologists, CT colonography readers should be cautious to avoid the impulse to rapidly read studies as this may result in a significant decrease in polyp detection rates (Burling et al. 2006b). The time allocated to reading these studies should be protected in a manner similar to the reading of screening mammograms.

Using the mammography analogy, it is likely that the sensitivity for polyp detection increases when studies are double read compared with single read examinations. A second reader does not necessarily have to be a trained radiologist – this role could potentially be filled by computer-aided detection (CAD). CAD is an automated computer software mechanism used to highlight abnormalities within a colon that may be missed by the radiologist. CAD could act as the first or second reader in combination with a trained radiologist (Johnson et al. 2007). The benefits of CAD have been shown in other radiological applications such as mammography and lung nodule detection. There is considerable interest among academic radiologists and commercial companies in this tool and, although not yet fully FDA approved or verified in multicentre trials, CAD is a rapidly developing tool that may become standard in CT colonography reading in the future (Graser et al. 2007; Hock et al. 2008; Summers et al. 2008; Taylor et al. 2008; Mang et al. 2007b).

A standard report format should also be agreed upon at a local level. If used by all reporting radiologists a standard printed report would help improve communication with the referring clinician or patient and help direct appropriate patient follow-up and management. Such a report would stratify patients into specified groups depending on the CT colonography findings. The factors that decide group designation would include polyp size, morphology, location and attenuation. A system has been proposed similar to the BI-RADS system used in mammography that is called C-RADS. Patients would be classified into groups C1 to C5 and the report would also include an E1 to E5 categorization based on the presence or absence of significant extra-colonic findings. This proposal, based on the coordinated efforts of the American College of Radiology and the Working group on Virtual Colonoscopy, was published in 2005 (Zalis et al. 2005).

The successful implementation of any new practice requires that there be adequate and proper utilization of that resource that justifies the expense of providing the equipment, training the staff, performing the studies and reading the datasets. This requires close collaboration and communication between radiologists and many different staff, including radiographers, secretarial and nursing staff in Radiology, primary care physicians, endoscopy staff and gastroenterologists. The success of any CT colonography service is close liaison between the radiology and gastroenterology departments. A good working relationship between the two groups allows free exchange of information and ideas, promotes patient referrals and, most importantly provides a clear mechanism for follow-up of any abnormal cases. It is up to the radiologist to promote the technique within their hospital by meeting local physician groups, particularly the gastroenterologists, and explaining the advantages and disadvantages, indications and contraindications of this new procedure. Easy same-day access to CT colonography following failed colonoscopy is appealing to both patients and gastroenterologists and is an effective way of introducing and promoting this technique at a local level. Gastroenterologists as a group are only too aware of the potential significance of CT colonography as a screening tool for colon cancer and its implications for both their future practice and ours. It is vital that we gain their confidence from the outset and that we are sufficiently familiar with current literature on colon cancer screening and CT colonography to address any issues or questions that may arise.

3.6 Patient Information, Referral and Follow Up

For patients and the population in general, particularly those considering a screening test, easy access to information regarding the procedure and clear communication with the providers is also important. There should exist within a department a means by which patients can be informed of the procedure, the necessary preparation, potential risks and complications, implications of a normal and abnormal result and what mechanism for follow-up exists. The most practical way of achieving this would be through printed literature on the test and access to a liaison staff member such as a nurse or radiographer who has been specifically trained.

There is merit in the suggestion made by Mark. E. Klein (Washington Radiology Associates) when he spoke at a previous international Virtual Colonoscopy conference that a department introducing a CT colonography service would be well advised to perform a pilot study on the first 40–50 patients with conventional colonoscopy correlation in each case. This gives the radiologist a valuable opportunity to become familiar with all aspects of the technique and to address organizational issues including the process of patient referrals, timing of appointments, the staffing and infrastructure required, optimal bowel preparation and distension, to become familiar with the reading software and issues related to interpretation and to consider mechanism for follow-up when required. Specific details relating to each of these topics will be dealt with in later chapters and have also been addressed in the literature (Kim et al. 2007; Pickhardt 2007; Lefere et al. 2007).

3.7 Cost and Financial Implications

The economic implications of setting up a CT colonography service must also be considered. Each department must consider whether or not it is financially viable for them to provide this service. Estimates suggest that, when all factors are considered, the real cost of providing a CT colonography examination is in the order of €250, however apart from a handful of healthcare providers there is currently no reimbursement for screening CT colonography. CT colonography in symptomatic patients is now increasingly reimbursed but coverage is somewhat limited and inconsistent. In light of the recently published joint guidelines from the American Cancer Society, the US Multi-Society Task Force on Colorectal Cancer, and the American College of Radiology (Levin et al. 2008a, b), one would hope that this would improve. Where this is not the case, Radiologists must be able to address and discuss these issues with their local health insurance companies to ensure that the interests of their patients are protected and that they are appropriately reimbursed for capital costs and their professional time.

3.8 Quality Assurance

Establishing a CT colonography service requires a major investment in time, cost and personal commitment. However maintaining a quality service and insuring high quality clinical standards is equally important, particularly when considering screening populations. This will involve setting standards, measuring competence, continuous medical education, clinical audit and quality control. Appropriate audit and quality control will assess the various systems involved in a CT colonography service from the time an appointment is made right through to patient follow-up so that potential deficiencies can be identified and appropriate changes implemented as required.

References

Levin B et al (2008a) Screening and surveillance for the early detection of colorectal cancer and adenomatous polyps, 2008: a joint guideline from the American Cancer Society, the US Multi-Society Task Force on Colorectal Cancer, and the American College of Radiology. Gastroenterology 134 (5): 1570–1595

Levin B et al (2008b) Screening and surveillance for the early detection of colorectal cancer and adenomatous polyps, 2008: a joint guideline from the American Cancer Society, the US Multi-Society Task Force on Colorectal Cancer, and the American College of Radiology. CA Cancer J Clin 58(3): 130–160

Kim DH et al (2007) CT colonography versus colonoscopy for the detection of advanced neoplasia. N Engl J Med 357(14): 1403–1412

Fenlon HM et al (1999) A comparison of virtual and conventional colonoscopy for the detection of colorectal polyps. N Engl J Med 341(20):1496–1503

Shinners TJ et al (2006) Patient-controlled room air insufflation versus automated carbon dioxide delivery for CT colonography. AJR Am J Roentgenol 186(6):1491–1496

Pickhardt PJ (2006) Incidence of colonic perforation at CT colonography: review of existing data and implications for screening of asymptomatic adults. Radiology 239(2):313–316

Burling D et al (2006a) Potentially serious adverse events at CT colonography in symptomatic patients: national survey of the United Kingdom. Radiology 239(2):464–471

Yee J et al (2003) Comparison of supine and prone scanning separately and in combination at CT colonography. Radiology 226(3):653–661

European Society of Gastrointestinal and Abdominal Radiology CT Colonography Group Investigator (2007) Effect of directed training on reader performance for CT colonography: multicenter study. Radiology 242(1):152–161

Rockey DC et al (2007) Standards for gastroenterologists for performing and interpreting diagnostic computed tomographic colonography. Gastroenterology 133(3):1005–1024

Soto JA, Barish MA, Yee J (2005) Reader training in CT colonography: how much is enough? Radiology 237(1):26–27

Johnson CD et al (2003) Prospective blinded evaluation of computed tomographic colonography for screen detection of colorectal polyps. Gastroenterology 125(2):311–319

Cotton PB et al (2004) Computed tomographic colonography (virtual colonoscopy): a multicenter comparison with standard colonoscopy for detection of colorectal neoplasia. JAMA 291(14):1713–1719

Pickhardt PJ et al (2003) Computed tomographic virtual colonoscopy to screen for colorectal neoplasia in asymptomatic adults. N Engl J Med 349(23):2191–2200

Spinzi G et al (2001) Computed tomographic colonography and conventional colonoscopy for colon diseases: a prospective, blinded study. Am J Gastroenterol 96(2):394–400

Johnson CD et al (2008) Accuracy of CT colonography for detection of large adenomas and cancers. N Engl J Med 359(12):1207–1217

McFarland EG et al (2008) Revised colorectal screening guidelines: joint effort of the American Cancer Society, U.S. Multisociety Task Force on Colorectal Cancer, and American College of Radiology. Radiology 248(3):717–720

Ferrucci JT (2000) CT colonography for colorectal cancer screening: lessons from mammography. AJR Am J Roentgenol 174(6):1539–1541

Fenlon HM (2002) CT colonography: pitfalls and interpretation. Abdom Imaging 27(3):284–291

Mang T et al (2007a) Pitfalls in multi-detector row CT colonography: a systematic approach. Radiographics 27(2):431–454

Dachman AH et al (2007) CT colonography: visualization methods, interpretation, and pitfalls. Radiol Clin North Am 45(2):347–359

Taylor SA et al (2007) European Society of Gastrointestinal and Abdominal Radiology (ESGAR): consensus statement on CT colonography. Eur Radiol 17(2):575–579

Burling D et al (2006b) CT colonography interpretation times: effect of reader experience, fatigue, and scan findings in a multi-centre setting. Eur Radiol 16(8):1745–1749

Johnson KT, Fletcher JG, Johnson CD (2007) Computer-aided detection (CAD) using 360 degree virtual dissection: can CAD in a first reviewer paradigm be a reliable substitute for primary 2D or 3D search? AJR Am J Roentgenol 189(4):W172–W176

Graser A et al (2007) Computer-aided detection in CT colonography: initial clinical experience using a prototype system. Eur Radiol 17(10):2608–2615

Hock D et al (2008) Virtual dissection CT colonography: evaluation of learning curves and reading times with and without computer-aided detection. Radiology 248(3):860–868

Summers RM et al (2008) Performance of a previously validated CT colonography computer-aided detection system in a new patient population. AJR Am J Roentgenol 191(1):168–174

Taylor SA et al (2008) Flat neoplasia of the colon: CT colonography with CAD. Abdom Imaging 34:173–181

Mang T et al (2007b) Effect of computer-aided detection as a second reader in multidetector-row CT colonography. Eur Radiol 17(10):2598–2607

Zalis ME et al (2005) CT colonography reporting and data system: a consensus proposal. Radiology 236(1):3–9

Pickhardt PJ (2007) Screening CT colonography: how I do it. AJR Am J Roentgenol 189(2):290–298

Lefere P, Dachman AH, Gryspeerdt S (2007) Computed tomographic colonography: clinical value. Abdom Imaging 32(5):541–551

The Eligible Patient: Indications and Contraindications

M. Raquel Oliva, Ayodale S. Odulate, and Koenraad J. Mortele

CONTENTS

M. Raquel Oliva, MD, PhD
Abdominal Imaging and Intervention Section, Brigham and Women's Hospital, Harvard Medical School, 75 Francis Street, Boston, MA 02115, USA
Ayodale S. Odulate, MD
Koenraad J. Mortele, MD
Brigham and Women's Hospital, Harvard Medical School, 75 Francis Street, Boston, MA 02115, USA

4.1 History

The development of computed tomography (CT) independently by both Godfrey N Hounsfield and Allan M Cormack in 1972 has forever changed the practice of medicine in detection, surveillance and treatment of disease. In the past 36 years, we have seen an explosion in technological innovation, particularly in the field of CT, yielding improved diagnosis and follow-up of diseases by radiologists.

In 1994, Vining and Gelfand introduced computed tomographic colonography (CTC), also referred to as virtual colonoscopy, as a tool to evaluate the insufflated colon (Vining et al. 1994). Early work in CTC involved patient populations with an increased risk of colon cancer with the goal of detecting colorectal cancer. Initial studies were performed with single detector CT scanners with thick collimated slices and were primarily read in the 2D axial plane. We have advanced significantly from the days of single detector scanners with 4, 8, 16, 64, and 128 multidetector-row scanners now available. Total volume imaging in a single breath-hold, as a result of multidetector-row scanning, has been shown to improve accuracy of polyp detection by decreasing motion artifact (Gryspeerdt et al. 2004). Also, due to significant software improvements, post-processing reformations are currently reconstructed in any plane in a matter of seconds (Bruzzi et al. 2001) and continued advancements in 3D software development have made virtual endoscopic flythrough of the colon applicable in clinical practice (Pickhardt et al. 2005).

The practical execution of CTC is still somewhat variable: patient bowel preparation, scanning acquisition parameters and post-processing software vary. Methods of interpretation also vary, with some proponents advocating a primary 3D read with 2D images evaluation for problem solving (Pickhardt et al. 2007) vs. a primary 2D read with 3D flythrough for problem solving (Dachman et al. 1998). No technique has yet proved to be superior to any other consistently and differences are seen regionally. Overall, however, the CTC literature has shown consistent improvement in the sensitivity and specificity of polyp and colorectal cancer detection as the technology has improved.

CTC as a screening tool for colon cancer continues to improve and is now a credible alternate and less-invasive tool to evaluate the colon, recently acknowledged by the American Cancer Society, the US Multi-Society Task Force on Colorectal Cancer, and the American College of Radiology (Levin et al. 2008). Initial studies in the mid to late 1990s evaluated patients at high risk for colon cancer with a single-slice scanner and demonstrated sensitivities of polyp detection ranging from 50 to 90% for polyps larger than 10 mm with specificities ranging from 70 to 90% (Van Dam et al. 2004). As the technology and application of CTC developed over time, the detection of colon cancer and polyps, even those smaller than 10 mm, improved (Yee et al. 2001). This has been validated in a large multicentric trial, in which 90% of the adenomas or cancers measuring 10 mm or more in diameter were identified in asymptomatic adults (Johnson et al. 2008). Gradually, CTC is being integrated into the algorithm for colon cancer screening worldwide.

This chapter explores the current indications and contraindications of CTC, and provides recommendations regarding which patients may benefit the most from CTC. Current reimbursable indications in the US by major third party payers are briefly described. Lastly, the current technologies under development with possible future indications are discussed.

4.2 Indications

Originally CTC was recommended for patients who were unwilling or unable to undergo optical colonoscopy. The indications accepted by the American College of Radiology practice guideline for the performance of CTC in adults included: screening individuals who are at average or elevated risk for colorectal carcinoma or who have a first-degree relative with a history of colorectal neoplasm; surveillance examination in patients with a history of previous colonic neoplasm, either benign or malignant; diagnostic examination in patients with known or prior colorectal carcinoma and in symptomatic patients including, but not limited to, those with abdominal pain, diarrhea, constipation, gastrointestinal bleeding, anemia, intestinal obstruction, and weight loss; following incomplete screening, surveillance, or diagnostic colonoscopy; and patients who require colonoscopy while on anticoagulant therapy (ACR 2006). Recently published Joint Guideline from the American Cancer Society, the US Multi-Society Task Force on Colorectal Cancer, and the American College of Radiology also recommended CTC as one of the possible screening tests for the early detection of colorectal adenomas and cancer (Levin et al. 2008) (Table 4.1).

Table 4.1. Guideline for using CT colonography for the early detection of colorectal adenomas and cancer in an asymptomatic patient

Screening CT colonography		
Indication	Age to begin (years)	Interval
Average-risk women and men	50	Every 5 years
Patient with first-degree relative age ≥60 years with a history of colorectal cancer or adenomatous polyp	40	Every 5 years
Patient with two second-degree relatives with history of colorectal cancer	40	Every 5 years
Patients with small rectal hyperplastic polyps[a]	–	Every 5 years

[a]An exception is patient with a hyperplastic polyposis syndrome

4.2.1 Screening CT Colonography

In the United States, colorectal cancer is the third most common cancer diagnosed in men and women and the second leading cause of death from cancer (Jemal et al. 2008). The 5-year survival is 90% if the disease is diagnosed while still localized but only 10% when metastases develop (Gennari et al. 2007). Approximately 75% of all colorectal cancers occur among persons with average risk, i.e., those without predisposing conditions to develop colorectal cancer, such as inflammatory bowel disease (IBD), familial adenomatous polyposis, hereditary nonpolyposis colorectal cancer, or a first-degree relative with a history of colorectal cancer or adenomatous polyp before the age of 60 years (Winawer et al. 1991; Ahsan et al. 1998). The age range for development of colon cancer is from the late forties to the seventies in average-risk patients. The high-risk patient population accounts for approximately 25% of the colorectal cancer incidence in the United States.

The proposed natural history of colon cancer in the average risk patient, as described in the National Polyp Study in 1990, confirmed the expected developmental course of colorectal cancer beginning with an adenomatous polyp, progressing to high-grade dysplasia, and then, frank carcinoma. However, the majority of the polyps resected measuring less than 10 mm in size represent hyperplastic polyps and other benign findings. Therefore, the goal of polypectomy should be adenoma resection. Research suggests there is about a 5-year interval between the stages of adenomatous polyp and adenoma with high-grade dysplasia, and another 5-year interval to develop frank cancer (O'Brien et al. 1990). The majority of adenomas that will develop into cancer are polypoid or villous in shape (Fig. 4.1). A small proportion of adenomas known as non-polypoid, flat or depressed lesions have been shown to be difficult to identify on optical colonoscopy and other colonic imaging modalities (Park et al. 2007). There is controversy and uncertainty of the prevalence of these non-polypoid lesions. Moreover, the lack of specific diagnostic criteria used in various studies makes it difficult to state what the true sensitivity of CTC for the detection of these flat lesions is (Fidler and Johnson 2008).

Positive predictive characteristics of an adenoma with increased propensity to develop into cancer are its size and the total number of adenomas. Polyps greater than 10 mm in diameter and more than three in number, regardless of their size, have been reported as risk factors for transformation into colorectal cancer through the "adenoma-carcinoma sequence," as described above. Overall, the literature suggests that the risk of an adenoma, measuring 5 mm or less in greatest dimension, to develop into cancer is significantly low, approximately 0.9% (O'Brien et al. 1990).

The goal of colorectal cancer screening is to reduce the morbidity and mortality of colon cancer by early detection and resection of adenomas and cancers (Frazier et al. 2000; Winawer and Zauber 2002). A Joint Guideline from the American Cancer Society, the US Multi-Society Task Force on Colorectal Cancer, and the American College of Radiology supports screening average-risk individuals starting at 50 years of age to detect and prevent CRC. Screening can be performed with tests that detect adenomatous polyps and cancer (flexible sigmoidoscopy every 5 years, or optical colonoscopy every 10 years, or double-contrast barium enema every 5 years, or CTC every 5 years) or tests that primarily detect cancer (annual guaiac-based fecal occult blood test with high test sensitivity for cancer, or annual fecal immunochemical test with high sensitivity for cancer, or stool DNA test with high sensitivity for cancer, at uncertain interval) (Levin et al. 2008). Patients classified as high-risk for developing colorectal cancer undergo screening at a much younger age and shorter interval, as specified by their personal risk factors.

Albeit imperfect with a documented adenoma miss rate ranging from 6 to 27% (depending on the size of the lesion), optical colonoscopy is still the gold standard for colon cancer screening (Rex et al. 1997). Colon cancers have also been missed by optical colonoscopy. A study performed in Canada reported a cancer miss rate of 4% in cancers originating in the right colon (Bressler et al. 2004). Several reasons

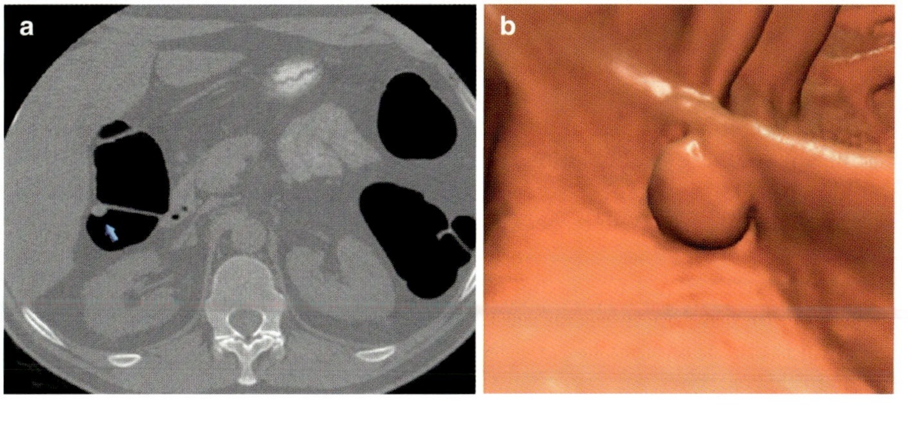

Fig. 4.1. Colonic adenoma: (a) axial CT image and (b) 3D image demonstrate a tubular adenoma with low-grade dysplasia in the transverse/ascending colon

exist why cancers are missed on optical colonoscopy: poor bowel preparation, slippage of the endoscope around flexures, redundant colon, misinterpretation of the findings and failure to biopsy (Leaper et al. 2004). A false negative optical colonoscopy may have serious implications, as patients may not have another colon screening test for a decade.

Optical colonoscopy is not without risk to patients, and significant morbidity and mortality has been reported (Garbay et al. 1996). The most common adverse outcome associated with optical colonoscopy includes hemorrhage and perforation. The rate of perforation of the colon is 0.2–0.4% after diagnostic colonoscopy, increases with polypectomy, and approximates 5% with hydrostatic balloon dilation of a colonic stricture (Zubarik et al. 1999).

A landmark multicentric study published by Pickhardt et al. compared CTC and optical colonoscopy in an asymptomatic average-risk patient population. As a screening study, comparable adenoma and colorectal cancer detection rates were reported (Pickhardt et al. 2003). In fact, the sensitivity and specificity per patient and per polyp were similar and not statistically different between CTC and optical colonoscopy for adenomas greater than 10 mm. The sensitivity of CTC for adenomatous polyps was 93.8% for polyps at least 10 mm in diameter, 93.9% for polyps at least 8 mm in diameter, and 88.7% for polyps at least 6 mm in diameter. The sensitivity of optical colonoscopy for adenomatous polyps was 87.5, 91.5, and 92.3% for the three sizes of polyps, respectively. The specificity of CTC for adenomatous polyps was 96.0% for polyps at least 10 mm in diameter, 92.2% for polyps at least 8 mm in diameter, and 79.6% for polyps at least 6 mm in diameter (Pickhardt et al. 2003). A recently published large, multicentric study of 2,531 asymptomatic adults showed that CTC screening identified 90% of patients with adenomas and cancers measuring 10 mm or more in diameter (Johnson et al. 2008). These findings support the previously published data regarding the role of CTC in screening patients with an average risk of colorectal cancer.

Detection rates for polyps less than or equal to 5 mm in diameter are lower and the debate over the significance of these smaller lesions continues. Again, the aim of colorectal cancer screening is to detect cancer and adenomas. With respect to adenomas, the term "advanced adenoma" has been used to describe clinically significant adenomas that have the greatest likelihood to develop into cancer. Current understanding is that adenomas larger or equal to 10 mm reside in this category.

CTC as a screening tool has the potential to have a wider public acceptance compared to optical colonoscopy. Acceptance of a screening study by a population is multi-factorial. Many physical and psychological barriers to colorectal cancer screening have been described. Surveys have reported patient's reluctance to undergo colorectal cancer screening because of time commitment associated with optical colonoscopy, use of colon cathartic, sedation requirements, prior painful experience and even embarrassment (Rozen et al. 2005). CTC is relatively fast without the need for sedation or a driver post procedure. Patients have described the post procedure discomfort less for CTC than with optical colonoscopy. Several studies have shown that patients' acceptance of CTC is greater than of optical colonoscopy or double contrast barium enema (Svensson et al. 2002; Taylor et al. 2003). Development of minimal bowel prep or prep-less CTC through fecal tagging and electronic cleansing appears to be within reach, thus making a truly prep-less colorectal screening test an attractive possibility (Lefere et al. 2002).

Currently CTC is indicated as a screening test to detect colorectal adenomatous polyps and cancer for asymptomatic individuals who are at average-risk for colorectal carcinoma, starting at 50 years of age; patients who have a first-degree relative aged 60 years or more with a history of colorectal cancer or adenomatous polyp, starting at 40 years of age; or patients with two second-degree relatives with colorectal cancer, starting at 40 years of age (Levin et al. 2008). CTC is also a screening option for patients with history of small rectal hyperplastic polyps, with the exception of patients with a hyperplastic polyposis syndrome, since they are at increased risk for adenomas and colorectal cancer and need to be identified for more intensive follow up (Levin et al. 2008) (Table 4.1).

The American College of Radiology guidelines for reporting CTC findings are as follows: surgical consultation when a mass is found; resection if a polyp measuring 10 mm or more is found or if there are three or more polyps 6 mm or larger; shorter interval follow up with CT colonography or optical colonoscopy if less than three polyps measuring 6–9 mm are noted, possibly in 3 years interval; and continue routine screening if no polyp measuring 6 mm or more is present (Zalis et al. 2005). However, the new Joint Guideline from the American Cancer Society, the US Multi-Society Task Force on Colorectal Cancer, and the American College of Radiology recommends optical colonoscopy if patients have one or more polyps measuring 6 mm or larger on CTC (Levin et al. 2008).

Therefore, currently in our practice, the CTC reporting guidelines recommend optical colonoscopy if there is a polyp measuring 6 mm or more, and recommend continued routine screening if no polyp measuring greater than 5 mm is present.

4.2.2 Diagnostic CT Colonography

The indications for diagnostic CTC closely follow those for optical colonoscopy (Rankin 1987). Patients with bowel related symptoms, such as abdominal pain, change in bowel habits, lower gastrointestinal bleeding, iron deficiency anemia, intestinal obstruction, and weight loss can undergo a diagnostic CTC.

When undergoing a diagnostic CTC, the patient is scanned in both the supine and prone positions, but unlike screening CTC, the patient is injected with intravenous iodinated contrast material during the supine acquisition (Chen et al. 1999). Injection of contrast aids in the differentiation of polyp vs. adherent stool. Studies have also demonstrated increased accuracy of polyp detection with the use of intravenous contrast material (Morrin et al. 2000). A contrast-enhanced scan may aid in the detection of extracolonic causes of the patients symptoms. Finally, diagnostic CTC has the ability to detect and stage colorectal cancer, unlike the other two alternatives, optical colonoscopy and double contrast barium enema.

Diagnostic CTC may be used to further evaluate findings on optical colonoscopy. Not infrequently, diagnostic CTC is performed in patients with suspicious intramural or extra-mural masses detected on optical colonoscopy (Fig. 4.2).

Occasionally, patients are unable to undergo optical colonoscopy due to presence of a colonic stricture, redundant sigmoid, or contraindications to sedation. Flexible sigmoidoscopy can be performed without sedation; however, the majority of the colon is not evaluated. Although double contrast barium enema evaluates the entire colon, many proponents of the new technology believe that CTC should be the study of choice for patients who are unable to undergo optical colonoscopy, as the sensitivity and specificity of polyp detection is higher for CTC compared to double contrast barium enema (Johnson et al. 2004; Toma et al. 2008).

4.2.3 Preoperative Assessment

The assessment of colon proximal to an obstructing colonic mass has been a shortcoming of optical colonoscopy. In the past, interoperative palpation or postoperative colonoscopy was performed with the possibility of a second surgery required for the missed synchronous cancer or adenoma. The sensitivity of hand palpation is fairly low and intraoperative insufflation of the colon increases the risk of peritoneal contamination.

Double-contrast barium enema remains in the algorithm for work-up of colorectal cancer in evaluation of the proximal bowel in case of an obstructing mass. This examination is not preferred, as the proximal colon often does not drain all of the contrast by the time of surgery. Patients are also at increased risk for postoperative morbidity if a reactive peritonitis develops secondary to insipissated barium contamination intraoperatively.

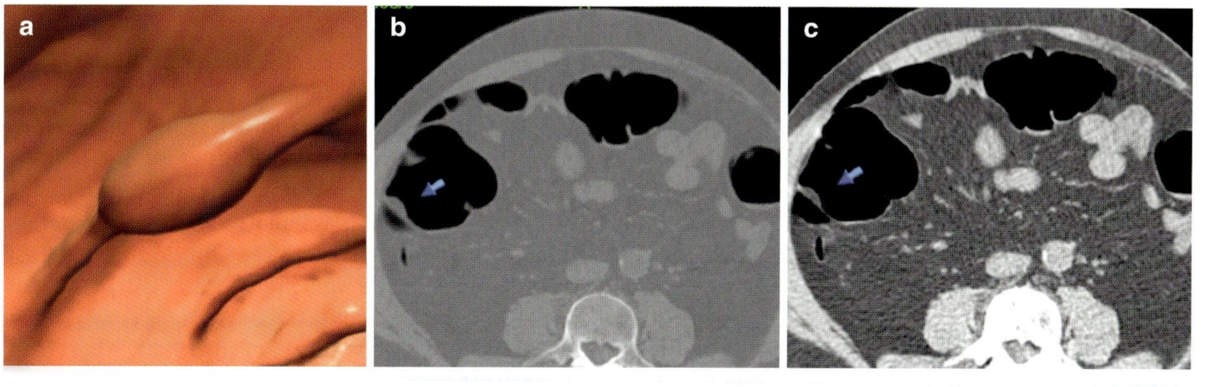

Fig. 4.2. Submucosal colonic lipoma: (a) 3D endoluminal view of the colon and (b) axial CT image with: window settings show a 12 mm lesion in the ascending colon; (c) axial CT image with soft tissue window settings demonstrate a fatty lesion consistent with a submucosal lipoma

The incidence of synchronous neoplasia in the colon has been described at a rate of 1.5–9% (Fenlon et al. 1999a). Adenomas harboring in the colon of patients with colon cancer have been reported at an incidence of 27–55% (Fenlon et al. 1999a). CTC has been shown to be a feasible and useful method for evaluating the entire colon before surgery in patients with occlusive carcinomas. CTC identified all of the cancers including two synchronous cancers proximal to the obstructing mass that were missed by double contrast barium enema (Fenlon et al. 1999b). In addition, CTC demonstrated 16 of 18 polyps in the proximal colon (Fenlon et al. 1999b).

4.2.4 Postoperative Colorectal Cancer Surveillance

Metachronous adenomas and neoplasms have been reported on surveillance colonoscopy at a fairly high rate (Fukutomi et al. 2002). The American Society of Clinical Oncology in 2005 updated a set of guidelines for the surveillance of the postoperative patient with colorectal cancer after thorough review of the literature on common surveillance protocols. Patient's follow-up exams should include: history and physical examination and risk assessment every 3–6 months for the first 3 years; carcinoembryonic antigen test every 3 months in patients with stage II or III disease for at least 3 years after diagnosis, if the patient is a candidate for surgery or systemic therapy; annual CT of the chest and abdomen for 3 years; colonoscopy at 3 years and then, if normal, once every 5 years thereafter, except for colorectal cancer patients with high-risk genetic syndromes, in which case shorter interval is recommended; and for patients who have not received pelvic radiation, flexible sigmoidoscopy of the rectum every 6 months for 5 years (Desch et al. 2005).

The role of CTC has been evaluated specifically in this patient population. Incomplete colonoscopies secondary to postoperative strictures and rigid mesentery have been reported. In 2002, Gollub et al. reported an optical colonoscopy failure rate of 4–29% in postoperative or postradiotherapy patients (Gollub et al. 2002). These patients would undergo a double contrast barium enema for complete evaluation of the colon. As discussed, CTC sensitivity for polyp detection is greater than double contrast barium enema and thus makes it a superior surveillance tool in this subset of patients.

The additional benefit of CTC for surveillance includes evaluation of the abdominal and pelvic viscera. The anastomosis can be specifically evaluated. In some surveillance algorithms, patients undergo colonoscopy and liver ultrasound. Laghi et al. reported on a group of patients undergoing surveillance with carcinoembryonic antigen test, liver ultrasound, colonoscopy and chest X-rays (Laghi et al. 2003). In his study, the patients underwent contrast-enhanced CTC and findings were directly compared to optical colonoscopy findings. CTC detected all polyps seen with optical colonoscopy with two false positives. This study also showed CTC to be able to diagnose liver metastases and lung base nodules. Therefore, contrast-enhanced CTC appears to be a valuable alternative surveillance tool in postoperative patients at increased risk for adenomas and cancer.

4.2.5 Incomplete Optical Colonoscopy

CTC has been shown to be superior to double contrast barium enema following incomplete optical colonoscopy and, in fact, failed colonoscopy was the first established indication for CTC. An incomplete colonoscopy is defined as failure to intubate up to the cecum. The reported rate of failed colonoscopy ranges from 8% to as high as 35%. Patients with a history of an incomplete colonoscopy have a significant increased risk of failing a second attempt. A multitude of reasons contribute to a failed optical colonoscopy: poor bowel preparation, redundant colon, strictures, history of failed colonoscopies and patient discomfort. Double-contrast barium enema was usually the next step in the algorithm of colon evaluation and in most cases performed the same day. On some occasions, however, double contrast barium enema is suboptimal as well, sometimes due to poor bowel prep, patient inability to move on the table or inadequate barium coating of the colonic mucosa secondary to an air block from the previous incomplete colonoscopy (Macari et al. 1999).

In patients with failed colonoscopy, Macari et al. reported, using CTC, a sensitivity of polyp detection of 87%, compared with 45% for double contrast barium enema. The specificity was also better for CTC than double contrast barium enema; 98 vs. 89%, respectively (Macari et al. 1999). Therefore, in patients who have failed optical colonoscopy, CTC rather than a second attempt of optical colonoscopy or double contrast barium enema may be prudent.

4.2.6 Inflammatory Bowel Disease Surveillance

Patients with ulcerative colitis and Crohn's disease have an increased risk of colorectal cancer the longer the disease progresses; an approximate 3% risk of colon cancer has been reported (Mpofu et al. 2006). Optimal surveillance strategies for colon cancer in patients with IBD have not been established. Furthermore, no clear evidence exists that surveillance improves colon cancer survival in this patient population (Mpofu et al. 2006).

There is, however, consensus that patients with IBD should undergo surveillance colonoscopy, although the interval in which this should be done and the optimal number and location of biopsies that should be obtained are uncertain. The American Society for Gastrointestinal Endoscopy (ASGE) recommends that patients with ulcerative colitis (UC) who have pancolitis should begin surveillance colonoscopy after 8 years of disease American Society for Gastrointestinal Endoscopy 1998. Four biopsies should be obtained every 10 cm from the cecum to the rectum. In addition, any suspicious lesions or masses should be biopsied. Colonoscopy should be repeated every 1–3 years. The finding of carcinoma or high-grade dysplasia is an indication for colectomy. Colectomy is also indicated for any degree of dysplasia associated with a lesion or mass. For patients with low-grade dysplasia confirmed by an expert pathologist, the ASGE acknowledges that most experts recommend colectomy. However, in patients in whom colectomy is not feasible or is unacceptable, frequent surveillance (e.g., every 3–6 months) is considered an acceptable alternative. For patients with left-sided colitis, the ASGE recommends that surveillance should begin after 15 years of disease. Surveillance is not indicated in ulcerative colitis limited to the rectum.

The American Gastroenterological Association acknowledges that the risk of colorectal cancer associated with Crohn's colitis is similar to that of ulcerative colitis to a comparable extent, with regard to duration and age of onset of inflammatory disease. As a result, the surveillance strategy discussed above for UC also applies for Crohn's colitis patients.

The recently published Joint Guideline from the American Cancer Society, the US Multi-Society Task Force on Colorectal Cancer, and the American College of Radiology recommends colorectal cancer screening with optical colonoscopy and biopsies every 1–2 years for patients with IBD (chronic ulcerative colitis and Crohn's colitis) (Levin et al. 2008). Since cancer risks begin to be significant about 8 years after the onset of pancolitis and 12–15 years after the onset of left-sided colitis, this is the time recommended to start screening (Levin et al. 2008).

However, in this patient population with history of colitis and possible prior segmental colonic resections, fistulas and strictures often develop at the anastomosis and make passage of the colonoscopy device very unlikely. Scarring of the mesentery may also cause rigidity and may lead to failed colonoscopies. Historically, patients would then go on to double-contrast barium enema for complete evaluation of the colon.

Ota et al. reported a study of 33 patients with Crohn's disease and compared CTC with optical colonoscopy and double contrast barium enema in the detection of lesions in the colon proximal to a stenosis (Ota et al. 2003). CTC was found to be superior to both double contrast barium enema and optical colonoscopy in the evaluation of the proximal colon. Colonoscopy was limited to mucosal evaluation and CTC had the added advantage of evaluating all of the bowel wall as well as extra-luminal disease.

Biancone et al. described a beneficial use of CTC in this particular subset of Crohn's patient with strictures and failed colonoscopies (Biancone et al. 2003). His study was performed in 16 patients who had undergone partial colectomy, including ileocolonic anastomosis, for Crohn's colitis to evaluate for recurrence at the anastomosis. Patients underwent both optical colonoscopy and CTC. CTC was found to be as accurate in the detection of recurrence at the site of anastomosis with the added evaluation of small bowel dilatation proximal to the stricture and degree of bowel wall thickening. A significant limitation of CTC was its inability to perform biopsies. In patients with IBD, CTC is a possible tool for further subdividing patient populations into those who have positive findings and need to go on to optical colonoscopy and biopsy and those who have negative findings and can continue to be screened at regular intervals.

4.3 Contraindications

The contraindications to CTC are few and, in general, different from those encountered with optical colonoscopy (Table 4.2). Weight and girth limitations of the scanner, artifact from metal prosthesis and claustrophobia are examples of limitations unique to CT. Absolute contraindications to instrumentation of the

Table 4.2. Contraindications for CT colonography

Contraindications for CTC	
Absolute	**Relative**
Physical weight limitations	Pregnancy
Acute abdomen	Hip joint replacements
Acute diverticulitis	
Recent pelvic or abdominal surgery	
Toxic megacolon	
Colonic hernia	
Incompetent ileocecal valve*	

colon include presence of an acute abdomen, recent abdominal or pelvic surgery, acute diverticulitis, and colonic hernia (Fig. 4.3). Relative contraindications include pregnant patients and an incompetent ileocecal valve.

4.3.1 Absolute Contraindications

Many CT scanners have a weight limit of 300–400 pounds and a circumferential girth limit of 60 cm. The colon of a patient with an acute abdomen should not be inflated with room air or CO_2, and consultation with a surgeon is most appropriate. Patients with active diverticulitis should not be referred to CTC. If an abscess or free air is suspected, CT of the abdomen and pelvis can be performed with oral and IV contrast. Insufflation of the colon is contraindicated and may cause perforation and widespread peritonitis. Similarly, if a patient has recently undergone pelvic or abdominal surgery, in the past 4 months, insufflation of the colon is contraindicated. Patients with a known history of colonic hernia or toxic megacolon should not undergo colonoscopy or CTC.

4.3.2 Relative Contraindications

Pregnancy is a relative contraindication to CTC. The radiation and absorbed dose to the fetus during the dual scan is the major issue. In the rare instance that a pregnant patient is suspected to have a colorectal cancer and there is a real risk of perforation with optical colonoscopy, CTC may be the safer alternative. The gestational age of the fetus is an important factor when contemplating risk. The relative risk of childhood cancers is 1.4 with an exposure of 10 mGy (Kusama and Ota 2002). Radiation doses are heavily regulated and the effective dose limit to the fetus is 0.5 rem (5 mSv) (Huda and Stone 2003). The effective dose of thin-section low dose CTC is approximately 5.0 mSv for men and 7.8 mSv for women. The effective dose to the fetus in uterus, however, is less

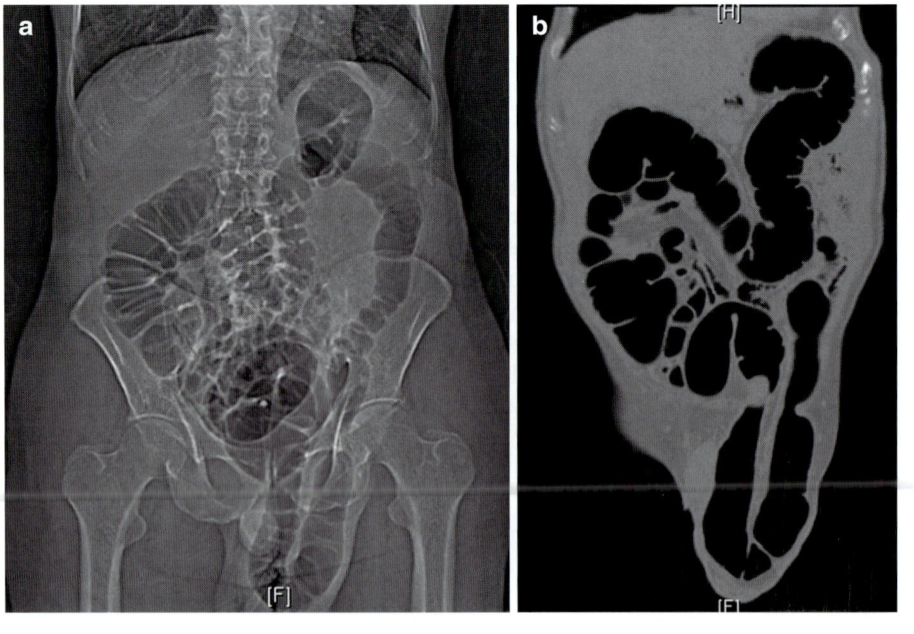

Fig. 4.3. Left inguinal colonic hernia: (**a**) scout image shows loop of bowel in a left inguinal hernia; (**b**) coronal reformatted CT image shows distended colon within a left inguinal hernia

than the stated dose of 7.8 mSv (Macari et al. 2002 and Iannaccone et al. 2003).

Patients with metallic hip joint replacements will have significant artifact in the pelvis with limited evaluation of colonic segments in this region. This is a relative contraindication depending on the clinical question asked. Intravenous iodinated contrast allergy is also a relative contraindication for diagnostic CTC as any patient with a history of a mild contrast allergy can be premedicated for the exam or not receive the injection. Claustrophobia is also a relative contraindication to CTC as patients can take an oral sedative prior to the study. An incompetent ileocecal valve is another relative contraindication for this study as distention of the colon may be suboptimal.

4.4 Current Reimbursable Indications

The first reimbursable indication for CTC was studying the colon following a failed colonoscopy. In the US, CTC is currently coded under the CPT category III code 0066T for screening and 0067T for diagnostic CTC (Knechtges et al. 2007). Reimbursement by Medicare and some third party payors for CTC is approved only for diagnostic CTC, following a failed colonoscopy and with specific ICD-9 codes. Medicare and Medicaid do not currently cover colon cancer screening with CTC and therefore patients have to pay out of pocket. Recently, however, the Centers for Medicare & Medicaid Services have initiated a national coverage analysis for the use of screening CTC for colorectal cancer, which will evaluate the available evidence for screening CTC and determine if a national coverage determination is warranted. Wisconsin to date, to the best of our knowledge, is the lone state that has successfully lobbied the local major third party payors and secured reimbursement for screening CTC.

4.5 Future Indications

The need for colon cleansing with bowel cathartics may be revisited with further development of electronic bowel cleansing software and prep-less fecal tagging protocols. This promises to significantly increase the overall percentage of patients willing to participate in colorectal cancer screening and, therefore, reduce morbidity and ultimately mortality related to colorectal cancer.

Polyp surveillance with CTC may be further refined and some patients ultimately spared from unnecessary polypectomy. Concerns regarding radiation dose may be further reduced with continued dose reduction software development.

4.6 Summary

CTC, now 15 years old, has made substantial progress in the detection of adenomas and colorectal cancer. Recent studies report comparable sensitivities and specificities to optical colonoscopy for polyps 10 mm or larger. The recently published American Cancer Society guideline has included CTC as one of the screening tests for colorectal cancer. CTC is currently approved by Medicare and some third-party players as a diagnostic study in patients with specific symptoms and after failed colonoscopy. Work continues to approve CTC as a colorectal cancer screening exam.

References

Ahsan H, Neugut A, Garbowshi G et al (1998) Family history of colorectal adenomatous polyps and increased risk for colorectal cancer. Ann Intern Med 128:900–905

ACR (2006) American College of Radiology practice guideline for the performance or computed tomography (CT) colonography in adults. ACR practice guideline, CT colonography 2005 (Res. 29). Amended 2006 (Res. 17, 35), pp 503–508

American Society for Gastrointestinal Endoscopy (1998) The role of colonoscopy in the management of patients with inflammatory bowel disease. Gastrointest Endosc 48: 689–690

Knechtges PM, McFarland BG, Keysor KJ et al (2007) National and local trends in CT colonography reimbursement: past, present, and future. J Am Coll Radiol 11:776–799

Biancone L, Fiori R, Tosti C et al (2003) Virtual colonoscopy compared with conventional colonoscopy for stricturing postoperative recurrences in Crohn's disease. Inflamm Bowel Dis 9:343–350

Bressler B, Paszat LF, Vinden C et al (2004) Colonoscopic miss rates for right-sided colon cancer: a population-based analysis. Gastroenterology 127:452–456

Bruzzi J, Moss A, Fenlon H (2001) Clinical results of CT colonoscopy. Eur Radiol 11:2188–94

Chen S, Lu D, Hecht J et al (1999) CT colonography: value of scanning in both the supine and prone positions. Am J Roentgenol 172:595–599

Dachman A, Kuniyoshi J, Boyle C et al (1998) CT colonography with three-dimensional problem solving for detection of colonic polyps. Am J Roentgenol 171:989–995

Desch CE, Benson AB 3rd, Somerfield MR, American Society of Clinical Oncology et al (2005) Colorectal cancer surveillance: 2005 update of an American Society of Clinical Oncology practice guideline. J Clin Oncol 33:8512–8519

Fenlon H, Nunes D, Schroy P et al (1999a) A comparison of virtual and conventional colonoscopy for the detection of colorectal polyps. N Engl J Med 341:1496–1503

Fenlon H, McAneny D, Nunes D et al (1999b) Occlusive colon carcinoma: virtual colonoscopy in the preoperative evaluation of the proximal colon. Radiology 210:423–428

Fidler J, Johnson C (2008) Flat polyps of the colon: accuracy of detection by CT colonography and histologic significance. Abdom Imaging 34:157–171

Frazier A, Lindsay M, Graham A et al (2000) Cost-effectiveness of screening for colorectal cancer in the general population. JAMA 284:1954–1961

Fukutomi Y, Moriwaki H, Nagase S et al (2002) Metachronous colon tumors: risk factor and rationale for the surveillance colonoscopy after initial polypectomy. J Cancer Res Clin Oncol 128:569–574

Garbay J, Suc B, Rotman N et al (1996) Multicentre study of surgical complications of colonoscopy. Br J Surg 83:42–44

Gennari L, Russo A, Rossetti C (2007) Colorectal cancer: what has changed in diagnosis and treatment over the last 50 years? Tumori 3:235–41

Gollub M, Ginsberg M, Cooper C et al (2002) Quality of virtual colonoscopy in patients who have undergone radiation therapy or surgery: how successful are we? Am J Roentgenol 178:1109–1116

Gryspeerdt S, Herman M, Baekelandt M et al (2004) Supine/left decubitus scanning: a valuable alternative to supine/prone scanning in CT colonography. Eur Radiol 14:768–777

Huda W, Stone RM (2003) Review of radiologic physics, 2nd edn. Lippincott Williams and Wilkins, Philadelphia

Iannaccone R, Laghi A, Catalano C et al (2003) Detection of colorectal lesions: lower-dose multi-detector row helical CT colonography compared with conventional colonoscopy. Radiology 229:775–781

Jemal A, Siegel R, Ward E et al (2008) Cancer statistics, 2008. CA Cancer J Clin 2:71–96

Johnson C, MacCarty R, Welch T et al (2004) Comparison of the relative sensitivity of CT colonography and double-contrast barium enema for the screen detection of colorectal polyps. Clin Gastroenterol Hepatol 2:314–321

Johnson CD, Chen MH, Toledano AY et al (2008) Accuracy of CT colonography for detection of large adenomas and cancers. N Engl J Med 12:1207–1217

Kusama T, Ota K (2002) Radiological protection for diagnostic examination of pregnant women. Congenit Anom 42: 10–14

Laghi A, Iannaccone R, Bria E et al (2003) Contrast-enhanced computed tomographic colonography in the follow-up of colorectal cancer patients: a feasibility study. Eur Radiol 13:883–889

Levin B, Lieberman DA, McFarland B et al (2008) Screening and surveillance for the early detection of colorectal cancer and adenomatous polyps, 2008: a joint guideline from the American Cancer Society, the US Multi-Society Task Force on Colorectal Cancer, and the American College of Radiology. CA Cancer J Clin 3:130–160

Leaper M, Johnston MJ, Barclar M et al (2004) Reasons for failure to diagnose colorectal carcinoma at colonoscopy. Endoscopy 36:499–503

Lefere P, Gryspeerdt S, Dewyspelaere J et al (2002) Dietary fecal tagging as a cleansing method before CT colonography: initial results polyp detection and patient acceptance. Radiology 224:393–403

Macari M, Berman P, Dicker M et al (1999) Usefulness of CT colography in patients with incomplete colonoscopy. AJR 173:561–564

Macari M, Bini EJ, Xue X et al (2002) Colorectal neoplasms: prospective comparison of thin-section low-dose multidetector row CT colonography and conventional colonoscopy for detection. Radiology 2:383–392

Morrin M, Farrell F, Kruskal J et al (2000) Utility of intravenously administered contrast material at CT colonography. Radiology 217:765–771

Mpofu C, Watson AJ, Rhodes JM (2006) Strategies for detecting colon cancer and/or dysplasia in patients with inflammatory bowel disease. Cochrane Database Syst Rev (2):CD000279; Review

O'Brien M, Winawer S, Zauber A et al (1990) The National Polyp Study. Patient and polyp characteristics associated with high grade dysplasia in colorectal adenomas. Gastroenterology 88:371–379

Ota Y, Matsui T, Ono H et al (2003) Value of virtual computed tomographic colonography for Crohn's colitis: comparison with endoscopy and barium enema. Abdom Imaging 28:778–783

Park SH, Lee SS, Choi EK et al (2007) Flat colorectal neoplasms: definition, importance, and visualization on CT colonography. AJR Am J Roentgenol 4:953–959

Pickhardt P, Choi J, Hwang I et al (2003) Computed tomographic virtual colonoscopy to screen for colorectal neoplasia in asymptomatic adults. N Engl J Med 349: 2191–2200

Pickhardt PJ, Lee AD, McFarland EG et al (2005) Linear polyp measurement at CT colonography: in vitro and in vivo comparison of two-dimensional and three-dimensional displays. Radiology 3:872–878

Pickhardt PJ, Lee AD, Taylor AJ et al (2007) Primary 2D versus primary 3D polyp detection at screening CT colonography. AJR Am J Roentgenol 6:1451–1456

Rankin GB (1987) Indications, contraindications, and complications of colonoscopy. In: Sivak MV (ed) Gastrointestinal Endoscopy. WB Saunders, Philadelphia, pp 873–878

Rex D, Cutler C, Lemmel G et al (1997) Colonoscopic miss rates of adenomas determined by back-to-back colonoscopies. Gastroenterology 112:24–28

Rozen P, Pignone M, Crespi M et al (2005) Workgroup V: professional education and advocacy. UICC International Workshop on Facilitating Screening for Colorectal Cancer, Oslo, Norway (29 and 30 June 2002). Ann Oncol 1:42–45

Svensson MH, Svensson E, Lasson A et al (2002) Patient acceptance of CT colonography and conventional colonoscopy: prospective comparative study in patients with or suspected of having colorectal disease. Radiology 2:337–345

Taylor S, Halligan S, Saunders B et al (2003) Acceptance by patients of multidetector CT colonography compared with barium enema examinations, flexible sigmoidoscopy, and colonoscopy. Am J Roentgenol 181:913–921

Taylor SA (2004) Beyond the future: The SIGGAR1 Trial. In: The Fifth International Symposium on Virtual Colonoscopy, Boston, MA, USA

Toma J, Paszat LF, Gunraj N et al (2008) Rates of new or missed colorectal cancer after barium enema and their risk factors: a population-based study. Am J Gastroenterol 12: 3142–3148

van Dam J, Cotton P, Johnson D et al (2004) AGA future trends report: CT colonography. Gastroenterology 127: 970–984

Vining D, Gelfand D, Bechtold R et al (1994) Technical feasibility of colon imaging with helical CT and virtual reality. Am J Rotenogr 162(suppl):104

Winawer S, Schottenfeld D, Flehinger B (1991) Colorectal cancer screening. J Natl Cancer Inst 83:243–253

Winawer S, Zauber A (2002) The advanced adenoma as the primary target of screening. Gastrointest Endosc Clin N Am 1212:1–9

Yee J, Akerkar G, Hung R et al (2001) Colorectal neoplasia: performance characteristics of CT colonography for detection in 300 patients. Radiology 219:685–692

Zalis ME, Barish MA et al (2005) CT colonography reporting and data system: a consensus proposal. Radiology 1: 3–9

Zubarik R, Fleischer DE, Mastropietro C et al (1999) Prospective analysis of complications 30 days after outpatient colonoscopy. Gastrointest Endosc 50:322–328

Patient Preparation for CT Colonography

J. Yee

CONTENTS

J. Yee, MD
University of California,
San Francisco, CA 94121, USA

5.1 Introduction

CT colonography or virtual colonoscopy has increasing support as a screening tool for colorectal polyps and carcinoma. This radiologic examination uses the patient data acquired from a helical CT scanner and combines it with computer software that post-processes the data to generate both two- and three-dimensional images of the colon for analysis. However, before the patient undergoes the CT scan, there are initial steps that must be taken to help obtain images of the colon that are of high diagnostic quality. The key element for a high-quality CT colonography examination is a well-cleansed and well-distended colon (Figs. 5.1 and 5.2). When the colon contains residual fluid and/or stool, this can cause false-negative and false-positive results. Residual material in the colon will also limit the diagnostic usefulness of computer-aided detection algorithms. If the colon is poorly distended, this too can lead to lesions being missed, and an area of collapse may simulate the apple-core appearance of a carcinoma. Patients are typically scanned in two opposing positions (supine and prone) so that portions of the colon that have residual material or poor distension in one position may be reevaluated in the opposing view. CT colonography may also be successfully performed using reduced bowel preparation with the aid of fecal and fluid tagging (Taylor et al. 2008). Investigation is currently under way evaluating the use of non-cathartic protocols in combination with fecal and fluid tagging for CT colonography.

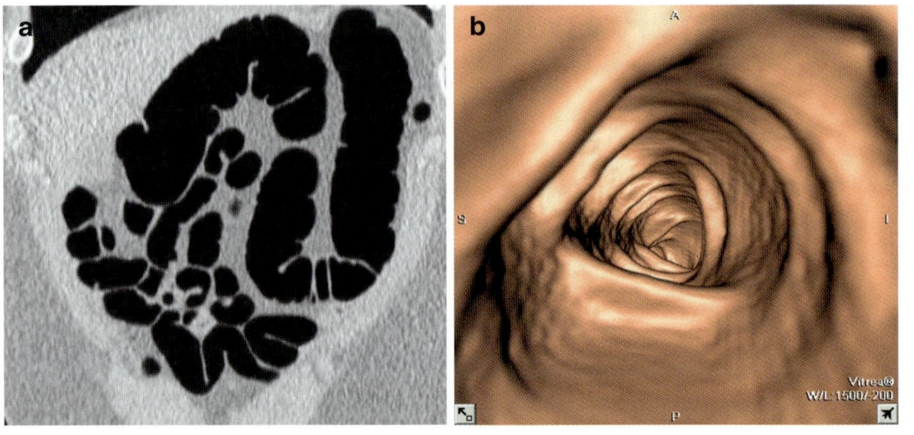

Fig. 5.1. (**a**) Coronal multiplanar reformat demonstrates a well-cleansed transverse colon with no layering fluid or residual solid stool. (**b**) Three-dimensional endoluminal view from the same patient showing normal haustral folds which are easily evaluated because of the absence of residual material

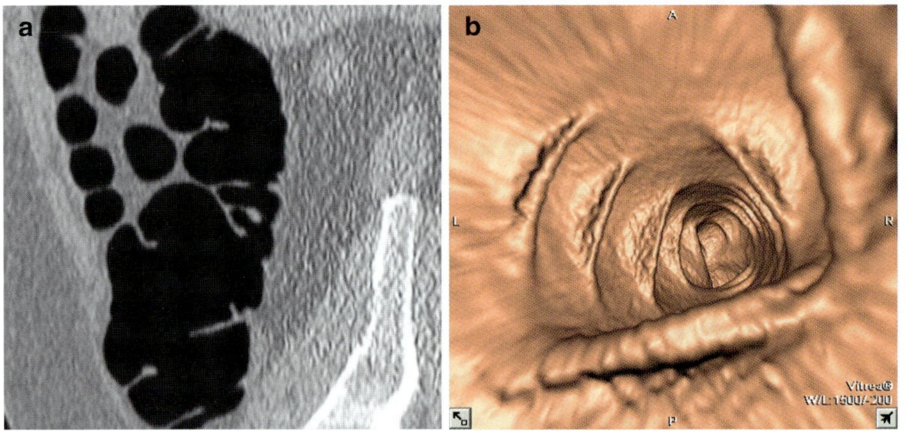

Fig. 5.2. (**a**) Excellent distension of the ascending colon and cecum on a sagittal multiplanar reformat optimizes diagnostic ability. (**b**) A well-distended segment in the same patient on the endoluminal view allows easy navigation

5.2 Colonic Preparation

Proper cleansing of the colon is essential if the radiologist is to identify colonic lesions accurately on CT colonography, particularly if fecal and fluid tagging is not employed. Remaining pools of fluid in the colon can hide polyps and cancer both on two-dimensional axial and reformatted images and on three-dimensional endoluminal views (Figs. 5.3 and 5.4). Residual solid stool may be misdiagnosed as a polyp, particularly if it is homogeneous and nonmobile. Large amounts of residual stool can obscure true colorectal polyps and even cancer. Bowel cleansing for CT colonography is currently similar to that used for other colon tests such as the barium enema and standard colonoscopy. There are two main strategies, the first being to maintain a clear liquid diet starting about 24 h before the CT scan. The second strategy is to clean the colon by having the patient ingest a cathartic or laxative that promotes emptying of the colon. Polyethylene glycol is an electrolyte lavage solution in a nonabsorbable medium that patients drink in large volumes to bring about colonic evacuation. Sodium phosphate and magnesium citrate are saline cathartics which are highly osmotic agents containing inorganic ions that draw fluid into the bowel lumen to induce peristalsis and elimination of bowel contents.

5.2.1 Polyethylene Glycol

Polyethylene glycol electrolyte lavage solution is often the agent preferred by gastroenterologists for colonic cleansing in patients prior to fiberoptic colonoscopy. One unit of the solution is composed of 236 g of polyethylene glycol as well as electrolytes such as sodium and potassium, and is administered orally in a large volume to empty the colon. The product typically comes in powder form in a large container and is mixed with about 4 L of water.

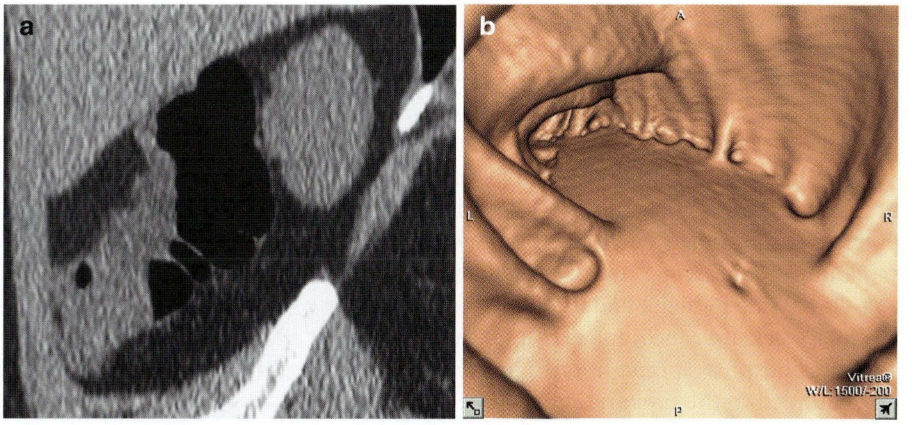

Fig. 5.3. (**a**) Suboptimal bowel preparation due to a large amount of residual fluid layering along the dependent wall of the colon as seen on this sagittal multiplanar reformatted view. (**b**) Poor cleansing with a large amount of layering fluid that obscures the colonic wall beneath it on this endoluminal view in the same patient

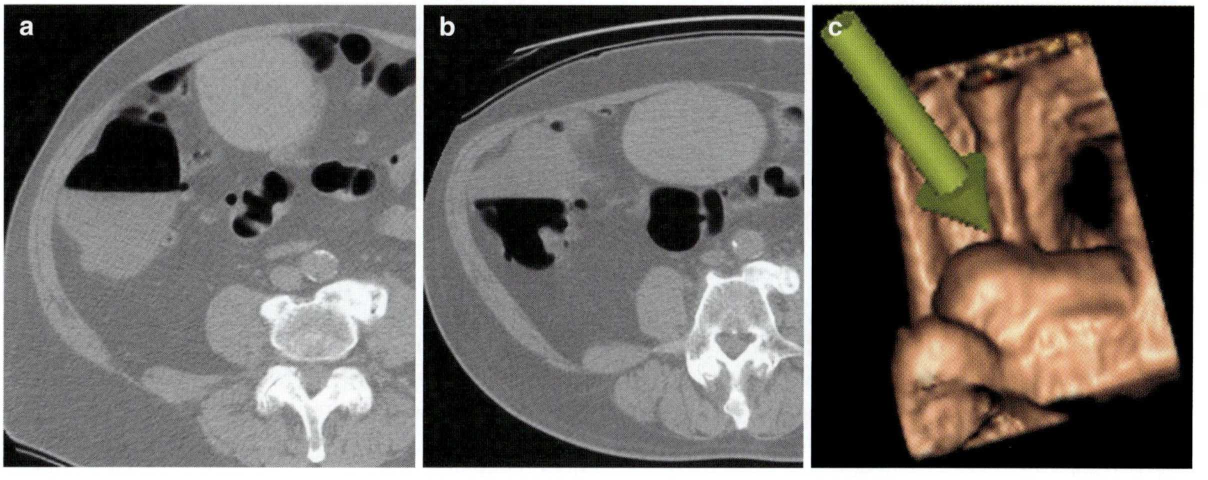

Fig. 5.4. (**a**) Supine axial view of the ascending colon demonstrates greater than 50% of the lumen filled with fluid. (**b**) Prone axial view in the same patient demonstrates the large adenomatous polyp that would have been missed if dual-position imaging had not been performed. (**c**) Prone three-dimensional cube view shows the same large irregular adenomatous polyp (yellow arrow)

Patients are instructed to drink the 4 L of polyethylene glycol solution within a 3-h period during the afternoon or early evening before the day of the procedure. Polyethylene glycol is not contraindicated in patients with renal failure or congestive heart failure. However, many patients, especially the elderly, have a difficult time ingesting this large volume during the limited period, and patient compliance may be a problem. Additionally, patients may experience abdominal discomfort, nausea and bloating. In a study of patients being prepared for surgery, 100 patients underwent bowel cleansing with polyethylene glycol and 100 patients received sodium phosphate. Although the quality of the colonic cleansing was similar in both groups, it was found that patients tolerated the sodium phosphate (65% stated they would take the same agent again, 95% completed the preparation) significantly better than the polyethylene glycol (25% would take the same preparation again, 37% ingested the entire amount) (Oliviera et al. 1997).

Polyethylene glycol is not an optimal bowel cleansing agent for CT colonography because it is a “wet preparation.” Although it is very effective in clearing solid material, polyethylene glycol often leaves a large amount of residual fluid which may compromise the diagnostic ability of the CT. Excess fluid in the colon does not often hinder the colonoscopy evaluation, since the gastroenterologist is able to aspirate or remove the extra fluid at the time of the procedure to reveal the underlying mucosa. Many of the studies that have been published evaluating the accuracy of CT colonography have used standard colonoscopy as the reference standard, which is typically performed on the same day. In these studies, patients have usually received polyethylene glycol for colonic cleansing. A reduced volume of polyethylene glycol as a possible drier but still effective in bowel preparation for CT Colonography is under investigation.

In a study evaluating the effect of different bowel preparations on residual fluid at CT colonography, 11 patients undergoing same-day CT colonography and screening colonoscopy received polyethylene glycol. Thirty-one patients undergoing CT colonoscopy within 1 week after incomplete colonoscopy received sodium phosphate preparation. Three readers who were blinded to the preparation used in the patients independently evaluated the quantity of residual fluid in six segments of the colon using a four-point scale: *1*, no residual fluid; *2*, less than 25% of the lumen filled with fluid; *3*, 25–50% of the lumen filled with fluid; and *4*, greater than 50% of the lumen filled with fluid. A statistically significant difference was found between the two groups, with the mean summed residual fluid score equal to 16.3 for the sodium phosphate group and a mean summed score of 26.9 for the polyethylene glycol group (Macari et al. 2001). In a prospective randomized study evaluating bowel cleansing methods prior to CT colonography in 50 patients, the overall quality of bowel cleansing was found to be better for sodium phosphate than with polyethylene glycol and the sodium phosphate preparation was better tolerated with significantly less nausea and less fecal incontinence (Ginnerup Pedersen et al. 2002).

Polyethylene glycol may be effective in specific patient populations. In a study of 86 Korean patients who typically maintain a high residue diet, wet and dry preparations for CTC were compared (Kim et al. 2006). Twenty-four patients received 4 L of polyethylene glycol prior to CTC and 62 patients received 90 mL (double-dose) of sodium phosphate. Image quality was found to be significantly better in the wet preparation group. Interpretation times were also significantly shorter in the wet preparation group although sensitivity for detection of 10 mm or larger polyps was comparable for the two groups.

5.2.2 Sodium Phosphate

Sodium phosphate (also known as phospho-soda) is a saline cathartic that is familiar to radiologists since it is often used as a cleansing agent prior to double-contrast barium enema. The laxative effect of sodium phosphate results from its osmotic properties which causes large outflow from the colon. A kit is commercially available containing a 1.5-oz or 45-mL bottle of monobasic and dibasic sodium phosphate, four bisacodyl tablets (5 mg each) and one bisacodyl suppository (10 mg). Bisacodyl is a contact laxative that stimulates parasympathetic reflexes to induce evacuation (Gelfand et al. 1991). Patients are instructed to mix the 45 mL of sodium phosphate with 4 oz (ca. 125 mL) of water and to ingest this with an additional 8 oz (ca. 250 mL) of water at about 6 p.m. the evening before the procedure. The time to onset of the laxative effect is about 1 h in general, and patients are instructed to remain close to a restroom. The four bisacodyl tablets are taken at about 9 p.m. the same evening and the bisacodyl suppository is administered on the morning of the procedure.

Reported complications from the use of sodium phosphate are rare and may result from induced hypovolemia, or patients can develop significant electrolyte disturbances, such as hypernatremia, hyperphosphatemia, hypocalcemia, and hypokalemia (Ehrenpreis et al. 1996; Vukasin et al. 1997). Sodium phosphate is contraindicated in patients with known renal failure, preexisting electrolyte abnormalities, congestive heart failure (particularly if on diuretic therapy), ascites, and ileus (Fass et al. 1993). Although some gastroenterologists and radiologists prescribe a "double dose" (3 oz or 90 mL) of sodium phosphate for colonic cleansing, this must be administered with caution, especially in older patients, given the increased potential for serious blood electrolyte abnormalities. The first dose of 45 mL is given the evening before and the second dose is administered the morning of the procedure, the two doses separated by about 10–12 h (Pickhardt et al. 2003). The US Food and Drug Administration (FDA) has released a warning about the potential toxicity of oral sodium phosphate as a colonic cleansing agent for colonoscopy (FDA 2002). There have been recent reports of metabolic acidosis, renal failure due to acute phosphate nephropathy, tetany, and death in patients taking more than the 45 mL dose of sodium phosphate (Khurana et al. 2008, Markowitzet al., 2005). To avoid serious adverse events, it has been advised that oral sodium phosphate be administered as recommended to patients without major comorbid conditions (Hookey et al. 2002).

In contrast to polyethylene glycol lavage solution, sodium phosphate is known as "dry preparation" since little fluid typically remains in the colon. In the setting of a dry colon, even small amounts of residual solid material may be seen as pseudo-polypoid lesions on CT colonography. There are multiple published studies evaluating the adequacy of bowel cleansing in patients using sodium phosphate versus polyethylene glycol. While some colonoscopy studies have found similar quality of bowel cleansing irrespective of the purgative agent used (Afridi et al. 1995; Golub et al. 1995; Marshall et al. 1993), other studies have found sodium phosphate to be more effective at cleansing the bowel than polyethylene glycol (Cohen et al. 1994; Kolts et al. 1993; Vanner et al. 1990). A meta-analysis including 1,286 patients from eight colonoscopist-blinded trials comparing sodium phosphate and polyethylene glycol lavage solution found that, overall, sodium phosphate is as effective as polyethylene glycol and is a more easily completed preparation. A cost saving of approximately $40 per colonoscopy was also identified with the use of sodium phosphate (Hsu and Imperiale 1998). A study evaluating the quantity of fluid retention and the adequacy of bowel wall coating in patients receiving sodium phosphate versus polyethylene glycol prior to having a barium enema found that there was no significant difference (O'Donovan et al. 1997).

5.2.3 Magnesium Citrate

Magnesium citrate is a saline cathartic that may also be used as a bowel cleansing agent prior to CT colonography. It prevents water resorption and also stimulates cholecystokinin, which causes increased fluid secretion into the small bowel (Bartram 1994). Magnesium citrate comes either in a powder form which is reconstituted with 8 oz (ca. 250 mL) of water or as a premixed solution in a 10-oz (ca. 310 mL) bottle. This is ingested in the late afternoon on the day prior to the procedure with an additional 8 oz (ca. 250 mL) of water. Bisacodyl tablets and suppository are typically used in conjunction with magnesium citrate similar to sodium phosphate.

An advantage of using magnesium citrate is that it is known as a low-sodium preparation. It contains 12 mg of sodium in its mixed form, compared with 5,004 mg of sodium for sodium phosphate. Although in rare instances sodium phosphate has been associated with clinically significant electrolyte disturbances, the use of magnesium citrate has not been found to cause any similar abnormalities. A study found that all patients receiving sodium phosphate had significant elevations in phosphorus levels followed by a decline in serum calcium levels compared with patients receiving magnesium citrate (Oliviera et al. 1997).

Magnesium citrate has been used with a reduced total volume of polyethylene glycol lavage solution prior to colonoscopy as a strategy to improve patient compliance and tolerance. This has also been found to improve the quality of colonic cleansing and to decrease the preparation time (Sharma et al. 1998). Magnesium citrate has also been evaluated in combination with bisacodyl as a mild cathartic for CTC (Jensch et al. 2008). Forty patients with an increased risk for colorectal carcinoma were prescribed a low-fiber diet starting 2 days before the CT scan. All patients received 80 mL of 40% weight/volume barium sulfate and 110 mL of diatrizoate meglumine as tagging agents. Group 1 received 20 mg bisacodyl orally, Group 2 received 30 mg bisacodyl orally, Group 3 received 20 mg bisacodyl and 8.2 mg magnesium citrate, and Group 4 received 30 mg bisacodyl and 16.4 mg magnesium citrate. Results showed that image readability was good or excellent in all groups except for one patient from Group 2 and two patients from Group 3. There was significantly more stool present in Group 2 compared to Group 4. Increasing amounts of laxative were associated with lower patient acceptance.

5.3 Colonic Distension

Proper distension of the colon is necessary to allow the radiologist the ability to visualize polyps and cancers that may impinge upon the lumen on CT colonography (Figs. 5.5 and 5.6). A segment of colon that is poorly distended or collapsed can simulate a malignant narrowing such as that caused by an annular carcinoma (Fig. 5.7). A well-trained technologist or nurse can assist in placing the rectal tube with care and performing the colonic insufflation, depending upon local guidelines. With the patient in a right-side-down decubitus position on the CT table, the rectal tube is placed. Various types of administration sets are available when performing manual insufflation, including a rectal tip attached to tubing and an insufflation bulb or a Foley catheter attached to an insufflation bulb. Preliminary insufflation in this position is suggested, allowing for the filling of the rectosigmoid and the descending colon. The patient is then turned to a supine position and insufflation continues to fill the transverse colon and then the right colon. In general it

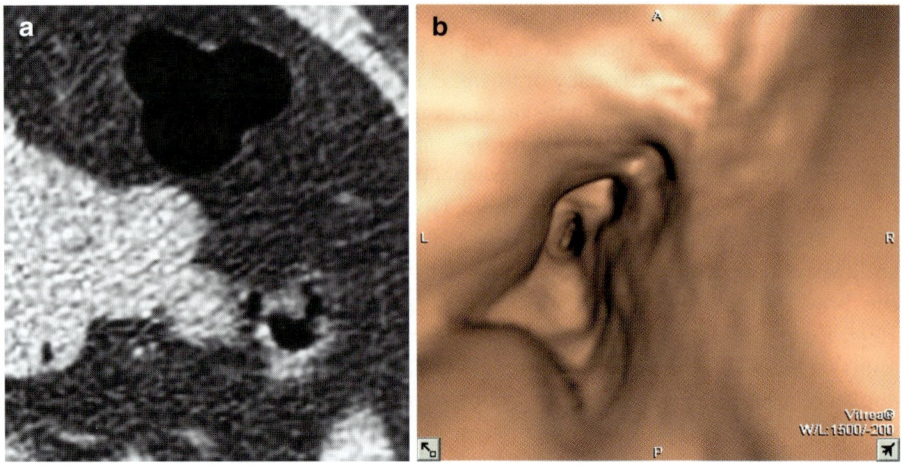

Fig. 5.5. (**a**) Poor distension of the descending colon limits the diagnostic ability for lesions on this axial image. (**b**) Endoluminal view in the same patient showing suboptimal distension which inhibits navigation through this segment

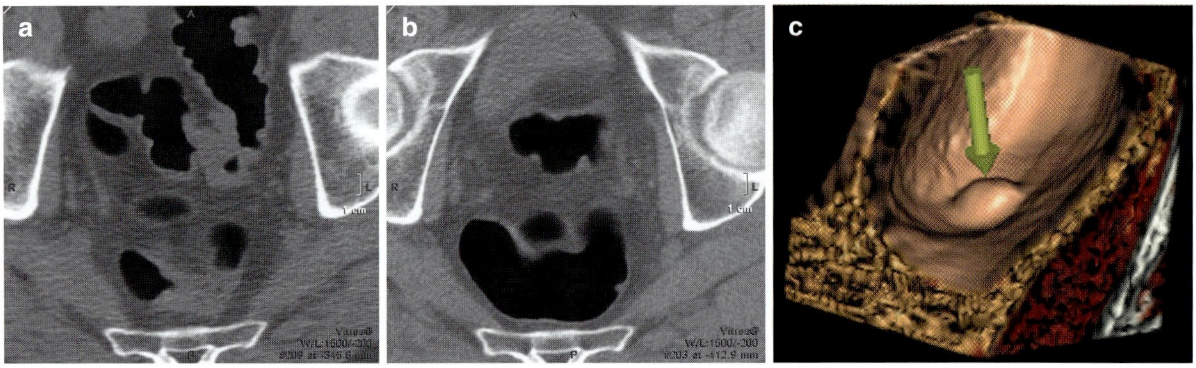

Fig. 5.6. (**a**) Collapse of a portion of the rectum in the supine position on an axial image. (**b**) Excellent distension of the rectum with the same patient in a prone position, demonstrating a small polyp along the left posterolateral colonic wall. (**c**) Three-dimensional cube view of the same polyp seen in the prone position

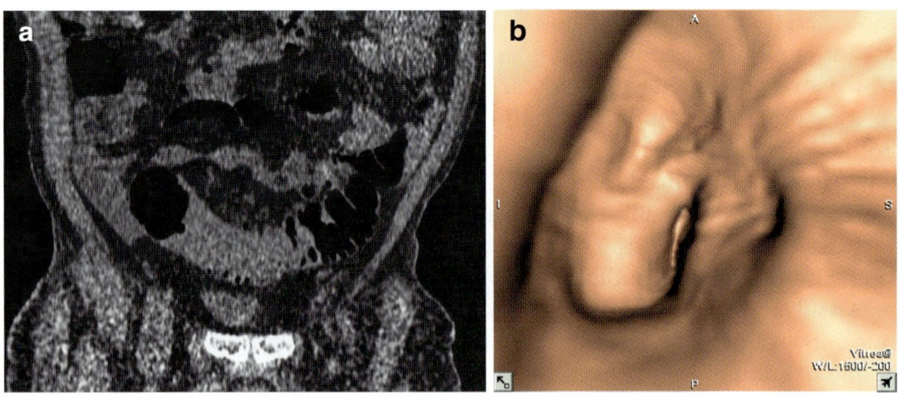

Fig. 5.7. (**a**) Collapse of a long length of the sigmoid on coronal multiplanar reformatted view simulating annular carcinoma. (**b**) Occlusion of the lumen on endoluminal view due to collapse of the sigmoid in the same patient. This appearance may also be caused by an occluding carcinoma, and proper colonic distension is essential for differentiation

will take at least 2–3 L of gas to adequately distend the colon. A CT scout view of the abdomen and the pelvis is obtained. If the entire colon, particularly the sigmoid, is not well distended, then repeat administration of the gas is performed according to maximum patient tolerance. Following supine axial image acquisition, the patient is turned prone and another CT scout image is obtained with additional gaseous insufflation if segments of colon with suboptimal distension are noted on the scout view.

5.3.1 Room Air

Currently room air is used most frequently to manually insufflate the colon for CT colonography. Its ease of use and familiarity to radiologists and technologists because of a similar route of administration per rectum for double-contrast barium enema examinations has made it easily adaptable for CT colonography. It is also readily available at no additional cost. A large component of room air is nitrogen, which is inert, so that there is no active diffusion across the bowel wall when the colon is distended with air. Thus, following retrograde insufflation of the colon with room air, the colon will remain filled until the air is passed distally. Occasionally patients may experience severe pain and distension up to several hours after the CT colonography examination because of excess residual air within the colon. In an evaluation of symptom rates, 7% of subjects experienced significant pain and 13% had severe distension following air insufflation of the colon for barium enema (Skovgaard et al. 1995).

5.3.2 Carbon Dioxide

Carbon dioxide (CO_2) has been used instead of atmospheric air for insufflation of the colon for colonoscopy as well as for barium enema examination because it has been found to decrease patient discomfort. CO_2 is readily resorbed through the colonic wall because of a steep diffusion gradient and it is then exhaled from the lungs. One hundred patients were randomized to undergo colonoscopy with insufflation with either air or CO_2. Post-procedural pain was reported in 45 and 31 of patients receiving air at 1 and 6 h, respectively, after colonoscopy compared with 7 and 9%, respectively in subjects insufflated with CO_2 (Sumanac et al. 2002). In a study of 142 subjects, approximately half of the patients received room air and the other half received CO_2 to distend the colon for barium enema. Patients who received CO_2 were found to have a reduced incidence of both immediate and delayed pain, from 31 to 12.5% and from 12.9 to 4.2% respectively (Robson et al. 1993). In another study of 151 patients undergoing barium enema, 86 received room air and 65 received CO_2 for colonic insufflation. Almost one-third of patients who received room air experienced pain versus only 11% of patients who underwent colonic distension with CO_2. While none of the CO_2 patients reported severe pain, five patients who received room air reported significant pain (Coblentz et al. 1985). In a comparative study, 105 patients undergoing barium enema received either manually administered air, CO_2, or a 50/50 mixture of the two gases. No difference in mucosal coating was found. Patients who received CO_2 had significantly less immediate and delayed pain than those who received air and less delayed pain than those insufflated with the 50/50 mixture. It was also found that air provided better distension than the other two gases although the difference did not attain statistical significance (Holemans et al. 1998). Another study identified less optimal colonic distension with manually administered CO_2 than with room air in 100 patients referred for barium enema. It was concluded that poor distension could lead to diagnostic errors and thus outweigh any advantages in patient acceptability when using CO_2 as an insufflation agent (Scullion et al. 1995).

More recently, CO_2 has also been used to distend the colon for CT colonography. The retrograde administration of CO_2 may be performed either manually, similar to retrograde air insufflation, or electronically using a specific commercially available mechanical device developed for CT colonography. Although manual administration of CO_2 may lead to suboptimal bowel distension as described above, our experience shows more reliable and consistent optimal bowel distension with the use of electronic CO_2 insufflation for CT colonography, which maintains a constant infusion of CO_2 into the colon up to a certain preset pressure. For colonoscopy, a pressure maintained at 35 mmHg with a CO_2 flow rate of 1 L/min has been proven safe (Phaosawasdi et al. 1986). For CO_2 administration during CT colonography, the maximum pressure setting allowed using the mechanical device is 25 mmHg. With a fixed flow rate of 3 L/min, the pressure is set at about 15 mmHg to start with and then slowly increased to a maximum of 25 mmHg depending upon patient tolerance. CO_2 instillation is continued in the supine and prone positions until completion of the scan. The total amount of CO_2 insufflated during CT colonography is typically about 4 L due to the relatively short procedural time. This amount is far less than during an average laparoscopic procedure of approximately 2 h using CO_2 flow rates of 5–15 L/min with a total CO_2 consumption of approximately 40 L (Taskin et al. 1998). No complications have been reported in the literature till date for intracolonic CO_2 insufflation.

The adequacy of colonic distention and patient tolerance were analyzed in a study of 47 patients who received electronic insufflation of carbon dioxide for CTC compared to 94 patients who received manual insufflation of carbon dioxide (Burling et al. 2006). There was significantly better colonic distention in patients receiving automated electronic insufflation with the best distention occurring in the distal supine colon. The effectiveness of automated carbon dioxide insufflation for colonic distention on CTC in patients with severe luminal narrowing due to cancer was evaluated in 36 patients (Kim et al. 2008). Thirty-eight patients without stenosis were included in the control group. All patients first underwent optical colonoscopy followed by CTC within 8 days. Results showed that there was no significant difference in distention between the stenotic and nonstenotic groups in any colonic segments in both supine and prone positions. No perforations occurred in either group. It was concluded that automated pressure-controlled carbon dioxide insufflation is as efficient for colonic distention in patients with malignant stenosis as in patients without stenosis.

5.4 Anti-Spasmodic Agents

Anti-spasmodic agents are used to relax the bowel wall and to minimize peristalsis. Glucagon has been employed for CT colonography in the USA, although its usefulness has not been substantiated. Butyl scopolamine is used in Europe for CT and MR colonography, where it has been found to be cheaper and more effective than glucagon as a spasmolytic agent. However, the utility of butyl scopolamine for CT and MR colonography is also controversial.

5.4.1 Glucagon

Glucagon is a polypeptide hormone normally produced by the pancreatic islets of Langerhans. It causes an increase in blood glucose, but is perhaps better known for its clinical use as a hypotonic agent for the stomach, small bowel, and colon. Glucagon relaxes the smooth muscle of the gastrointestinal tract and is thought to improve bowel distension and decrease patient discomfort due to spasm. The effectiveness of glucagon is dependent upon location, and it has been found to be most effective on the duodenum and least effective on the colon (Chernish and Maglinte 1990). Although uncommon, the most frequently encountered side effects of glucagon are nausea, vomiting and headache. One study found that 4% of patients experienced nausea following the intravenous administration of glucagon prior to CT colonography (Morrin et al. 2002). Rarely, generalized allergic-type reactions such as urticaria, respiratory distress and hypotension may occur. Glucagon is contraindicated in patients with pheochromocytoma, insulinoma, poorly controlled diabetes or a known hypersensitivity to glucagon.

Glucagon was used in the past, and is still being used at some sites, as a spasmolytic agent for CT colonography. Many of the older published trials evaluating the performance of CT colonography for polyp detection were performed on subjects who had received 1 mg of glucagon intravenously. The routine use of glucagon for colonic evaluation had been adopted from barium enema practice. Some studies have found decreased discomfort during and after barium enema when glucagon is given prior to the procedure (Bova et al. 1993; Meeroff et al. 1975). However, it has also been reported that there was no improvement in colonic distension on double-contrast barium enema after the administration of glucagon and that there was also no improvement in colon polyp detection rates on double-contrast barium enema with glucagon administration (Thoeni et al. 1984). Important differences exist between the barium enema examination and CT colonography when considering the usefulness of glucagon for these studies. Liquid barium may cause colonic spasm during the barium enema examination, but this does not occur during CT colonography. Additionally CT colonography is a much more rapid study than barium enema. Colonic insufflation with air is important during the scan phase of the CT, which is very short and occupies less than 15 s in each position, whereas a distended colon is needed for at least 15 min after glucagon is administered for the barium enema examination.

Trials specifically evaluating the value of intravenous glucagon for CT colonography have been conducted. CT colonography was performed in 60 patients following manual air insufflation of the colon up to maximum patient tolerance. Thirty-three patients received 1 mg of glucagon immediately prior to the CT scan and the remaining patients did not (Yee et al. 1999a). Segmental as well as overall colonic distension was evaluated. The colon was divided into eight segments in both supine and prone positions for a total of 16 segments per patient. It was found that glucagon administration did not significantly improve colonic distension in supine or prone positions. In patients receiving glucagon, 222 segments (84.1%) were considered adequately distended while in patients not receiving glucagon, 187 segments (86.6%) were adequately distended. No statistically significant differences were identified between the glucagon group and the nonglucagon group for overall colonic distension scores in the prone, supine, or combined positions.

Another study also found that colonic distension at CT colonography is improved by dual positioning but not by the administration of intravenous glucagon (Morrin et al. 2002). In a study of 96 patients, 74 subjects received 1 mg of glucagon intravenously immediately prior to CT scanning and 22 patients did not. A five-point scale was used to score the adequacy of distension, with a rating of *1* collapsed and *5* excellent distension. There was no statistically significant difference between glucagon and nonglucagon groups (mean distension scores 3.6 and 3.9, respectively). We do not administer glucagon routinely for CT colonography at our institution, but we use it in specific cases where there is significant patient discomfort or evidence of colonic spasm on the scout CT view. Initial investigation has also found that glucagon does not appear to improve the sensitivity of CT colonography for the detection of colorectal polyps (Yee et al. 1999b).

5.4.2 Hyoscine *n*-Butylbromide

Hyoscine *n*-butylbromide (Buscopan) is an anticholinergic agent that has been used as a muscle relaxant for the barium enema examination as well as for CT and MR colonography in Europe. It has not received approval for use in the USA. Buscopan has a different mechanism of action than glucagon and is less expensive. Hypotonia of the colon is induced by its action on the postganglionic parasympathetic receptors in smooth muscle. Contraindications to the use of anticholinergic agents include glaucoma, severe prostatic hyperplasia, unstable heart disease, bowel obstruction or ileus, and myasthenia gravis. Anticholinergics can cause side effects such as tachycardia, dry mouth, acute urinary retention, and acute gastric dilatation.

In a study comparing various antispasmodic agents for barium enema, 106 patients received a placebo, 109 patients received 1 mg intravenous glucagon, and 109 patients received 20 mg intravenous Buscopan prior to the enema (Goei et al. 1995). Results showed that Buscopan performed better than glucagon for colonic distension, although about 5% of patients who received Buscopan experienced blurry vision. The routine use of Buscopan for CT colonography is controversial. In a study of 73 patients undergoing CT colonography, 36 patients received 20 mg of Buscopan intravenously and 37 subjects received no muscle relaxant immediately prior to scanning. Intravenous Buscopan was not found to improve the adequacy of colonic distension, and there was no significant improvement in the accuracy of polyp detection (Rogalla et al. 2005). It was concluded that the routine use of intravenous Buscopan for CT colonography was not supported. Another study performed on 136 patients randomized subjects to receive either 20 or 40 mg of Buscopan or no muscle relaxant prior to CT colonography (Bruzzi et al. 2003). Significantly improved distension was found in the cecum and in the ascending and transverse colon in the supine position and in the ascending and descending colon in the prone position. No incremental advantage was found with the larger dose of 40 mg. This study also found that the use of a rectal balloon catheter did not improve distension. A recently published study compared patients not receiving an antispasmodic agent with patients receiving 1 mg of glucagon intravenously and subjects receiving 20 mg of Buscopan intravenously immediately prior to supine-only CT colonography (Taylor et al. 2003). Mean colon volumes and radial distensibility were significantly better with Buscopan only when comparing patients who received Buscopan with patients who did not receive any muscle relaxant. The value of Buscopan for CT colonography using dual positioning remains controversial.

References

Afridi SA, Barthel JS, King PD et al (1995) Prospective, randomized trial comparing a new sodium phosophate-bisacodyl regimen with conventional PEG-ES lavage for outpatient colonoscopy preparation. Gastrointest Endosc 41:485–489

Bartram CI (1994) Bowel preparation–principles and practice. Clin Radiol 49:365–367

Bova JG, Jurdi RA, Bennett WF (1993) Antispasmodic drugs to reduce discomfort and colonic spasm during barium enemas: comparison of oral hyoscyamine, IV glucagon, and no drug. AJR 161:965–968

Bruzzi JF, Moss AC, Brennan DD et al (2003) Efficacy of IV buscopan as a muscle relaxant in CT colonography. Eur Radiol 13:2264–2270

Burling D, Taylor SA, Halligan S et al (2006) Automated insufflation of carbon dioxide for MDCT Colonography: distention and patient experience compared with manual insufflation. AJR 186:96–103

Chernish SM, Maglinte DDT (1990) Glucagon: common untoward reactions–review and recommendations. Radiology 177: 145–146

Coblentz CL, Frost RA, Molinaro V et al (1985) Pain after barium enema: effect of CO_2 and air on double-contrast study. Radiology 157:35–36

Cohen SM, Wexner SD, Binderow SR et al (1994) Prospective, randomized, endoscopic-blinded trial comparing precolonoscopy bowel cleansing methods. Dis Colon Rectum 37:689–696

Ehrenpreis ED, Nogueras JJ, Botoman VA et al (1996) Serum electrolyte abnormalities secondary to Fleet's phospho-soda colonoscopy prep. Surg Endosc 10:1022–1024

Fass R, Do S, Hixson LJ (1993) Fatal hyperphosphatemia following Fleet phospho-soda in a patient with colonic ileus. Am J Gastroenterol 88:929–932

Food and Drug Administration (2002) Science background: safety of sodium phosphates oral solution. Center for Drug Evaluation and Research, Food and Drug Administration, Washington, DC

Gelfand DW, Chen MYM, Ott DJ (1991) Preparing the colon for the barium enema examination. Radiology 178:609–613

Ginnerup Pedersen B, Christiansen TE, Mortensen FV et al (2002) Bowel cleansing methods prior to CT colonography: a prospective, comparative, randomized blinded study. Acta Radiol 43:306–311

Goei R, Nix M, Kessels AH et al (1995) Use of antispasmodic drugs in double contrast barium enema examination: glucagon or buscopan? Clin Radiol 50:553–557

Golub RW, Kerner BA, Wise WE et al (1995) Colonoscopic bowel preparations–which one? A blinded, prospective, randomized trial. Dis Colon Rectum 38:594–599

Holemans JA, Matson MB, Hughes JA et al (1998) A comparison of air, CO_2 and air/CO_2 mixture as insufflation agents for double contrast barium enema. Eur Radiol 8:274–276

Hookey LC, Depew WT, Vanner S (2002) The safety profile of oral sodium phosphate for colonic cleansing before colonoscopy in adults. Gastrointest Endosc 56:895–902

Hsu CW, Imperiale TF (1998) Meta-analysis and cost comparison of polyethylene glycol lavage versus sodium phosphate for colonoscopy preparation. Gastrointest Endosc 48: 276–82

Jensch S, deVries AH, Pot D et al (2008) Image quality and patient acceptance of four regimens with different amounts of mild laxatives for CT Colonography. AJR 191:158–167

Khurana A, McLean L, Atkinson S et al (2008) The effect of oral sodium phosphate drug products on renal function in adults undergoing bowel endoscopy. Arch Intern Med 168:593–597

Kim SH, Choi BI, Han JK et al (2006) CT Colonography in a Korean population with a high residue diet: comparison between wet and dry preparations. Clin Radiol 61:483–494

Kim SY, Park SH, Choi EK et al (2008) Automated carbon dioxide insufflation for CT Colonography: effectiveness of colonic distention in cancer patients with severe luminal narrowing. AJR 190:698–706

Kolts BE, Lyles WE, Achem SR et al (1993) A comparison of the effectiveness and patient tolerance of oral sodium phosphate, castor oil, and standard electrolyte lavage for colonoscopy or sigmoidoscopy preparation. Am J Gastroenterol 88: 1218–1223

Macari M, Lavelle M, Pedrosa I et al (2001) Effect of different bowel preparations on residual fluid at CT colonography. Radiology 218:274–277

Markowitz GS, Stokes MB, Radhakrishnan J et al (2005) Acute phosphate nephropathy following oral sodium phosphate bowel purgative: an under-recognized cause of chronic renal failure. J Am Soc Nephrol 16:3389–3396

Marshall JB, Pineda JJ, Barthel JS et al (1993) Prospective, randomized trail comparing sodium phosphate solution with polyethylene glycol-electrolyte lavage for colonoscopy preparation. Gastrointest Endosc 39:631–634

Meeroff JC, Jorgens J, Isenberg JI (1975) The effect of glucagon on barium enema examinations. Radiology 115:5–7

Morrin MM, Farrell RJ, Keogan MT et al (2002) CT colonography: colonic distention improved by dual positioning but not intravenous glucagon. Eur Radiol 12:525–530

O'Donovan AN, Somers S, Farrow R et al (1997) A prospective blinded randomized trial comparing oral sodium phosphate and polyethylene glycol solutions for bowel preparation prior to barium enema. Clin Radiol 52: 791–793

Oliviera L, Wexner SD, Daniel N et al (1997) Mechanical bowel preparation for elective colorectal surgery–a prospective, randomized, surgeon-blinded trial comparing sodium phosphate and polyethylene glycol-based oral lavage solutions. Dis Colon Rectum 40:585–591

Phaosawasdi K, Cooley W, Wheeler J et al (1986) Carbon dioxide-insufflated colonoscopy: an ignored superior technique. Gastrointest Endosc 32:330–333

Pickhardt P, Choi JR, Hwang I et al (2003) Computed tomographic virtual colonoscopy to screen for colorectal neoplasia in asymptomatic adults. Radiology 349: 2191–2200

Robson NK, Lloyd M, Regan F (1993) The use of carbon dioxide as an insufflation agent in barium enema–does it have a role? Br J Radiol 66:197–198

Sharma VK, Chockalingham SK, Ugheoke EA et al (1998) Prospective, randomized, controlled comparison of the use of polyethylene glycol electrolyte lavage solution in four-liter versus two-liter volumes and pretreatment with either magnesium citrate or bisacodyl for colonoscopy preparation. Gastrointest Endosc 47:167–171

Skovgaard N, Sloth C, Von Benzon E et al (1995) The role of carbon dioxide and atmospheric air in double-contrast barium enema. Abdom Imaging 20:436–439

Sumanac K, Zealley I, Fox BM et al (2002) Minimizing post-colonoscopy abdominal pain by using CO_2 insufflation: a prospective, randomized, double-blind, controlled trial evaluating a new commercially available CO_2 delivery system. Gastrointest Endosc 56:190–194

Scullion DA, Wetton CWN, Davies C et al (1995) The use of air or CO_2 as insufflation agents for double contrast barium enema: is there a qualitative difference? Clin Radiol 50: 558–561

Taskin O, Buhur A, Birincioglu M et al (1998) The effects of duration of CO_2 insufflation and irrigation on peritoneal microcirculation assessed by free radical scavengers and total glutathione levels during operative laparoscopy. J Am Assoc Gynecol Laparosc 5:129–133

Rogalla P, Lembcke A, Ruckert JC et al (2005) Spasmolysis at CT colonography: butyl scopolamine versus glucagon. Radiology 236:184–188

Taylor SA, Halligan S, Goh V et al (2003) Optimizing colonic distention for multi-detector row CT colonography: effect of hyoscine butylbromide and rectal balloon catheter. Radiology 229:99–108

Taylor SA, Slater A, Burling DN et al (2008) CT colonography: optimization, diagnostic performance and patient acceptability of reduced-laxative regimens using barium-based fecal tagging. Eur Radiol 18:32–42

Thoeni RF, Vandeman F, Wall SD (1984) Effect of glucagon on the diagnostic accuracy of double-contrast barium enema examinations. AJR 142:111–114

Vanner SJ, MacDonald PH, Paterson WG et al (1990) A randomized prospective trial comparing oral sodium phosphate with standard polyethylene glycol-based lavage solution (Golytely) in the preparation of patients for colonoscopy. Am J Gastroenterol 4:422–427

Vukasin P, Weston LA, Beart RW (1997) Oral Fleet phospho-soda laxative-induced hyperphosphatemia and hypocalcemic tetany in an adult. Dis Colon Rectum 40: 497–499

Yee J, Hung RK, Akerkar GA et al (1999a) The usefulness of glucagon hydrochloride for colonic distention in CT colonography. AJR 173:1–4

Yee J, Hung RK, Steinauer-Gebauer AM et al (1999b) Colonic distention and prospective evaluation of colorectal polyp detection with and without glucagon during CT colonography [abstract]. Radiology 213(Suppl):256

The Prerequisite: Faecal Tagging

Philippe Lefere and Stefaan Gryspeerdt

CONTENTS

6.1 Introduction

As described in the previous chapter, preparing the colon is a sine qua non to adequately perform state-of-the-art CT colonography. The option of an intensive preparation to obtain a colon as clean and dry as possible has been approved in 2005 in a consensus statement by several CT colonography experts and is currently still the method of choice to prepare the colon for CT colonography (Barish et al. 2005). Indeed, in a well-distended, clean, and dry colon, conspicuity of tumoral lesions should be at its best. However, the real world is not that simple. Indeed, two large trials of >600 patients have shown that an intensive cathartic preparation might be insufficient in obtaining good results of polyp detection (Cotton et al. 2004; Rockey et al. 2005). Both the Cotton and Rockey trials obtained very disappointing results with a sensitivity of <60% for adenomas ≥6 mm. Of the many flaws these two trials have been inflicted with, the lack of fecal tagging was considered a major shortcoming (Ferrucci and Working Group on CT Colongraphy 2005a and author reply Ferrucci 2005b). Furthermore, to date, the U.S. Department of Defence trial obtained the best results of polyp detection in a large asymptomatic population of 1,233 patients at average risk for colorectal cancer using a preparation combining a low-residue diet and oral laxatives with fecal tagging (Pickhardt et al. 2003a, b). Since the publication of this landmark study, fecal tagging was gradually accepted as an indispensable part of the colonic preparation for CT colonography. This propensity for fecal tagging was confirmed in the ESGAR-CTC consensus statement published in 2007 (Taylor et al. 2007) and in the recent ACRIN 6664 trial fecal tagging was part of the preparation (Johnson et al. 2008).

Philippe Lefere, MD
Stefaan Gryspeerdt, MD
Department of Radiology, Stedelijk Ziekenhuis, Bruggesteenweg 90, 8800 Roeselare, Belgium

The purpose of this chapter is: (1) to explain what fecal tagging is; (2) to demonstrate why this type of preparation is important; (3) to explain how fecal tagging is performed; (4) to explain how to use this method in daily clinical practice; (5) to show imaging findings; and (6) to shortly discuss future challenges.

6.2 What Is Fecal Tagging?

Fecal tagging means labeling of fecal residue in the colon. Stool tagging refers to labeling of residual stool, while fluid tagging refers to labeling of residual fluid. The technique is based on the oral ingestion of positive contrast material (barium and/or iodine) as part of the preparation prior to CT colonography. The orally ingested contrast material impregnates the residual stool and mixes with the residual fluid in the colon. By doing so, the residual stool and fluid, remaining in the colon after the preparation, have a hyperdense or white aspect on the two-dimensional CT images. The hyperdense residual stool is in strong contrast to the soft tissue density of the normal colonic structures and tumoral lesions. The hyperdense fluid allows inspection of normal structures beneath it and reveals the normal colonic structures and the lesions as a filling defect.

6.3 Rationale: Why We Do It!

The rationale of developing a preparation with fecal tagging was twofold: (1) improving diagnosis; and (2) improving patient compliance.

6.3.1 Improving Diagnosis

The use of sodium phosphate or magnesium citrate to cleanse the colon has been extensively explained in the previous chapter. Both products produce a clean and dry colon. However, despite the intensive colonic cleansing, the radiologist interpreting CT colonography is still faced with considerable problems. Indeed, because of the possible isodense aspect of fecal residue, residual stool may mimic polyps and residual

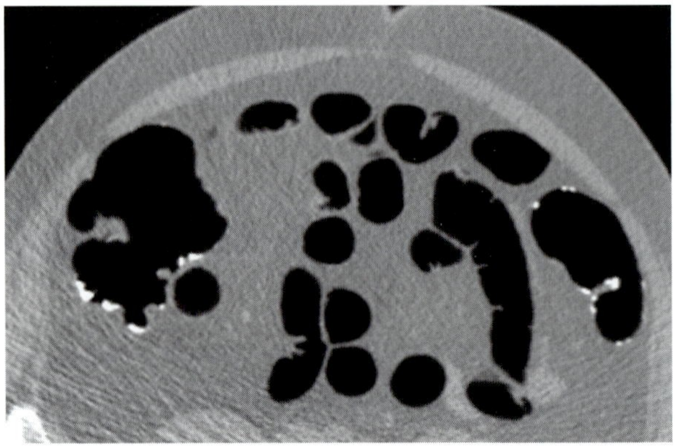

Fig. 6.1. The residual stool in the ascending and descending colon is tagged and appears white on the two-dimensional images, facilitating diagnosis

fluid may hide normal and pathologic conditions in the colon. A polyp with a long pedicle may mimic stool, because of an important positional shift when turning from supine to prone position (Fenlon 2002; Macari and Megibow 2001). Despite the fact that the imaging characteristics of stool are well established (central air inclusion, shift with dual positioning), problems still occur if the stool presents as an immobile soft tissue structure, possibly corresponding to stool, or a polyp with abutting stool or frankly a polyp. As such, a false-positive diagnosis may lead to a superfluous optical colonoscopy. On the other hand, false-negative findings may be created by solid residue and/or fluid hiding a lesion. The solution to solve this problem is offered by fecal tagging enabling an efficient differentiation between fecal residue and colonic lesion. Comparing fecal tagging with non-tagging, Lefere et al. (2002) could demonstrate an improvement in specificity (Fig. 6.1).

6.3.2 Improving Patient Compliance

Intensive cleansing of the colon mostly causes interruption of normal daily activity. In fact, preparations for full structural examinations of the colon are based on the intensive use of cathartics and produce more or less heavy diarrhea. Besides these, major inconveniences such as nausea, vomiting, and dizziness frequently occur. This important discomfort is known as a major barrier to comply with standard screening recommendations (Morrin et al. 1999) resulting in less than one half of the population participating to a colorectal cancer screening program (van Dam et al. 2004; Bromer and Weinberg 2005). To avoid preparation-related side effects and to increase patient compliance, a reduced cathartic cleansing in combination with fecal tagging has been developed (LEFERE et al. 2002). In fact, as the fecal residue is labeled in the colon, more residues can be left over in the colon without compromising the diagnostic performance of CT colonography. This offers the opportunity of reducing or eliminating the cathartic cleansing part of the preparation and should enable considerable improvement of patient compliance for examinations of the colon (see below).

6.4 How to Do Fecal Tagging!

6.4.1 Basic Principles

Current state-of-the-art CT colonography requires a combination of a dietary preparation, a full cathartic preparation, and fecal tagging to prepare the patient for CT colonography. In order to not unnecessarily complicate the procedure and to reduce the inconveniences for the patients, it is important to reduce the preparation to only 1 day. Similarly, it is important to try reducing the interruption of the normal daily activity by administering the laxatives after 5 p.m. The dietary preparation consists of a low-residue diet and is meant to reduce the fat intake and the fecal volume. This can be achieved with a clear liquid diet, consisting of commercially available energy drinks, or with a classic low-residue diet. This diet consists of a list of allowed and forbidden food items. The cathartic preparation cleanses the colon to eliminate the fecal residue. In CT colonography, it is particularly important to obtain a dry colon using a dry preparation (see previous chapter). Finally, fecal tagging facilitates interpretation of the images.

How to combine these three different aspects of the CT colonography preparation in a harmonious and efficient entity? Several tagging regimens have been extensively tested. Two large trials obtained very good results combining a low-residue diet with intensive cathartic cleansing and fecal tagging (KIM et al. 2007; JOHNSON et al. 2008). First of all, Kim et al. combined a clear liquid diet with bisacodyl and sodium phosphate as cleansing agents and a combination of barium and iodine for fecal tagging. Comparing CT colonography with optical colonoscopy in two large cohorts of >3,000 patients, CT colonography scored very well making the authors conclude that CT colonography is ready for colorectal cancer screening. Second, in the ACRIN 6664 trial, several preparations were used (JOHNSON et al. 2008). One of them consisted of the combination of a classic low-residue diet, sodium phosphate or magnesium citrate and bisacodyl as cleansing agents and barium and iodine as tagging agents. A highly concentrated 40% (w/v) barium suspension was used. The high concentration allowed reducing the barium volume to drink (LEFERE et al. 2005). Examples of preparations are presented in Table 6.1.

The advantages of these preparations are related to the performance of CT colonography. Indeed, in both

Table 6.1. Examples of preparations. For faecal tagging a choice can be made between different barium concentrations. Available concentrations are 40%, 4% and 2.1% w/v. We instruct to drink an additional glass of water at 5, 6, 7 and 8 pm. Abbreviations: CLD = clear liquid diet; CLRD: classic low residue diet.

Kim et al. (2007)	Johnson et al. (2008)	Lefere et al. (2005)
8 am: CLD	8 am: CLRD®	8 am: CLRD
12 am: CLD	8 am: barium 40 %, 20 ml	8 am: barium 40 %, 20 ml
12 am: bisacodyl 5 mg 2 tab	12 am: CLRD	12 am: CLRD
3 pm: phosphosoda 45 ml	12 am: barium 40 %, 20 ml	12 am: barium 40 %, 20 ml
6 pm: barium 2.1%, 250 ml	5 pm: CLRD	5 pm: CLRD
9 pm: gastrografin 60 ml	5 pm: barium 40 %, 20 ml	5 pm: barium 40 %, 20 ml
	6 pm: phosphosoda or mag citrate	6 pm: mag citrate
	7 pm: bisacodyl 5 mg, 2 tab	7 pm: bisacodyl 5 mg, 4 tab
	8 pm: gastrografin 30 ml	

trials very good results of lesion detection were obtained. As the colon is very clean and dry, the choice can be made between primary 2D or primary 3D approach for interpretation. Furthermore, as the colon is very well prepared, same day optical colonoscopy can be performed without additional preparation enabling immediate removal of polyps detected at CT colonography. Possible disadvantages are related to the side effects of the cathartic preparation with interruption of the normal daily activity (nausea, vomiting) causing a burden for patient compliance. Patient compliance becomes particularly important when screening for colorectal cancer (see below).

6.4.2 What Product to Use?

As mentioned, two products are available for fecal tagging: barium and iodine. Barium mixes well with solid stool and is used for fecal tagging. Because of its high weight, barium settles out in water and does not mix well with the fluid contents of the colon. Barium is usually administered as a suspension. When using low concentrations such as 2.1% (w/v) (=2.1 g of barium/100 mL) volumes up to 500 mL have to be administered (Kim et al. 2007). Using a higher concentration of 40% (w/v), Lefere et al. (2005) could reduce the volume to drink to 50 mL. Iodinated contrast is water-soluble, mixes well with fluid, and is the preferred product for fluid tagging. Diatrizoate meglumine and diatrizoate sodium (Gastrografin®) is preferred in Europe over its non-ionic counterparts, which are usually more expensive to use Thomeer et al (2003), Iannaccone et al. (2004), Faecal tagging with non-ionic iodine has bee successfully applied by Zalis et al (2003 and 2006).

Besides the ability and efficacy of labeling the colonic contents, the choice of the product will also depend on its safety profile.

What are the side effects of these products? Is there any known hypersensitivity?

Frequently, side effects, such as nausea, vomiting, and diarrhoea, have been described with the use of iodinated contrast. When used in combination with a full cathartic cleansing, it is difficult to determine whether these side effects are caused by iodine or by the full cathartic cleansing. However, in their study on laxative-free CTC, using 200 mL of sodium and meglumine diatrizoate, Iannaccone et al (2004). described these side effects in 10% of patients. In the few reports comparing ionic and non-ionic iodinated contrast, there is no significant difference in side effects (Kinnunen et al. 1989; Laerum et al. 1991). Barium has been reported with a better patient acceptability and with fewer side effects (Carr et al. 1985; Chambers et al. 1984).

Although very rare, an anaphylactic reaction due to iodine-allergy cannot be excluded. In the Manual on Contrast Media, published by the American College of Radiology, known prior moderate or severe reaction to iodinated contrast media (high and low osmolality) is a contra-indication for oral administration American College of Radiology Committee on Drugs and Contrast Media (2005). The reason is that a small portion (1–2%) of oral iodinated contrast is absorbed in the human body and, as anaphylactic reactions are not dose-related, even a very small amount absorbed in the gastrointestinal tract may cause a fatal reaction. Serious reactions with intra-venous iodinated contrast occur in 1–2/1,000 and 1–2/10,000 patients with high-osmolality and low-osmolality contrast media, respectively. Therefore, the use of iodinated contrast for fecal tagging in patients with a history of hypersensitivity for intravenous or oral iodine should be considered a contra-indication. In these cases, barium fecal tagging has to be performed (see below).

Barium is inert and has a negligible absorption of 0.000002% in the GI tract. The extremely rare reactions to barium suspensions have been attributed to the additives in the barium suspension. Serious reactions with barium suspensions occur in 1/1,000,000 to 1/2,500,000 cases, making barium at least 100 times safer than the iodinated contrast (Seymour et al. 1997; Skucas 1997).

6.4.3 Implementation in Clinical Practice

6.4.3.1 Instruction Folder

It is accepted that availability of written information improves patient compliance (Murphy and Coster 1997). To proceed fluently with the preparation and to avoid misinterpretation of the instructions and/or misuse of the provided items, the patients receive an information folder. This folder provides them with all the practical information necessary to bring this preparation to a good end by: (1) showing all items of the preparation on a picture; (2) explaining how to proceed with the meals; (3) explaining how to ingest the contrast material; (4) explaining how to proceed with the cathartic cleansing; (5) giving advice when to drink additional water. A short explanation concerning the adenoma–carcinoma sequence underscoring the importance of screening for colorectal cancer encourages the patients to follow the preparation meticulously.

6.4.3.2
Indications

In daily clinical practice, the radiologist needs a solution for different scenarios:

6.4.3.2.1
After Incomplete Colonoscopy

Optical colonoscopy may be incomplete for two different reasons: because of an obstructing malignant tumor or because of colonic redundancy, dolichocolon or benign colonic disease as diverticulosis. Gryspeerdt et al. (2005) compared CT colonography performed immediately after incomplete optical colonoscopy (thus after a standard colonoscopy cleansing with polyethylene glycol) with CT colonography performed after fecal tagging. In the latter case, CT colonography was not performed on the day of incomplete colonoscopy, but some days later after a new preparation with fecal tagging. In the group of patients prepared with fecal tagging, there was significantly less residual fluid. This resulted in a statistically significant improvement of the colonic distention. Furthermore, fecal tagging was efficient in all patients. Following these results, the following strategy was developed. In case of an obstructing tumor, the best option is to immediately perform CT colonography with administration of i.v. contrast. This allows for immediate tumor staging and for detecting synchronous tumoral lesions in the colon. A good method is to start in prone position without i.v. contrast at a low dose (50 mAs) and to perform a second acquisition with i.v. contrast at a normal abdominal CT dose. As polyps tend to take up contrast, they might become hyperdense and when submerged, be recognized in the fluid.

In case of tortuosity or diverticular disease, we can consider that optical colonoscopy probably will fail on a next attempt and that CT colonography needs to be performed under the best conditions as possible. Indeed, in these cases, CT colonography will mostly be the unique diagnostic tool and the treatment will depend on the radiologist's interpretation. Hence, exact and accurate decision-taking might be vital for direct treatment or surgery. In our opinion, it is very meaningful in these cases to perform a new CT colonography a few days later after a new preparation with fecal tagging as described above.

According to Laghi (personal communication), after incomplete colonoscopy, same day fecal tagging and CT colonography can be performed by administering 60 mL of iodinated contrast some 2 h before starting the examination.

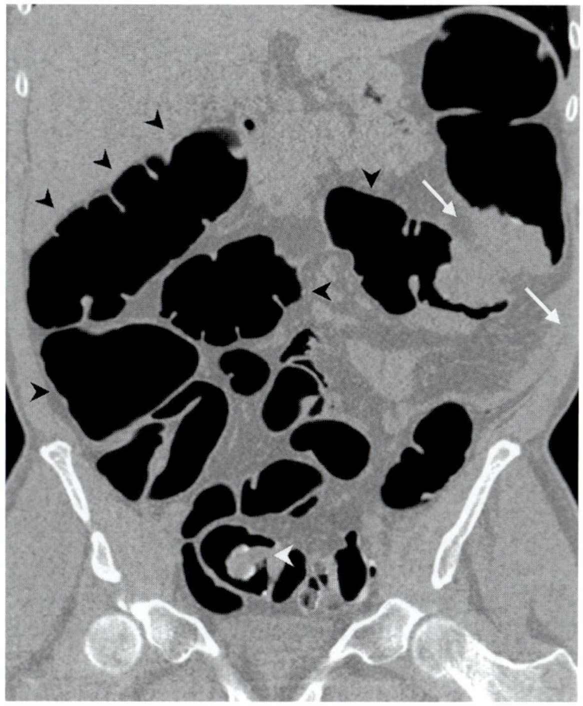

Fig. 6.2. Despite the large obstructing tumor in the transverse colon near the splenic flexure (*white arrows*), the proximal colon is clean (*black arrowheads*). There is a large stalked polyp in the sigmoid covered by a thin barium layer (*white arrowhead*). Ultra-low dose on a 64-slice scanner: 140 kV–10 mAs

6.4.3.2.2
The Symptomatic Patient

In case the patient presents with symptoms (see Chap. 2), diagnostic performance largely primes over patient compliance. The patient is seeking for help and is aware that very probably something is wrong in his abdomen or with his colon. In these cases, patient compliance almost becomes a non-issue. These patients need a full bowel preparation with or without fecal tagging and eventually with i.v. contrast according to local practice (procedure, see above). In case of an obstructing tumor, faecal tagging is not hampered. In these cases patients present with efficient tagging and the colon mostly is relatively clean. (Fig 6.2). in our experience none of these patients have suffered from post-procedural colonic impaction with baroliths.

6.4.3.2.3
The Asymptomatic Patient

In case of screening for colorectal cancer, the patient has no complaints and is not at all aware of possible disease. It is only by information received from his

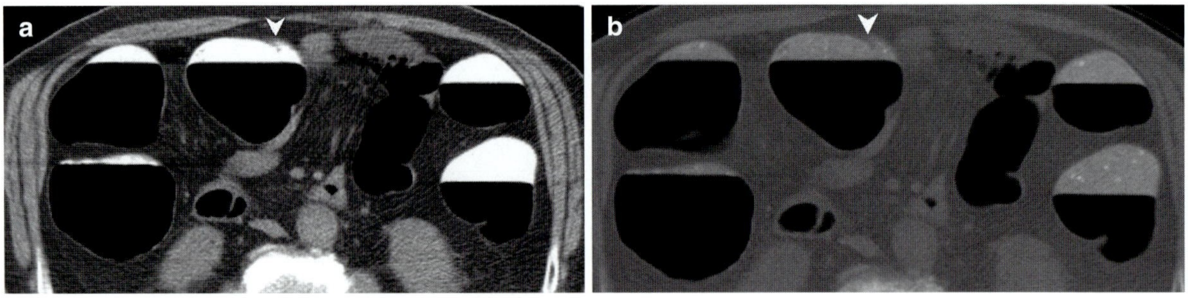

Fig. 6.3. a, b. Fluid tagging in soft tissue (**a**) and bone window (**b**) settings. The bone window setting enables visualization of the colonic wall and semicircular folds (*arrowhead*) through the dense fluid

clinical doctor or through journals or the Internet that he has some notion of screening the colon for colorectal cancer. In the majority of these patients, compliance becomes as important as diagnostic performance. As currently no CT colonography methods based on a reduced preparation have been validated in a large clinical trial, this group of patients still needs the classic triad of a low-residue diet, a full cathartic bowel preparation, and fecal tagging. The development of a laxative-free preparation is, however, considered a major objective and is subject to important research (see below).

6.4.3.2.4
The Frail and Elderly Patient

In these patients, it is important to reduce the preparation-related side effects. Furthermore, in these patients CT colonography is performed to detect lesions ≥1 cm or cancers. Therefore, in this category of patients CT colonography can be performed after preparation with a reduced amount of laxatives or even without laxatives (=laxative-free).

6.5
Imaging Findings

6.5.1
Reading the Data Sets

After the examination, the obtained images are sent to a dedicated workstation with regular CT colonography software. It is important to stress that no dedicated electronic cleansing or stool subtraction software is needed to adequately read and interpret the data sets. Reading is performed using either a primary 2D read with 3D problem-solving method or primary 3D reading with 2D problem-solving. In 2D rendering, we read the data sets using lung window (W/L: 1,500/–200 HU) and soft tissue (W/L: 400/100 HU) settings. In case the tagged residue has a high density, it is advised using additional bone window settings (W/L: 3,500/400). This will improve visualization of a negative filling defect in the tagged residue. The negative filling defect can be an anatomic structure or a lesion. This is particularly helpful in the case of dense fluid (Fig. 6.3a, b).

6.5.2
Stool Tagging

6.5.2.1
Tagged Stool

With fecal tagging, the residual stool appears as a bright hyperdense or white spot or mass in the colonic lumen with or without air inclusion, making it easy to recognize (Fig. 6.4a, b). This bright stool almost lights up when scrolling through the 2D images simplifying interpretation as there is no concern to mistake it as a lesion. In that way, the time consuming comparison between supine and prone position to detect an eventual positional shift of the residual stool becomes superfluous. This shortens the reading time considerably, avoids false-positives and improves polyp conspicuity. When reading the tagged data sets, looking for non-tagged "material" is imperative. This non-tagged material is highly suspicious and should be considered a lesion unless it has the specific characteristics of residual stool (Fig. 6.5). Even in case of an obvious change between supine and prone position, a polyp has to be excluded. In fact, polyps with a long stalk may show a considerable change in location with

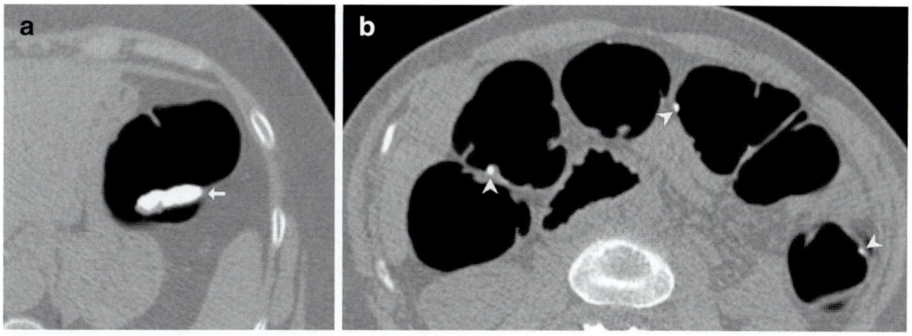

Fig. 6.4. a, b Examples of stool tagging (*arrow* and *arrowheads*). Confusion with a true lesion is excluded. No comparison between supine and prone images is necessary to exclude a lesion

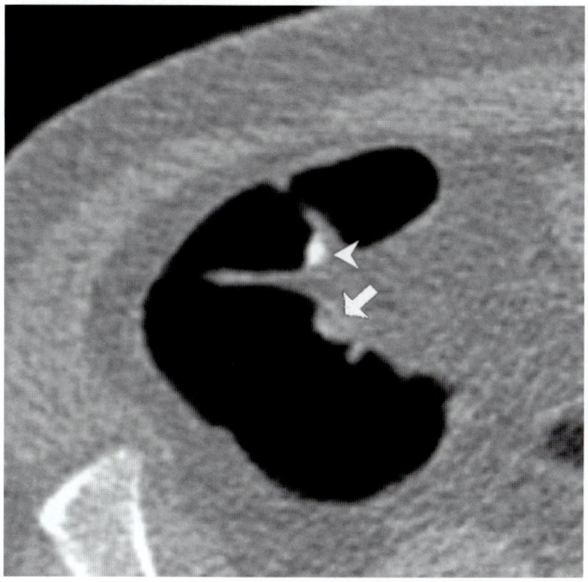

Fig. 6.5. Patient with right-sided sigmoid. There is tagged stool (*arrowhead*). There is also non-tagged "material" (*arrow*). This should be considered a lesion unless the contrary is proved. A correct diagnosis of an 8 mm sessile polyp was made

dual positioning. A similar lesion was mistaken as stool and caused a false-negative (one of the two missed lesions >1 cm) in the landmark study of Fenlon et al. (1999) Segmental mobility of the colonic segments may also cause a pseudochange in position causing a lesion to appera as non-tagged stool (fig 12)(Chen et al 2006). The density of the tagged stool varies between 100 and 3,000 HU. It is striking that there is a wide intra- and inter-patient variability. There is no apparent reason to explain this variability.

As with optical colonoscopy, tagged stool frequently abuts a lesion. This makes polyps more conspicuous for detection (Figs. 6.6 and 6.7). In these cases, polyp conspicuity is improved using soft tissue settings.

6.5.2.2 Non-Tagged Stool

In a minority of cases, a small amount of stool remains non-tagged.

6.5.2.2.1 Non-Tagged Stool <6 mm

Non-tagged stool <6 mm is too small to cause any concern, as it is generally accepted that polyps <6 mm do not need to be removed. Hence, pseudopolypoid lesions <6 mm caused by non-tagged residual stool should not be taken into consideration. This non-tagged stool appears as pinpoint filling defects abutting the colonic wall or is frequently floating in barium pools without touching the colonic wall (Fig. 6.8).

6.5.2.2.2 Non-Tagged Stool >6 mm

In case of larger non-tagged stool, it is important to look for the typical imaging findings of stool (Figs. 6.9 and 6.10). This stool may also present with: (1) moving to the dependent part of the colon with dual positioning; (2) presenting with an air inclusion (abdominal window setting); (3) presenting with a hyperdense peripheral ring and central hypodensity or air inclusion; (4) having a hooked appearance; (5) having no attachment to the colonic wall.

6.5.3 Fluid Tagging

Tagged fluid typically is hyperdense or white. This enables visualization of the colonic wall and eventual lesions through the fluid on the 2D images and solves the issue of the drowned segment. In fact, semicircular folds as well as tumoral lesions appear as negative

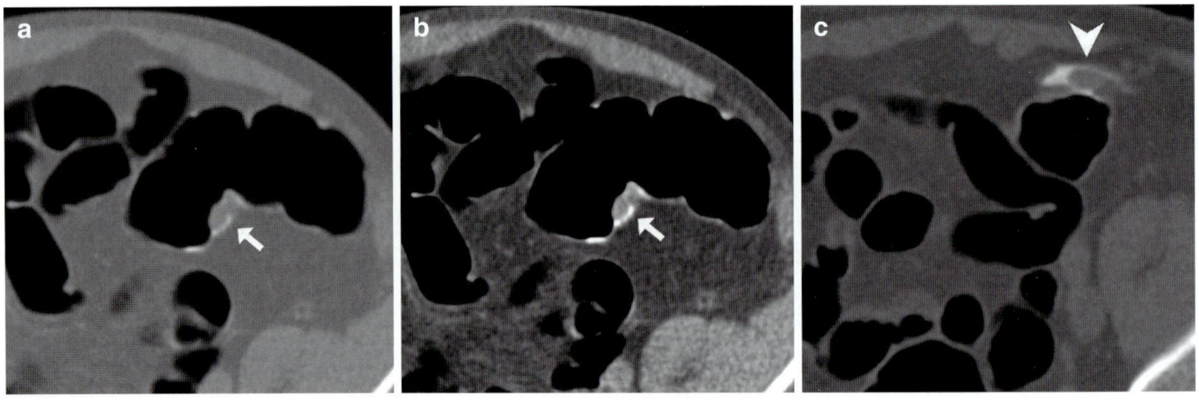

Fig. 6.6. (**a**) Supine view of the sigmoid in lung window settings (W/L 1,500/–200) showing a stalked polyp abutting the colonic wall, surrounded by a barium layer (*white arrow*). (**b**) Same image in soft tissue settings (W/L 400/100) showing improved conspicuity of the lesion. (**c**) The prone acquisition shows that the corresponding segment is collapsed. The lesion is still visible as a negative filling defect as it is surrounded by tagged fluid (*white arrowhead*)

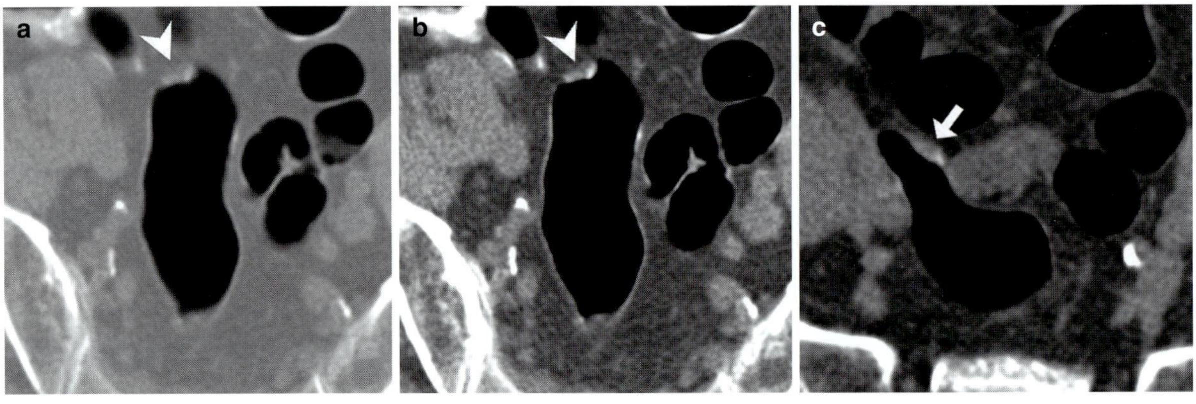

Fig. 6.7. (**a**) Small amount of barium abutting a lesion (*arrowhead*) in the sigmoid and hence improving polyp conspicuity. (**b**) Improved depiction of the lesion in soft tissue settings. (**c**) The prone view shows a partially collapsed sigmoid. The barium again delineates the lesion improving visualization (*white arrow*)

filling defects in the fluid (Figs. 6.3 and 6.11). This avoids false-negative findings. When tagged fluid is present in a collapsed segment, a lesion can sometimes be distinguished as a negative filling defect (Fig. 6.6). The semicircular folds show their typical appearance fading out in the colonic wall when scrolling through the axial slices. The density of the fluid varies between 100 and 1,000 HU (Fig. 6.12).

6.5.4 Miscellaneous Findings

6.5.4.1 Mucous Filaments

Mucous filaments appear as thin threadlike structures crossing the colonic lumen or lying on one or more semicircular folds. They can occur after a preparation without or with fecal tagging. In the latter case, these filaments can be tagged or non-tagged. They can change in shape with dual positioning. However, they may simulate the stalk of a polyp. It is important to not misinterpret it as a polyp and vice versa (Fig. 6.13). In that case, they are not connected to the head of a polyp. However, sometimes a semicircular fold simulates the head of a polyp on 2D images. Care has to be taken not to misinterpret a polyp with a thin stalk as a mucous filament (Fig. 6.14).

6.5.4.2 Foam

Fecal residue with a foamy appearance is mostly detected in the cecum or ascending colon. It appears as an amorphous inhomogeneous mixture mostly of

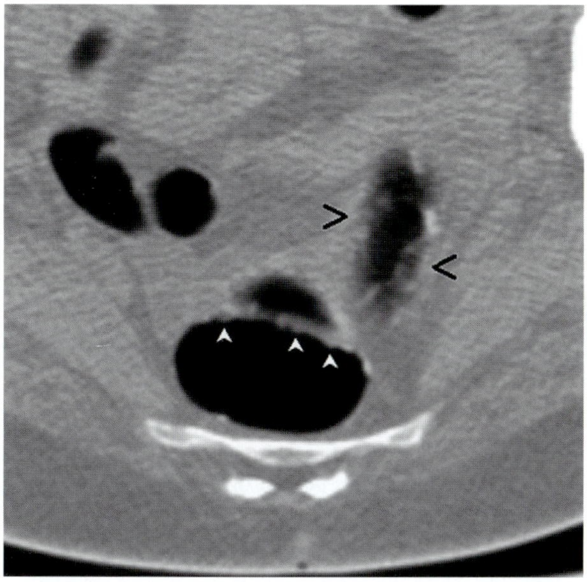

Fig. 6.8. Supine view of the rectosigmoid showing tiny non-tagged residue in the rectum (*white arrowhead*) and sigmoid (*open black arrowhead*). This stool is too small to cause any diagnostic problem

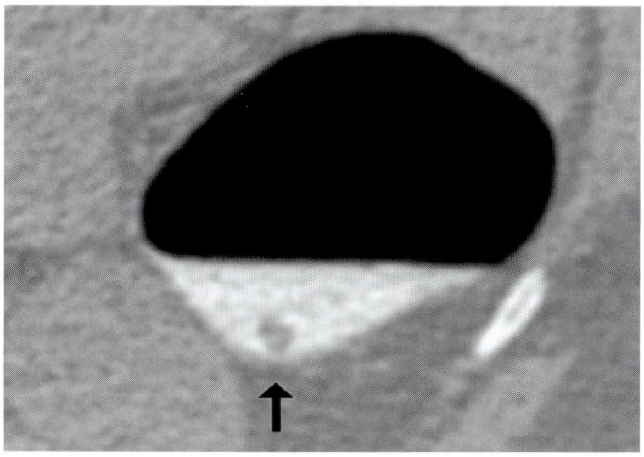

Fig. 6.9. Ultra low-dose scan (64 slice) showing tagged fluid level with floating non-tagged 6 mm residue (*arrow*). There is no contact with the colonic wall, so no confusion with a polyp is possible

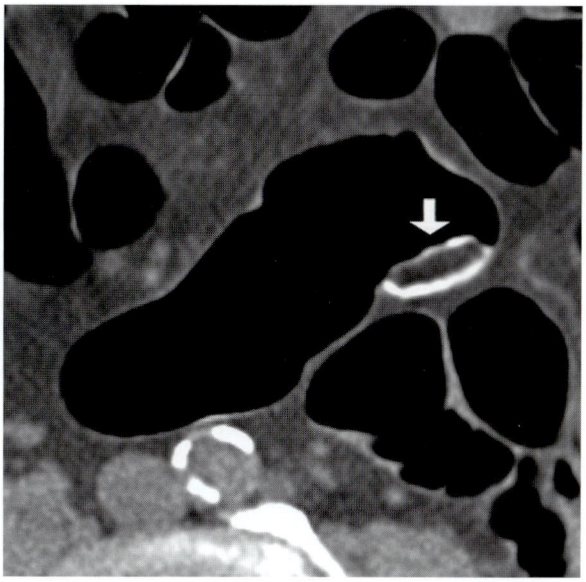

Fig. 6.10. Non-tagged stool >1 cm in the sigmoid (*arrow*). This non-tagged material shows the characteristics of non-tagged stool: completely surrounded by barium, hooked appearance, some minute air inclusions

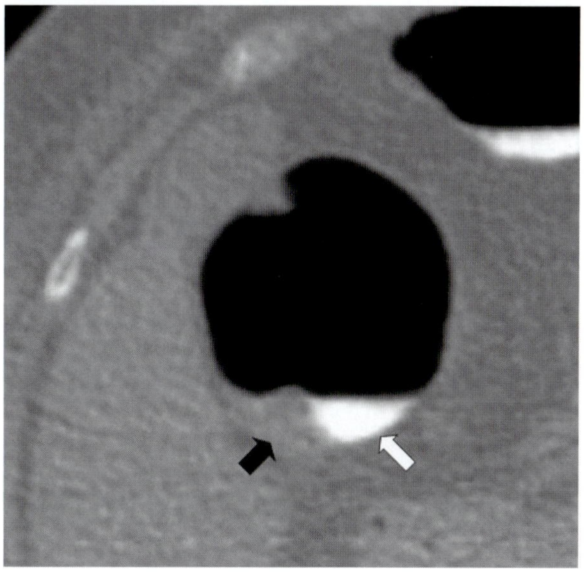

Fig. 6.11. Tagged fluid (*white arrow*) reveals a sessile polyp as a negative filling defect (*black arrow*)

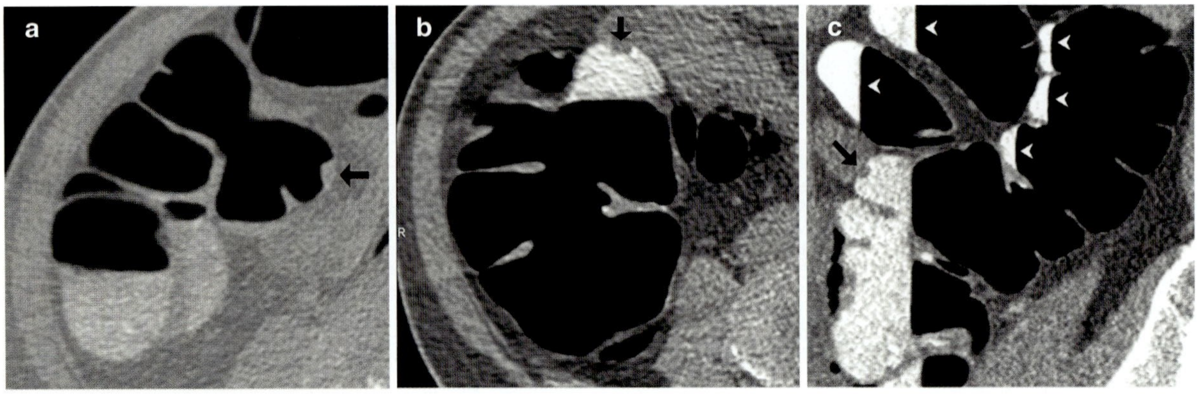

Fig. 6.12. (**a**) Supine image of the ascending colon obtained at ultralow dose (64 slice) showing sessile 8 mm polyp (*black arrow*). (**b**) Prone view shows the lesion covered by fluid. Because the fluid is tagged, the lesion appears as a negative filling defect (*arrow*). (**c**) The sagittal reformatted image confirms this finding (*arrow*). This image shows different densities of tagged fluids in the same patient (*white arrowheads*) Cecal mobility causes a slight change in position of the polyp.

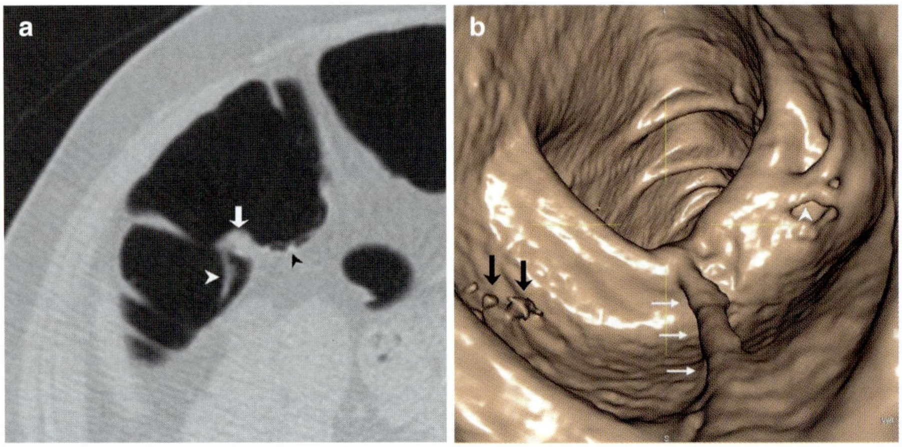

Fig. 6.13. (**a**) Supine view of the transverse colon showing a mucous filament (*white arrowhead*) attached to a prominent semicircular fold (*white arrow*), mimicking a stalked polyp. Some partially tagged foam (*black arrowhead*). (**b**) Corresponding endoluminal view showing the filament mimicking the stalk of a polyp (*white arrows*). The filament has an irregular shape. The foam is also visible (*black arrows*)

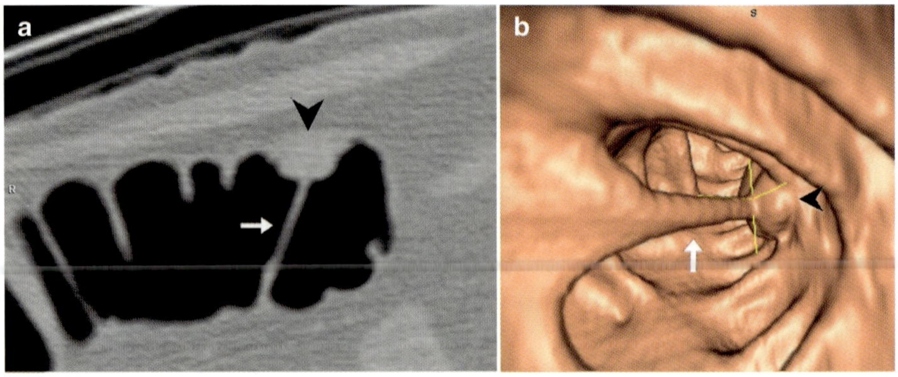

Fig. 6.14. (**a**) Polyp with a long thin stalk (*white arrow*) and with the head on the anterior colonic wall at the level of the transverse colon (*black arrowhead*). (**b**) Corresponding endoluminal view showing the stalk (*white arrow*) and the head (*black arrowhead*) of the polyp

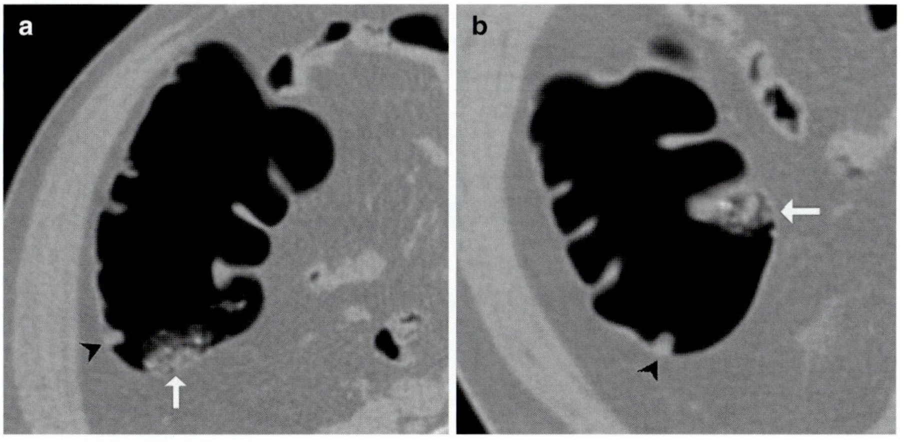

Fig. 6.15. (**a**) Non-tagged foam with some tiny tagged residue besides a possible sessile polyp (*black arrowhead*) in the ascending colon (supine view). (**b**) Corresponding prone view: the foam has moved to the anterior border of the ascending colon (*white arrow*). The sessile lesion remains unchanged (*black arrowhead*) and should be considered a sessile polyp. The lesion was confirmed on optical colonoscopy

air bubbles and stool. They occur in both preparations without and with fecal tagging. In the latter case, the foam is tagged or non-tagged. This foam may distract the reader's attention or cover a lesion making the detection difficult (Fig. 6.15).

6.6 The Future: Laxative-Free CT Colonography

6.6.1 Principles

It is known that the adherence of an asymptomatic patient population to a colorectal cancer screening program is low because of the embarrassment caused by the intensive cathartic cleansing of the colon. As with fecal tagging, the residue can easily be differentiated from true tumoral lesions, the idea was conceived to reduce the cathartic part of the preparation to improve patient compliance. This improved patient compliance was confirmed by Lefere et al. (2002). They compared the patient discomfort experienced the day before CT colonography in two groups of 50 patients. The former group was prepared with an intensive cathartic cleansing, while the latter was prepared with a combination of a reduced cathartic cleansing and fecal tagging (16 g of magnesium citrate vs. the full dose of 24 g + 750 mL of a 2.1% barium suspension). There were significantly less side effects (such as nausea, vomiting, and abdominal cramps) in the group prepared with the reduced cathartic cleansing and fecal tagging. This resulted in an improved final opinion. Further improvement of patient compliance was obtained by reducing the volume of barium to drink to 50 mL using a higher concentrated 40% (w/v) suspension (Lefere et al. 2005).

The next step, i.e. performing CT colonography after a preparation without cathartic cleansing, is obvious. This method has been called laxative-free CT colonography (Lefere et al. 2005). It is clear that this method would dramatically increase patient compliance. Both the radiological and gastroenterological community agree that laxative-free CT colonography is the way to go for if good results of lesion detection are obtained (Rex 2000). Furthermore, this would stop the discussion whether CT colonography could ever replace optical colonoscopy as a screening tool for colorectal cancer. Several methods have been developed. These methods are based on fecal tagging and are still in the research stadium. A truly prepless method (i.e. no diet, no fecal tagging, and no cathartic cleansing) has not yet been developed.

6.6.2 Results

Iannaccone et al. (2004) examined successfully 203 patients with laxative-free CT colonography. They performed fecal tagging over 2 days with a total of 200 mL of diatrizoate meglumine and diatrizoate sodium. The patients were also on a low-residue diet for 2 days. They obtained very good results of polyp detection: 86% for lesions ≥6 mm (79 lesions), 95.5%

for lesions ≥8 mm (45 lesions), 100% for lesions ≥1 cm (24 lesions). Using gastrografin, they had side effects in 10% of patients underscoring the laxative action of gastrografin. This was also the experience of Jensch et al. (2008). In their study of 168 patients, all patients had some form of diarrhea.

Therefore, the use of barium as the sole tagging agent should be considered as a truly laxative-free method. This method was successfully applied by Johnson et al. (2008). Using barium as the sole tagging agent, they obtained a sensitivity of 88 and 93% for lesions 6–9 mm and ≥1 cm, respectively. In this study, electronic cleansing was also successful.

6.7 Conclusion

Combing a low-residue diet with intensive cathartic cleansing of the colon and fecal tagging is considered essential to perform state-of-the-art CT colonography. Developing a robust method of laxative-free CT colonography could prove invaluable in developing CT colonography as a screening method for colorectal cancer.

References

American College of Radiology Committee on Drugs and Contrast Media (2005) Manual on contrast media, version 5.0 (iodinated gastrointestinal contrast media: indications and guidelines). American College of Radiology, Reston, pp 37–39

Barish MA, Soto JA, Ferrucci JT (2005) Consensus on current clinical practice of virtual colonoscopy. AJR Am J Roentgenol 184:786–792

Bromer MQ, Weinberg DS (2005) Screening for colorectal cancer–now and the near future. Semin Oncol 32:3–10

Carr DH et al (1985) Comparison of barium and diatrizoate bowel labelling agents in computed tomography. Brit J Radiol 58:393–394

Chambers SE et al (1984) A comparison of dilute barium and dilute water-soluble contrast in opacification of the bowel for abdominal computed tomography. Clinic Radiol 35: 463–464

Chen DC, Dachman AH (2006) Cecal mobility: a potential pitfall of CT colonography. AJR Am J Roentgenol. 186:1086-1089

Cotton PB, Durkalski VL, Pineau BC et al (2004) Computed tomographic colonography (virtual colonoscopy): a multicenter comparison with standard colonoscopy for detection of colorectal neoplasia. JAMA 291:1713–1719

Fenlon HM, Nunes DP, Nunes DP et al (1999) A comparison of virtual and conventional colonoscopy for the detection of colorectal polyps. NEJM 341:1496–1502

Fenlon HM (2002) CT colonography: pitfalls and interpretation. Abdom Imaging 27:284–291

Ferrucci J; Working Group on CT Colongraphy (2005a) CT colonography for detection of colon polyps and cancer. Lancet 365:1464–1465; author reply 1465–1466

Ferrucci JT (2005) Colonoscopy: virtual and optical–another look, another view. Radiology 235:13–16

Gryspeerdt S, Lefere P, Herman M et al (2005) CT colonography with fecal tagging after incomplete colonoscopy. Eur Radiol 15:1192–1202

Iannaccone R, Laghi A, Catalano C et al (2004) Computed tomographic colonography without cathartic preparation for the detection of colorectal polyps. Gastroenterology 127:1300–1311

Jensch S, de Vries A, Peringa J et al (2008) CT colonography with limited bowel preparation: performance characteristics in an increased-risk population. Radiology 247:122–132

Johnson CD, Chen MH, Toledano AL et al (2008) Accuracy of CT colonography for detection of large adenomas and cancers. N Engl J Med 359:1207–1217

Kim DH, Pickhardt PJ, Taylor AJ et al (2007) CT colonography versus colonoscopy for the detection of advanced neoplasia. N Engl J Med 357:1403–1412

Kinnunen J et al (1989) Omnipaque and gastrografin in gastrointestinal follow-through examinations. Röntgenblätter 42:228–231

Laerum F et al (1991) Iodinated contrast and the gastrointestinal tract. Invest Radiol 26:177–181

Lefere P, Gryspeerdt S, Dewyspelaere J et al (2002) Dietary fecal tagging as a cleansing method before CT colonography: initial results polyp detection and patient acceptance. Radiology 224(2):393–403

Lefere P, Gryspeerdt S, Marrannes J et al (2005) CT colonography after fecal tagging with a reduced cathartic cleansing and a reduced volume of barium. AJR Am J Roentgenol 184:1836–1842

Macari M, Megibow AJ (2001) Pitfalls of using three-dimensional CT colonography with two-dimensional imaging correlation. AJR Am J Roentgenol 176:137–143

Macleod AJ, Duncan KA, Pearson RH et al (1998) A comparison of Fleet Phospho-soda with Picolax in the preparation of the colon for double contrast barium enema. Clin Radiol 53:612–614

Morrin MM, Farrell RJ, Kruskal JB et al (1999) Virtual colonoscopy: a kinder, gentler colorectal cancer screening test? Lancet 354:1048–1049

Murphy J, Coster G (1997) Issues in patient compliance. Drugs 54:797–800

Pickhardt PJ, Choi JR, Hwang I et al (2003a) Computed tomographic virtual colonoscopy to screen for colorectal neoplasia in asymptomatic adults. N Engl J Med 349: 2191–2200

Pickhardt PJ, Pineau BC, Paskett ED et al (2003b) Virtual colonoscopy using oral contrast compared with colonoscopy for the detection of patients with colorectal polyps. Gastroenterology 125:304–310

Rex DK (2000) Virtual colonoscopy : time for some tough questions for radiologists and gastroenterologists. Endoscopy 32:260–263

Rockey DC, Paulson E, Niedzwiecki D et al (2005) Analysis of air contrast barium enema, computed tomographic colonography, and colonoscopy: prospective comparison. Lancet 365:305–311

Seymour PC et al (1997) Anaphylactic shock during a routine upper gastrointestinal series. AJR 168:957–958
Skucas J (1997) Anaphylactoid reactions with gastrointestinal contrast media. AJR 168:962–964
Taylor S, Laghi A, Lefere P et al (2007) European society of gastrointestinal and abdominal radiology (ESGAR): consensus statement on CT colonography. Eur Radiol 17:575–579
Thomeer M, Carbone I, Bosmans H et al (2003) Stool tagging applied in thin-slice multidetector computed tomography colonography. JCAT 27:132–139
van Dam J, Cotton P, Johnson CD et al (2004) AGA future trends report: CT colonography. Gastroenterology 127: 970–984
Zalis ME, Perumpillichira J, Del Frate C et al (2003) CT colonography: digital subtraction bowel cleansing with mucosal reconstruction–initial observations. Radiology 226: 911–917
Zalis ME, Perumpillichira, Magee c et al (2006) Tagging-based electronically cleansed CT colonography: evaluation of patient comfort and image readability. Radiology 239: 149–159

How to Get the Colon Distended?

David Burling, Stuart Taylor, and Steve Halligan

CONTENTS

David Burling, MD
Steve Halligan, MD
Intestinal Imaging Unit, Level 4V, St Mark's Hospital, Watford Road, Harrow, Middlesex HA1 3UJ, UK
Stuart Taylor, MD, MRCP, FRCR
Department of Imaging, University College Hospital, 2F Podium, 235 Euston Road, London NW1 2BU, UK

7.1 Introduction

The importance of achieving optimal colonic distention prior to CT colonography cannot be overstated, and the editors have justifiably devoted an entire chapter to the subject. Optimal luminal distention enables the reader to rapidly and confidently assess the colon, and undoubtedly improves diagnostic accuracy (Chen et al. 1999; Fletcher et al. 2000; Yee et al. 2003). Conversely, inadequate distention may obliterate the colonic lumen and result in wall/haustral fold thickening (Fig. 7.1), thereby variously hiding or mimicking colorectal neoplasia (Fig. 7.2a, b) (Fletcher et al. 1999; Macari Megibow 2001; Fenlon 2002). Interpretation times are increased when the colon is poorly distended, but of greater importance is the potential to miss significant colonic pathology

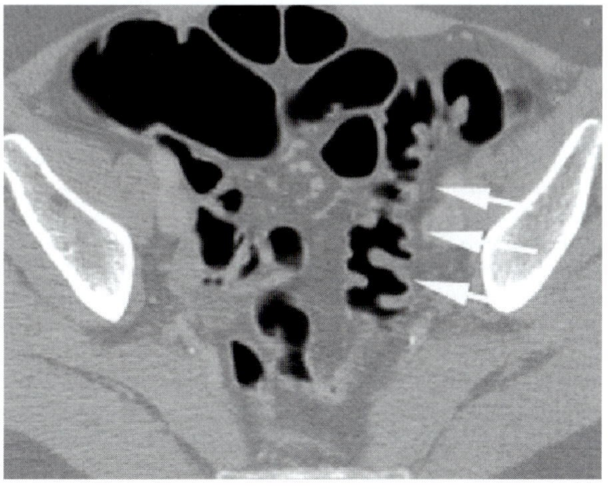

Fig. 7.1. A poorly distended sigmoid colon (*arrows*) resulting in bulbous haustral folds on this supine scan demonstrates how inadequate distention can thwart confident and time-efficient interpretation. Subsequent optical colonoscopy was unremarkable

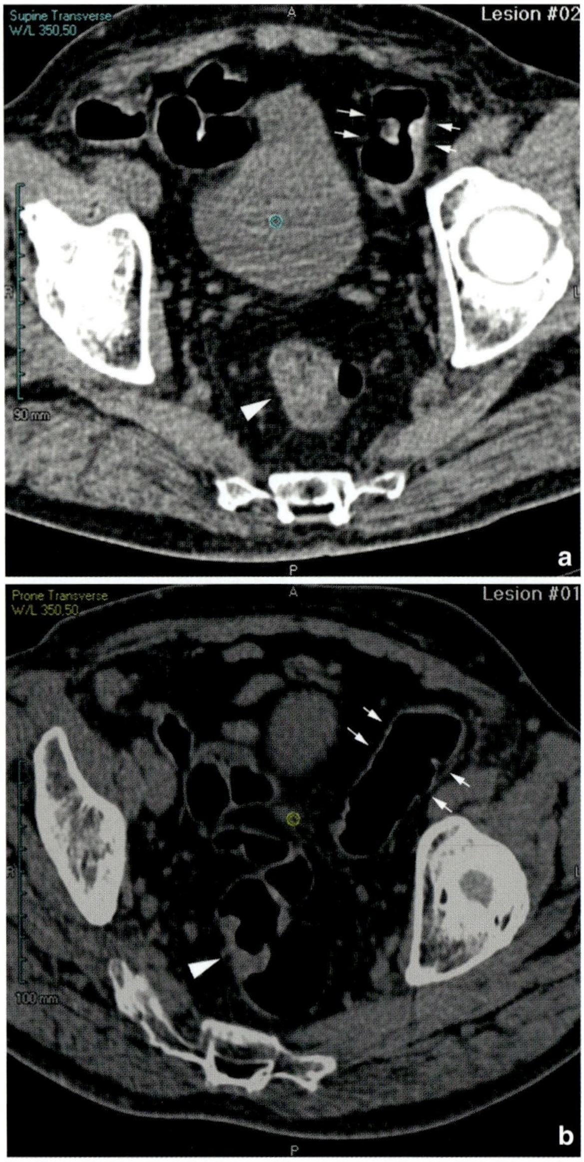

Fig. 7.2. Supine (**a**) and prone (**b**) axial images of a 64-year-old man, obtained using a four multi-detector row scanner, demonstrating the diagnostic dilemma posed by inadequate distention and the benefit of dual scan positioning. The supine scan demonstrates a possible cancer in the sigmoid colon (*arrows*) with a collapsed recto-sigmoid colon (*arrowhead*). In contrast, the prone scan, in which optimal distention is achieved, reveals that the area of concern in the sigmoid is normal (*arrows*), but a rectosigmoid cancer is revealed (*arrowhead*) (courtesy Laghi and Iannaccone)

(Fig. 7.3a–c), occasionally rendering the examination non-diagnostic (i.e. necessitating repeat examination or endoscopic referral) or sometimes frankly misleading. For example, a review of missed significant lesions from a large prospective multicenter trial of CT colonography (Rockey et al. 2005; Paulson et al. 2004) found that suboptimal distention, along with poor preparation, was implicated as a contributing factor in 16 of 28 (57%) false-negative examinations.

Several strategies have been proven to improve distention, the most notable being dual patient positioning (i.e. obtaining separate prone and supine acquisitions). Use of faster multi-detector row scanners and administration of intravenous spasmolytics (see section below) also help. However, despite these strategies, suboptimal distention is unfortunately still frequently encountered in day-to-day clinical practice.

Unlike bowel purgation, which is largely determined by intrinsic patient-related factors such as compliance and bowel transit time, colonic distention is greatly influenced by the actions of the colonographic practitioner present at the time of examination. On first inspection, distending the colon may appear a relatively simple and trivial procedure and, intuitively, skills acquired for barium enema should be easily transferrable to CT colonography. However, the colonographer is disadvantaged. Unlike barium enema, where real-time fluoroscopic screening is utilized to ensure satisfactory segmental distention, colonic insufflation prior to CT colonography is not performed under direct visualization: A scout view must suffice. As a result, inadequate distention may only be fully appreciated once full data acquisition is complete. Furthermore, the aim for CT colonography is not simply adequate inflation but optimal distention, preferably resulting in "pencil-thin" colonic wall and haustral folds. Colonic neoplasia is generally best seen when the colon is well distended, a statement that holds true for both primary 2D and 3D analysis (Pickhardt et al. 2004). Indeed, sessile and flat lesions with minimal protrusion into the lumen or causing subtle focal wall thickening may be invisible without optimal distention.

The purpose of this chapter is to provide an evidence-based review of strategies and techniques intended to safely optimize colonic distention, and to draw readers' attention to current areas of controversy.

7.2 Patient Preparation

Although less invasive than endoscopic procedures, like any medical investigation, CT colonography undoubtedly generates a degree of patient apprehension. As for barium enema, patients should be fully

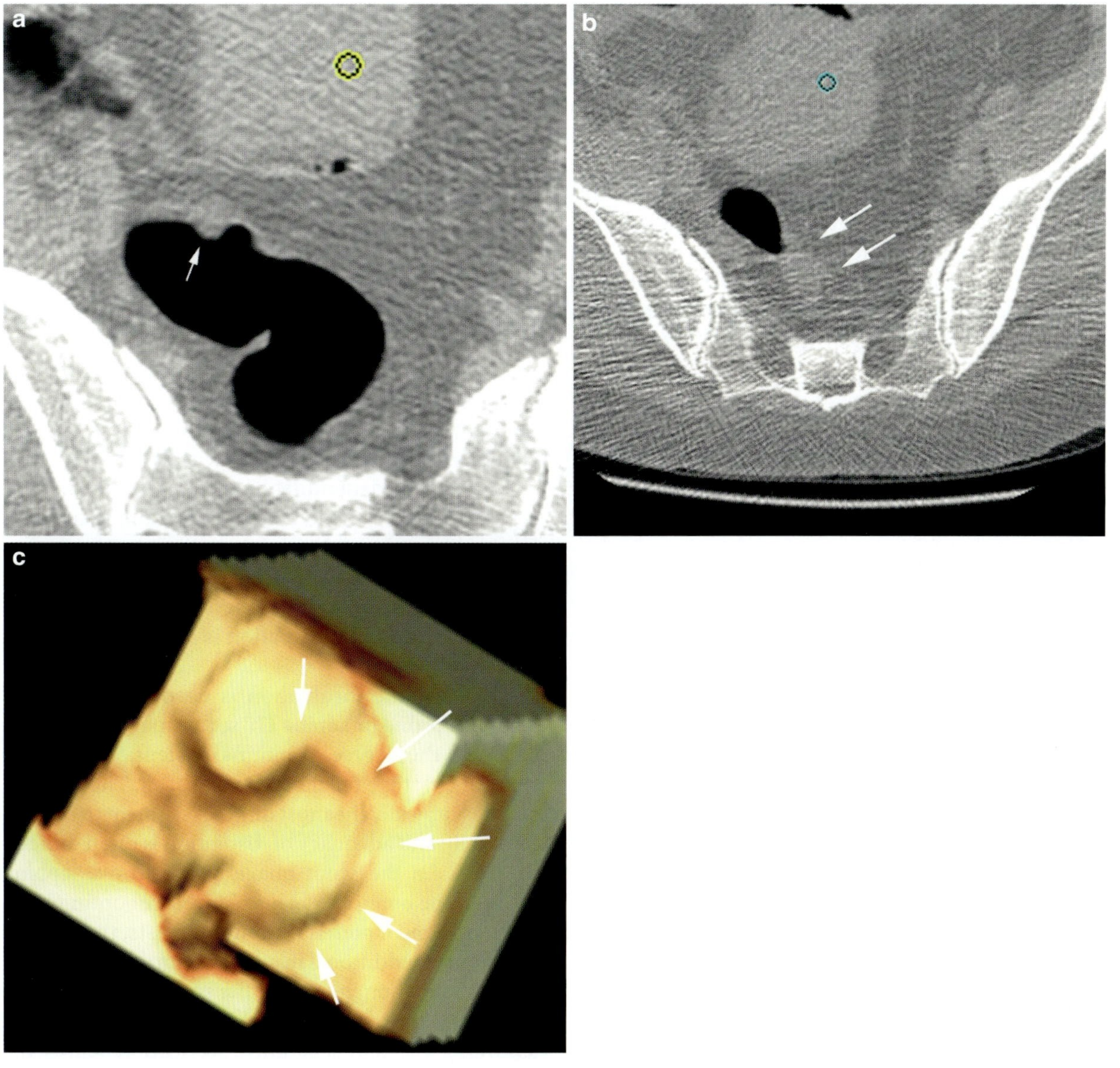

Fig. 7.3. A 12-mm rectosigmoid polyp in a 69-year-old woman is difficult to detect, as it lies partially submerged in fluid (*arrow*). (**a**) Unfortunately, it is concealed on the supine acquisition due to segmental collapse (*arrows*) (**b**) but the volume rendered, endoluminal display confirms its presence (*arrows*) (**c**)

apprised of what is going to happen to them and what is required of them (Rubesin et al. 2000). A simple, easily understood description of the examination should ideally be made available in advance, followed by a brief reminder just before the examination itself. An appropriate discussion will prepare patients for rectal catheter insertion, the feeling of abdominal bloating, and potential mild discomfort due to retained gas. Prior to entering the CT scanner room, patients should be encouraged to empty their bowel for a final time.

Once the patient is lying on the CT scanner table, a suitably qualified practitioner may choose to perform a rectal examination. This may be helpful for several reasons; detecting an occlusive tumor will avoid a potentially difficult and unsafe rectal catheter insertion and anal sphincter tone can be assessed quickly, which may influence the choice of catheter or method of insufflation. Digital rectal examination may also aid subsequent interpretation, which can be particularly challenging at the anorectal junction because of the frequent presence of hemorrhoids and redundant rectal mucosa. Despite these potential advantages, rectal examination can be uncomfortable and also embarrassing for patients. Moreover, radiographic technologists now frequently perform CT colonography examinations and are likely to be much less experienced at digital rectal examination, despite competence at catheter insertion. One compromise would be to perform a rectal examination in specific patient groups, for example those with symptoms highly suggestive of rectal cancer or in whom initial colonic insufflation is difficult, or in patients suspected of having poor anal tone (see section below).

7.3 Colonic Insufflation Methods

Colonic distention prior to CT colonography entails gently administering gas (air or carbon dioxide) via a rectal catheter using either manual or automated insufflation techniques. Both gases and insufflation methods are widely used and all have their advocates; some favor the least expensive and simplest method, i.e. room air insufflation by manual compression of a plastic insufflator bulb while others prefer carbon dioxide delivered by automated insufflation devices. Until relatively recently, there has been a lack of objective evidence to recommend one method over another but there is now data emerging that will help to guide future practice (Burling et al. 2006; Rogalla et al. 2004; Yee et al. 2002).

7.3.1 Manual Insufflation

The easiest and cheapest method for distending the colon is to use room air, often insufflated via a hand-held plastic bulb. Typically, patients lie on the CT scanner table in a left lateral position facing away from the operator. A lubricated rectal catheter attached to an insufflator bulb via a connecting tube is then inserted into the rectum and taped to the patients' buttocks. The patient is encouraged to retain any gas and avoid passing flatus by clenching their anus. Colonic insufflation is then performed by gently and intermittently squeezing the plastic bulb typically over a period of 1–2 min. Rapid successive bulb squeezes should be avoided, as they may precipitate rectosigmoid spasm causing patient discomfort, and limiting insufflation (Rubesin et al. 2000). Insufflation can be performed by either the patient or operator.

Insufflation is continued until the operator believes that the colon is optimally distended; most experts judge this by noting patient tolerance (Barish et al. 2005), stopping when the patient feels uncomfortable or bloated. In the presence of a competent ileocecal valve, this generally occurs following the introduction of approximately 2 L of gas, usually after 30–40 compressions (Morrin et al. 2002; Macari 2004). Limiting insufflation to a fixed volume or number of bulb compressions is not recommended because individual patients' colonic volume and tolerance vary. Some practitioners advise repositioning the patient part way through insufflation into either the prone or supine position (Chen et al. 1999; Taylor et al. 2003a, b), depending on which scan acquisition is performed first (see below), for example first filling the non-dependent right colon in the lateral decubitus position and then the remaining distal colon after repositioning. Assessment of right-sided filling by abdominal palpation is also recommended anecdotally.

Once colonic insufflation is deemed sufficient, a standard prone or supine CT scout image is acquired to assess the degree of luminal distention and anatomical coverage for the following scan. The sigmoid colon is typically the most difficult segment to distend optimally and adequacy of distention is often difficult to assess on the scout image owing to overlapping loops in the anteroposterior plane. If suboptimal distention is encountered or doubt persists, the authors recommend additional insufflation immediately prior to CT acquisition, repeating the scout image if necessary. Once the first acquisition has been obtained (and assuming a second is planned: see section below), the rectal catheter is left in situ and the patient repositioned. Once repositioned, and providing the patient is comfortable, the authors suggest further insufflation with approximately ten bulb compressions. We do not recommend insufflation while the patient is turning as this tends to precipitate anal leakage. Some workers advocate removing the rectal tube at this point because it may theoretically obscure rectal pathology. A repeat scout image is then performed routinely prior to the second CT acquisition (prone or supine), but we have found that patients rarely require additional insufflation following this (unless anal incontinence is present).

The ease and simplicity of this method is such that some patients can effectively insufflate their own colon using the hand-held bulb (Pickhardt et al. 2003).

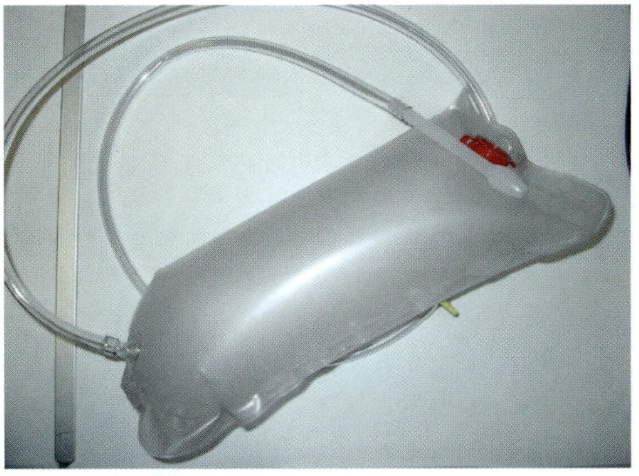

Fig. 7.4. Standard enema bag containing approximately 3 L of carbon dioxide for manual insufflation

However, success will depend greatly on the patient population concerned, and this approach requires well-motivated individuals, perhaps more applicable to a younger screening population (Pickhardt et al. 2003). Notably, the authors who proposed this method initially now routinely utilize automated insufflation in their clinical practice (Kim et al. 2007).

A standard enema bag filled with approximately 3 L of gas is an alternative to the plastic bulb insufflator, Fig. 7.4, and has the additional advantage of permitting manual insufflation of carbon dioxide. The bag (filled with air or carbon dioxide via a gas cylinder) is sealed with a plastic clip and attached to a rectal catheter via a connecting tube. Once the rectal catheter is in situ, the clip is released and the bag is gently compressed over 2–3 min, emptying its contents into the colon. Slow and gentle insufflation improves patient tolerance and ultimately allows greater volumes of gas to be administered. If the bag is empty and more gas required, then the plastic seal can be opened and room air introduced.

Carbon dioxide may also be insufflated directly from a gas cylinder via a tube with side hole for digitally controlling volume and pressure (Rogalla et al. 2004). Clearly, the pressure of insufflated gas must be carefully controlled using this method.

7.3.2 Automated Insufflation

Automated insufflation devices are now widely utilized across Europe and the USA, despite the additional equipment costs. Advocates suggest that insufflating carbon dioxide at controlled flow rates and pressures is convenient for the operator, and improves distention and patient compliance.

Early experience comparing a crudely modified laparosopic insufflator to manual bulb insufflation of room air showed equivocal effects on luminal distention (Ristvedt et al. 2003). More recently, two studies (Yee et al. 2002; Iafrate et al. 2004) compared specifically designed automated CO_2 insufflation devices with manual insufflation of room air. The first showed a modest improvement in distention using automated insufflation, particularly in the left colon (Yee et al. 2002). The second showed that the insufflation methods were equivocal for luminal distention but that examination times were significantly longer (although less ileal reflux was encountered) using the automated device (Iafrate et al. 2004). These data might suggest that only a modest benefit, if any, is derived from using an automated device. However, one significant advantage of automated insufflation is that administration has been specifically designed for use with carbon dioxide. As discussed below, there is good evidence from the colonoscopic and barium enema literature that demonstrates greater patient comfort when using carbon dioxide as opposed to air, because of its relatively rapid absorption through the colonic mucosa (Grant et al. 1986; Church and Delaney 2003). Recent data also suggest that automated insufflation produces significantly better distention when compared with manual insufflation of carbon dioxide, again particularly in the left colon (Burling et al. 2006; Rogalla et al. 2004).

At the time of writing, the authors are aware of only one commercially available device specifically designed for colonic insufflation (Fig. 7.5, Protocol colon insufflation system, BRACCO UK Ltd). This system controls the flow rate of carbon dioxide, which can be increased in a step-wise fashion from 1 to 3 L/min, to prevent spasm (1 L/min for the first 0.5 L, 2 L/min from 0.5 to 1.0 L, and then 3.0 L/min thereafter). The total volume of gas administered is displayed and updated continuously, and if intracolonic pressure (measured at the rectal catheter tip) increases beyond the limit set by the user (up to a maximum of 25 mmHg), the system automatically shuts down to prevent further insufflation, thereby reducing the risk of colonic perforation. Insufflation automatically ceases when a total of 4 L of gas has been administered and then for every 2 L administered beyond this. To recommence insufflation, the operator needs to manually override this additional safety feature by pressing the start button again.

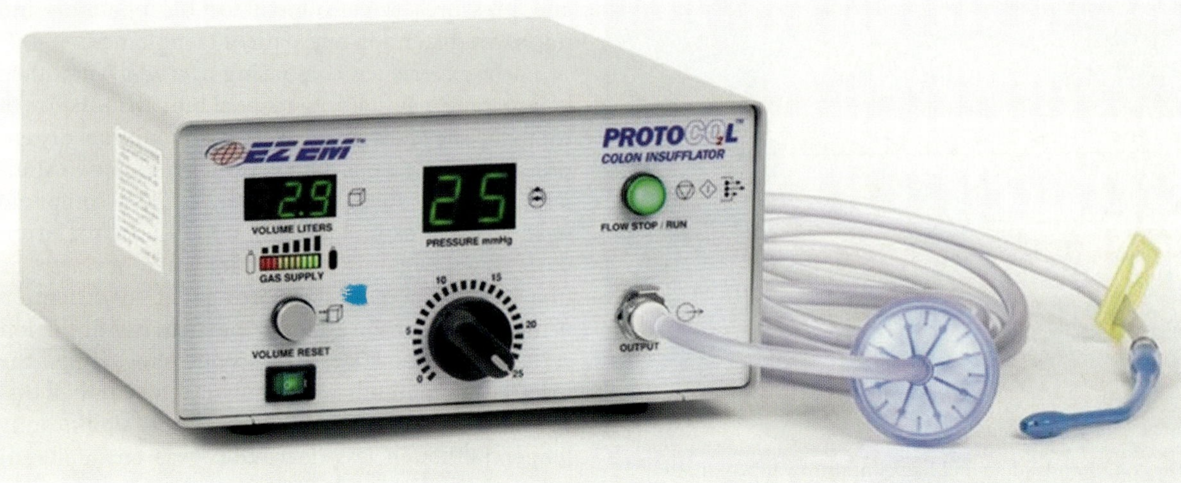

Fig. 7.5. Automated colonic insufflator, connected to a thin rectal catheter, displaying the intraluminal rectal pressure and total volume of carbon dioxide administered

The company's recommended technique is to insufflate the patient in the supine position. The pressure limit is set at 15 mmHg initially, increasing to 25 mmHg depending on the patient's tolerance. Three liters of carbon dioxide are instilled (again depending on the patient's tolerance), at which point the patient is asked if he/she can perceive gas on the right side of his/her abdomen – if not, insufflation is continued until he/she do, or until he/she feels uncomfortable. A CT scout is then performed to confirm adequate distention prior to data acquisition. For the prone acquisition, propping up the patient's chest with a pillow or foam wedge helps to optimize distention of the transverse colon. The authors use a slightly modified technique (described below), setting the pressure limit at 25 mmHg initially and pausing insufflation if the patient becomes uncomfortable. In our experience, the volume of gas administered during automated insufflation varies widely between patients (for example between 2.6 and 8.0 L with a median of approximately 4 L). Larger volumes are occasionally necessary, mostly due to anal incontinence, small bowel reflux, and/or colonic redundancy, but are paradoxically associated with significantly poorer distention. Clearly, these individuals are a challenging group to distend optimally and although the total volume of insufflated gas is a useful guide to the eventual adequacy of distention, practitioners should not limit their insufflation merely according to the total volume apparently administered. Interestingly, we have found no demonstrable learning curve when using the automated device, suggesting that once familiar with the device's controls, practitioners can independently achieve satisfactory results despite little prior experience.

7.4 Carbon Dioxide or Air?

As mentioned above, many practitioners suggest that carbon dioxide is superior to air, largely based on barium enema and colonoscopy literature, which suggests that it causes less discomfort because of its rapid mucosal absorption (Grant et al. 1986; Church et al. 2003). A recent study (Iafrate et al. 2004) also showed improved patient tolerance for CT colonography using automated carbon dioxide administration vs. manually administered room air, although it is not clear whether the benefit was derived from using the automated device or carbon dioxide gas. Using a validated patient satisfaction questionnaire, the authors recently compared automated vs. manual carbon dioxide insufflation and found virtually no difference between the two methods (Burling et al. 2006), suggesting that in the study by Iafrate et al. (2004), the use of carbon dioxide gas was the dominant factor. An additional advantage of rapid mucosal absorption is that it significantly reduces the technical difficulties associated with a distended colon if performing colonoscopy immediately after CT colonography.

The choice of insufflated gas is ultimately dependent on the preference of the individual practitioner. Patients almost certainly prefer carbon dioxide but the administration is relatively complicated and more expensive than bulb insufflation of room air. In an international survey of practitioners who were asked which gas they would advocate, 50% expressed no preference at all (Barish et al. 2005). Of the remainder, two-thirds preferred carbon dioxide over air.

7.5 Choice of Rectal Catheter

There is wider scope for using more flexible and thinner catheters during CT colonography than during barium enema because of the requirement to transmit only gas and because the consequences of anal incontinence are less dramatic. The choice of rectal catheter will mainly depend on local availability, method of insufflation, and individual patient, but there is some evidence suggesting that thin tubes are adequate for most circumstances.

Perhaps, the simplest catheter is a thin plastic or rubber tube, for example a standard 14F rectal tube (Jaques Nelaton rectal catheter; Rusch, Bucks) or a Foley catheter. The former was shown to be as effective as a standard inflatable rectal balloon catheter (Trimline DC; E-Z-EM, Westbury, NY) for achieving adequate distention (Taylor et al. 2003a, b). Alternatively, the Foley catheter is almost ubiquitous and can be used effectively when attached to a bulb insufflator. The soft tip allows safe and virtually painless insertion and it has a relatively small inflatable balloon, which can be used to assist continence if necessary.

However, routine use of an inflated rectal balloon catheter is discouraged for barium enema following evidence that the risk of rectal perforation is increased (Blakeborough et al. 1997), usually due to tearing the rectal wall either during insertion of the stiff catheter or due to the radial force applied by inflating the balloon. Practitioners should generally avoid standard barium enema balloon rectal catheters during CTC owing to their wide bore (2 cm diameter) and because insufflation of the large (100 mL when filled) balloon cannot be performed under flouroscopic control. Furthermore, as noted above, air insufflation using inflated large bore rectal balloon catheters has been associated with an increased risk of colonic perforation. Most experts recommend choosing the most appropriate catheter according to an individual's requirements; for example, most patients can be optimally scanned using a thin, flexible rectal tube whereas those with anal incontinence may require judicious use of a small volume inflated balloon catheter. In the latter situation, most complications can be avoided by performing a rectal examination (see section above), careful catheter insertion, and gentle balloon inflation.

Automated insufflation systems demand specific tubes that are designed to plug into the front of the device. These thin flexible, plastic tubes have a small (30 mL) balloon, which is used routinely in many centers.

Some groups advocate removing the tube for the second acquisition to enhance patient comfort and to facilitate subsequent rectal assessment. However, this issue is less relevant with thin catheters. Even if using larger catheters, the advantage of being able to insufflate additional gas likely outweighs any potential benefit of early removal.

7.6 Single vs. Multidetector Row Scanners

Multidetector row scanners are now almost universal in many countries and allow considerably reduced scan times, facilitating single breath-hold studies for the majority of patients. As a consequence, image misregistration has been practically eliminated and respiratory artifact reduced significantly (Hara et al. 2001). Moreover, distention also seems to be improved – a study by Hara et al. (2001) showed that suboptimal distention in at least one colonic segment was significantly more common with single-detector row CT (40 of 77 patients, 52%) compared with multi-detector row CT (26 of 160 patients, 19%). This finding was presumably because patients do not have to retain gas for as long and mucosal absorption is less critical.

7.7 Patient Positioning

Despite unanimous consensus in favor of dual position scanning amongst 27 international experts in 2003 (Barish et al. 2005), a minority still promulgate single position scanning.

However, the evidence in support of dual position scanning is overwhelming (Yee et al. 2003; Fletcher et al. 2000; Chen et al. 1999; Morrin et al. 2002). All these studies have found that colonic segments obscured by either fecal residue/fluid or poor distention will often be revealed by redistribution in the opposing position; for example, the rectum is usually optimally distended with the patient lying prone whereas the transverse colon is usually best distended on the supine acquisition since it is least dependent in this position. Unsurprisingly, improved segmental visualization significantly increases polyp detection. An early study (Chen et al. 1999) using manual insufflation to distend the colon with room air showed that the majority of colonic segments (59%) were inadequately distended if only one acquisition (prone or supine) was assessed. However, when data from both acquisitions were combined, a large majority of segments (87%) were adequately distended overall and polyp detection rates were increased. Later studies (Yee et al. 2003; Fletcher et al. 2000) confirmed these findings and demonstrated significantly improved polyp detection with dual position scanning owing to improved overall distention and therefore segmental visualization.

Advocates of single position scanning stress the additional radiation burden of scanning patients twice routinely, and choose to perform an additional scan only if visualization is deemed inadequate on the initial study. By necessity, this approach requires constant supervision. Moreover, studies of luminal visualization (Yee et al. 2003; Chen et al. 1999; Morrin et al. 2002) suggest that a second scan will be required frequently. Scanning routinely in a single position will require optimal distention throughout the colon (which is difficult to achieve in a single patient position, owing to the effects of gravity and peristalsis) and high-quality tagging of feces and fluid (possibly coupled with electronic subtraction). However, at the time of writing, an overwhelming proportion of authorities would strongly recommend routine dual position data acquisition.

Almost all published descriptions of CT colonography technique recommend acquiring the supine data set first, followed by the prone scan (Ristvedt et al. 2003; Yee et al. 2003; Gluecker et al. 2003; Svensson et al. 2002). This recommendation is likely a result of insufflation being performed in the supine position, which subsequently dictates the initial scan acquisition. Also, if intravenous contrast is utilized, this is frequently administered with the first scan and usually the supine position is chosen for convenience despite some evidence suggesting distention may be better overall on the prone scan (Morrin et al. 2002). However, in the authors' experience, the grade of distention is independent of the initial scan position (Burling et al. 2006). Left lateral decubitus positioning is an effective alternative to the prone position for the second CT acquisition (following the supine scan), particularly for immobile and elderly patients, or patients with respiratory disease (Gryspeerdt et al. 2004).

7.8 Intravenous Spasmolytics

There are two intravenous spasmolytics available for CT colonography; hyoscine butylbromide and glucagon hydrochloride. Both produce hypotonia in smooth muscle within the colonic wall (and elsewhere) and are used widely to improve distention during double contrast barium enema. However, while both agents have been shown to improve patient experience during barium enema, only hyoscine butylbromide reliably improves distention (Goei et al. 1995; Bova et al. 1993). As a result, it is widely utilized for barium enema across Europe (hyoscine butylbromide is not licensed for use in the USA).

The use of spasmolytics prior to CT colonography has been investigated widely. In one randomized study (Taylor et al. 2003a, b), intravenous administration of 20 mg hyoscine butylbromide immediately prior to gas insufflation was associated with significantly improved distention in all colonic segments proximal to the sigmoid. Moreover, for all segments combined, the colon was over six times more likely to be adequately distended compared to the situation where no spasmolytic was used. Interestingly, there was no additional benefit gained by increasing the dose administered to 40 mg. A smaller study (Bruzzi et al. 2003) also showed significantly improved transverse and descending colonic distention in patients given hyoscine butylbromide, but only in patients with diverticular disease. The authors postulated that hyoscine butylbromide might relieve diverticulosis-related spasm. More recently, data has been presented comparing hyoscine butylbromide and glucagon hydrochloride to no spasmolytic (Rogalla et al. 2004). These authors found that both spasmolytics were beneficial, an effect most marked when using hyoscine butylbromide. In contrast, two previous studies failed to demonstrate any benefit when glucagon hydrochloride was administered prior to CT colonography (Yee et al. 1999; Morrin et al. 2002).

While the authors would recommend routine use of hyoscine butylbromide prior to CT colonography, some caution needs to be exercised prior to administration. Glaucoma, cardiac ischemia, and urinary retention may all be precipitated and minor self-limiting effects of dry mouth and blurred vision are also associated.

Consequently, patients should be questioned about any relevant medical history and advised not to drive for a short time following administration.

7.9 Perforation Risk

Following its introduction, CT colonography has become an established, safe, non-invasive method of examining the whole colorectum. However, two reports of colonic perforation during CTC challenged its status as a safer alternative to colonoscopy (Coady-Fariborzian et al. 2004; Kamar et al. 2004). Both cases occurred in patients who could be considered "high risk"; one had severe colitis (Coady-Fariborzian et al. 2004) for which optical colonoscopy was considered too risky, and the second patient had recent deep endoscopic biopsy, likely corresponding to the site of perforation (Kamar et al. 2004). Nevertheless, data soon emerged in the radiological literature showing that these complications were not isolated.

Two large surveys of CTC-active centers from Israel and the UK, accompanied by two commentaries including a survey of US experts were published in the same journal in 2006 (Radiology April 2006; Sosna et al (2006); Burling et al (2006); Pickhardt (2006)) and have provided greater insight into the potential complications associated with CTC. The Israeli survey conducted by Sosna et al. (2006) identified seven cases of colonic perforation in 11,870 patients, an incidence of 0.06%. Six of the cases (84%) were in patients with symptoms of colorectal cancer whereas one patient was asymptomatic (a screening examination). All had potentially contributory causes including an obstructing inguinal hernia in three (0.03%), severe diverticulosis in two (0.02%), obstructing cancer in one (0.01%), and one patient had both inguinal hernia and diverticulosis. Notably, diverticulosis is an established risk factor for perforation at optical colonoscopy (Tran 2001). Furthermore, two patients had undergone prior "incomplete" colonoscopy and biopsy suggesting strongly that perforation may have occurred at the time of optical colonoscopy. CT is exquisitely sensitive for detecting extraluminal gas, and six of these cases were detected immediately after the examination resulting in surgery for four patients. The seventh patient, not identified until 48 h later, did not require surgery.

The author's own study (Burling et al. 2006) identified 13 serious adverse effects in 17,067 consecutive, unselected patients from the UK (0.08%), of which 9 were perforations. Four of these were asymptomatic whereas five had associated symptoms. Potentially attributable causes were found in four including inadvertent intubation of a rectal stump in a patient with a prior history of colonic resection; forceful catheterization by an inexperienced technologist resulting in perforation of a normal rectal wall; coexistent ulcerative colitis; and retrogradely obstructing (following colonic insufflation) sigmoid cancer. Notably, the perforations in the four asymptomatic patients were diagnosed while reporting the CTC between 6 h and 4 days after the procedure and were treated conservatively with no adverse effects. Therefore, the symptomatic perforation rate (perforation leading to symptoms for example abdominal pain) was 1 in 3,413 patients, i.e. 0.03%. Only one patient required laparotomy and no deaths were recorded. The authors concluded that the symptomatic perforation rate for CTC was approximately four times lower than conventional colonoscopy, i.e. 0.03 vs. 0.13%, respectively.

Pickhardt et al. undertook a US survey which included more than 20,000 patients. The overall complication rate was 1 in 5,481 patients (0.02%) with perforation in two patients (a rate of 1 in 10,962; 0.009%) and only one of these was symptomatic (1 in 21,923; 0.005%) (Pickhardt 2006). Both cases had undergone manual insufflation of room air and one had a potentially attributable cause; annular carcinoma of the sigmoid, ultimately requiring surgery for cecal perforation. It should be noted that the demographics of the US and UK data are likely to vary substantially, with US patients being younger and fitter (i.e. screening subjects) whereas the UK patients were examined to investigate symptoms of colorectal cancer and are thus older and frailer.

From these combined data, most experts agree that CTC is relatively safe and perforation can be potentially avoided in most cases. Where perforation does occur, it can be rapidly and accurately detected to optimize patient management. As the colon is frequently empty except for gas, the consequences of perforation are less than for barium enema, where barium peritonitis is a grave complication. More recently, the relative safety of CTC has been emphasized further in a large study by Kim and colleagues (Kim et al. 2007). This audit compared the perforation rate in two parallel screening populations of approximately 3,000 patients each undergoing either CTC or conventional colonoscopy. No perforations were encountered in the CTC group, whereas seven were identified in the conventional colonoscopy population (perforation rate of 1 in 452; 0.2%).

7.10 Recommended Technique

It is clear from the above discussion that the practitioner has many options available when attempting to optimize colonic distention prior to data acquisition. While some techniques have an established evidence-base, others are largely a matter of personal preference. Whatever regime is chosen, it is clear that good distention is absolutely pivotal to the ultimate success of any CTC examination. The following section will provide the reader with details of the authors' preferred methods.

Written patient information is provided and posted to the patient along with the bowel preparation approximately 2 weeks prior to examination. On the day of the examination, the radiologist or radiology resident greets the patient, checks they have understood what the procedure involves, they have no contraindications to hyoscine butylbromide or intravenous contrast, and are happy to proceed. They are asked to evacuate the rectum just prior to entering the scanner room. In an attempt to improve compliance, patients are warned routinely that they will experience abdominal bloating and mild discomfort while stressing the importance of good colonic distention for the accurate interpretation of their scan. They are also reassured that such discomfort generally improves significantly when the patient turns prone for the second scan acquisition.

The authors favor carbon dioxide for insufflation and in the past have slowly administered this via gentle compression of a filled enema bag as described in the sections above. However, we now utilize an automated insufflator delivering carbon dioxide via a narrow caliber catheter, reserving a balloon catheter for the very occasional patient with anal incontinence. The patient is asked to lie supine initially so that an intravenous catheter can be sited if intravenous contrast is to be used, and for administration of buscopan if not contraindicated. The patient is then asked to lie in the left lateral decubitus position and a lubricated rectal catheter, already attached to the insufflation device, is inserted. For all patients, the maximum pressure shutdown dial is set initially at 25 mmHg. Insufflation is commenced and after approximately 1.5 L has been introduced, the patient is turned into the supine position. Distention is then continued titrated to patient tolerance and sustained if rectal pressure remains low (i.e. below 15 mmHg), providing the patient does not complain of undue abdominal discomfort. Once either the patient is mildly uncomfortable or intraluminal pressure consistently remains above 25 mmHg (such that further insufflation is automatically prevented, which usually occurs following administration of between 2 and 4 L of gas), a first CT scout image is acquired. If distention is deemed optimal by the supervising radiologist, then the full supine scan is acquired in a single breath-hold. As long as the patient is comfortable, the authors prefer to leave the insufflator device switched on during scanning, but turn down the pressure limit to 15 mmHg so that this minimal rectal pressure is maintained. If the patient is uncomfortable, the device is paused to ensure that no further gas is insufflated until such time as the patient is happy for it to be recommenced. If distention is suboptimal despite the device recording rectal pressures exceeding 25 mmHg, the catheter is checked and repositioned because it may be that its tip is occluded against the rectal wall. If unsuccessful, we will either then reposition the patient (e.g. prone) or gently manually palpate the abdomen to encourage redistribution of gas.

Once the supine study has been acquired, the rectal catheter is left in situ and the patient asked to turn prone. A second scout is performed and if distention is then deemed suboptimal, the pressure limit is increased to 25 mmHg to encourage further insufflation. A further scout is then performed and when this demonstrates optimal insufflation, the second acquisition is obtained. The examination is then complete and the rectal catheter removed. The patient is reassured that much of the insufflated gas will be absorbed (rather than expelled), and that any abdominal cramping should ease within a few minutes.

7.11 Conclusion

There are several strategies available to the practitioner for optimizing colonic distention and if used appropriately, the time and effort invested will be rewarded by easier and more accurate interpretation for the radiologist. The authors recommend that ongoing quality assurance measures are adopted by all departments performing CT colonography to identify and minimize failure rates due to inadequate distention. Finally, safety concerns about CT colonography emphasize the need for appropriate training and care when undertaking rectal catheterization and colonic insufflation.

References

Barish MA, Soto JA, Ferrucci JT (2005) Consensus on current clinical practice of virtual colonoscopy. AJR 184:786–792

Blakeborough A, Sheridan MB, Chapman AH (1997) Retention balloon catheters and barium enemas: attitudes, current practice and relative safety in the UK. Clin Radiol 52: 62–64

Bova JG, Jurdi RA, Bennett WF (1993) Antispasmodic drugs to reduce discomfort and colonic spasm during barium enemas: comparison of oral hyoscyamine, i.v. glucagon and no drug. AJR 161:965–968

Bruzzi JF, Moss AC, Brennan DD et al (2003) Efficacy of IV Buscopan as a muscle relaxant in CT colonography. Eur Radiol 13:2264–2270

Burling D, Halligan S, Slater A, et al Potentially serious adverse events at CT colonography in symptomatic patients: national survey of the United Kingdom. Radiology 2006; 239: 464–471

Burling D, Taylor SA, Halligan S et al (2006) Automated insufflation of carbon dioxide for MDCT colonography: distension and patient experience compared with manual insufflation. AJR 186:96–103

Chen SC, Lu D, Hecht JR et al (1999) CT colonography: value of scanning in both the supine and prone positions. AJR 172:595–599

Church J, Delaney C (2003) Randomized controlled trial of carbon dioxide insufflation during colonoscopy. Dis Colon Rectum 46:322–326

Coady-Fariborzian L, Angel LP, Procaccino JA (2004) Perforated colon secondary to virtual colonoscopy: report of a case. Dis Colon Rectum 47:1247–1249

Fenlon HM (2002) CT colonography: pitfalls and interpretation. Abdom Imaging 27:284–291

Fletcher JG, Johnson CD, Maccarty RL et al (1999) CT colonography: potential pitfalls and problem solving techniques. AJR 172:1271–1278

Fletcher JG, Johnson CD, Welch TJ et al (2000) Optimization of CT colonography technique: prospective trial in 180 patients. Radiology 216:704–711

Gluecker T, Johnson D, Harmsen W et al (2003) Colorectal cancer screening with CT colonography, colonoscopy, and double contrast barium enema examination: prospective assessment of patient perceptions and preferences. Radiology 227:378–384

Goei R, Nix M, Kessels AH et al (1995) Use of antispasmodic drugs in double contrast barium enema examination: glucagon or buscopan? Clin Radiol 50:553–557

Grant DS, Bartram CI, Heron CW (1986) A preliminary study of the possible benefits of using carbon dioxide insufflation during double contrast barium enema. Br J Radiol 59(698):190–191

Gryspeerdt SS, Herman MJ, Baekelandt MA (2004) Supine/left decubitus scanning: a valuable alternative to supine/prone scanning in CT colonography. Eur Radiol 14:768–777

Hara AK, Johnson CD, MacCarty RL et al (2001) CT colonography: single versus multi-detector row imaging. Radiology 219:461–465

Iafrate F, Laghi A, Paolantonio P et al (2004) Colonic distension using mechanical CO_2 insufflator versus manual air distension. In: Radiological Society of North America scientific assembly and annual meeting program, Oak Brook, III: Radiological Society of North America, p 432

Kamar M, Portnoy O, Bar-Dayan A et al (2004) Actual colonic perforation in virtual colonoscopy: report of a case. Dis Colon Rectum 47:1242–1244

Kim DH, Pickhardt PJ, Taylor AJ et al (2007) CT colonography versus colonoscopy for the detection of advanced neoplasia. N Engl J Med 357:1403–12

Macari M, Megibow AJ (2001) Pitfalls of using 3D CT colonography with 2D imaging correlation. AJR 176:137–143

Macari M (2004) Techniques for CT colonography. In: Fifth international symposium virtual colonoscopy course handbook, Boston, pp 45–48

Morrin M, Farrell R, Keogan M et al (2002) CT colonography: colonic distension improved by dual positioning but not intravenous glucagons. Eur Radiol 12:525–530

Paulson EK, Foster WL, Thonpson WM et al (2004) Causes of errors in CT colonography (CTC) and air contrast barium enema (ACBE) in detection of colonic lesions 1 cm or larger (abstract). In: Radiological Society of North America scientific assembly and annual meeting program, Oak Brook, III: Radiological Society of North America, p 618

Pickhardt PJ, Choi JR, Hwang I et al (2003) Computed tomographic virtual colonoscopy to screen for colorectal neoplasia in asymptomatic adults. NEJM 349:2191–200

Pickhardt PJ (2004) Differential diagnosis of polypoid lesions seen at CT colonography (virtual colonoscopy). Radiographics 24:1535–1556

Pickhardt PJ. Incidence of colonic perforation at CT colonography: review of existing data and implication for screening of asymptomatic adults. Radiology 2006; 239: 313–316

Ristvedt S, McFarland E, Weinstock L et al (2003) Patient preferences for CT colonography, conventional colonoscopy, and bowel preparation. Am J Gastroenterol 98:578–585

Rockey DC, Paulson EK, Niedzwiecki D et al (2005) Analysis of air contrast barium enema, computed tomographic colonography, and colonoscopy: prospective comparison. Lancet 365:305–311

Rogalla P, Bauknecht HC, Hein PA et al (2004). Pressure-controlled colonic insufflation for CT colonography. In: Radiological Society of North America scientific assembly and annual meeting program (abstract), Oak Brook, III: Radiological Society of North America, p 432

Rubesin S, Levine MS, Laufer I et al (2000) Double-contrast barium enema examination technique. Radiology 215: 642–650

Sosna J, Blachar A, Amitai M, et al Colonic perforation at CT colonography: assessment of risk in a multicenter large cohort. Radiology 2006; 239: 457–463

Svensson MH, Svensson E, Lasson A et al (2002) Patient acceptance of CT colonography and conventional colonoscopy: prospective comparative study in patients with or suspected of having colorectal disease. Radiology 222: 337–345

Taylor SA, Halligan S, Goh V et al (2003a) Optimizing colonic distension for multi -detector row CT colonography: effect of hyoscine hydrobromide and rectal balloon catheter. Radiology 229:99–108

Taylor SA, Halligan S, Saunders BP et al (2003b) Acceptance by patients of multidetector CT colonography compared with barium enema examinations, flexible sigmoidoscopy, and colonoscopy. AJR 181:913–921

Tran DQ, Rosen L, Kim R, Riether RD, Stasik JJ, Khubchandani IT. Actual colonoscopy: what are the risks of prerforation? Am Surg. 2001; 67(9):845–7; discussion 847–8
Yee J, Hung RK, Akerkar GA et al (1999) The usefulness of glucagon hydrochloride for colonic distension in CT colonography. AJR 173:169–172
Yee J, Galdino G, Kumar N et al (2002) Comparison of colonic distention using electronic CO_2 insufflation and manual atmospheric insufflation on CT colonography (abstract). In: RSNA Scientific Assembly and Annual Meeting program, Oak Brook
Yee J, Kumar N, Hung R et al (2003) Comparison of supine and prone scanning separately and in combination at CT colonography. Radiology 226:653–661

Right Parameters

Andrea Laghi

CONTENTS

Andrea Laghi, MD
Department of Radiological Sciences, Sapienza – Università di Roma, Polo Pontino, ICOT Hospital, Latina, Italy

8.1 Introduction

CT colonography (CTC) is a diagnostic examination of the colon, based on a volumetric acquisition of the entire abdomen and pelvis within a single breath-hold (Vining et al. 1994). The use of a multidetector-row scanner (MDCT) is mandatory, with 4 rows to be considered as the minimum requirement; data acquisition with single-row spiral CT (SSCT) equipments is no longer recommended (Taylor et al. 2007).

Benefits of MDCT technology are volume coverage, scanning time, and longitudinal spatial resolution (Saini 2004; Laghi et al. 2001). The acquisition of a volume including the entire abdomen and pelvis can be obtained in around 20 s with a 16-row MDCT and in less than 10 s with a 64-row scanner. The use of submillimeter collimation (possible with 16-row MDCT and above) allows the acquisition of isotropic voxels with a higher quality of tri-dimensional reconstructions (Cody and Mahesh 2007). However, benefits in terms of image quality are counterbalanced by radiation, which still remains a major issue, making the optimization of dedicated study protocols, with regard to clinical indication, necessary (Luz et al. 2007; Hamberg et al. 2003). Scanning protocols are in continuous evolution because of the evolving technology (256 and 320 rows scanners have recently entered the market).

Despite initial confusion due to different study techniques, a general consensus about fundamental parameters has been reached, on behalf of the European Society of Gastrointestinal and Abdominal Radiology (ESGAR) (Taylor et al. 2007). Scanning parameters to be considered when optimizing a CTC study are as follows: collimation, image reconstruction thickness, pitch, kVp, and mAs. Pitch, kVp, and mAs will be discussed together with the issue of radiation exposure.

8.2 Scanning Parameters: Collimation and Image Reconstruction Thickness

Collimation is the parameter that has been mostly affected by the introduction of MDCT technology and it represents the major benefit over SSCT. The use of thin collimations for CTC is mandatory, since the size of detectable lesions depends fundamentally on this parameter: it is well known that a lesion smaller than the collimation cannot be detected because of partial volume artifacts (Rogalla and Meiri 2001). Thus, the problem is not only to choose the adequate collimation, but also to define the size of the "target" lesion. In the case the target is a polyp 5 mm or larger, 3 mm collimation is sufficient; but in the case the target lesion is smaller than 5 mm, a thinner collimation might be necessary.

With the advent of MDCT technology, the discussion about the collimation started and ended with 4-row MDCT scanners, where a compromise between a thin collimation (1 mm) with a relatively long acquisition time (around 40–50 s) and thus potentially incompatible with the breath-hold of an elderly or uncooperative patient, and a fast examination, around 20 s, but with a collimation of 2.5 mm was still necessary (Mc Collough 2002; Power and Pryor 2002). Some *in vitro* studies (Laghi et al. 2003; Wessling et al. 2003) comparing different protocols, with collimations ranging between 1 and 3 mm have shown no statistically significant differences in the identification of polyps ≥10 mm, but a clear advantage of thin collimation for the detection of diminutive lesions (≤5 mm). In particular, in the case of lesions ranging in size between 3 and 5 mm, increase in slice thickness from 1 to 5 mm caused a drop in sensitivity from 96 to 74% (Fig. 8.1) (Rogalla and Meiri 2001). Moreover, thin collimation is also beneficial for specificity, making, for example, the differentiation between polyps and fecal residues easier, thanks to the identification of tiny air bubbles within the stool residue (Taylor et al. 2003). Furthermore, in the era of computer-aided detection (CAD) systems, it has been recently demonstrated that the use of thinner slice thickness and reconstruction index can maximize per-polyp detection rate of CAD (Kim et al. 2008).

Further developments of MDCT technology have made this discussion obsolete, since with 16-row MDCT scanners and above, it is possible to use routinely a submillimeter collimation (0.5, 0.625, and 0.75 mm, depending on different vendors) (Rottgen et al. 2003; Luz et al. 2004; Tolan et al. 2007). With the present scanners the problem is exactly the opposite: it means to try to use thicker collimation (adding contiguous detectors; i.e., 0.625 + 0.625 mm = 1.25 mm) to reduce the number of acquired images per data set.

In any case, independently of collimation, slice thickness should be set at 1 mm, making this value an accurate identification of small polyps possible (Fig. 8.2) (see Table 8.1). The use of 1 mm thickness allows to limit the number of images per data set at 400–500 per scan.

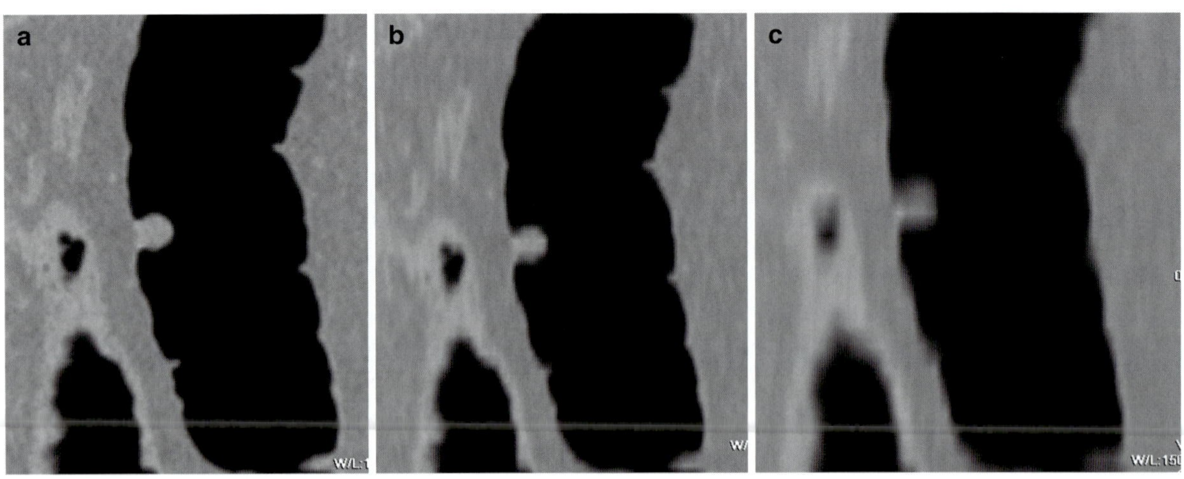

Fig. 8.1. Multiplanar sagittal reconstruction of a sessile polyp studied at 1 mm (**a**), 2.5 mm (**b**), and 5 mm (**c**). Please note the progressive degradation of image quality as the slice thickness increases

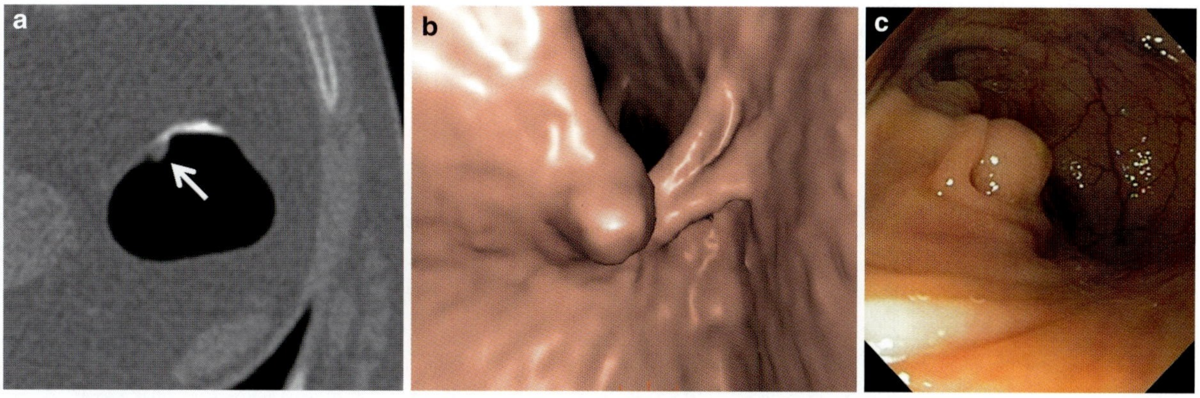

Fig. 8.2. Adenomatous polyp of the anterior wall of the descending colon, as shown on (**a**) axial image (*arrow*) and (**b**) virtual endoscopic view. Optical colonoscopy of the same lesion, showing a perfect correlation with virtual endoscopy (**c**)

Table 8.1. Main scanning parameters

		4 Rows	> 4 Rows	64	Notes
kVp			120		140 in obese subjects
mAs	Prone Supine Supine with i.v. contrast agent		≤50 ≤100 100–200		
Collimation (mm)		≤3	1–1.5	0.5–1.2	
Reconstruction thickness (mm)		1	1	0.8–1	
Pitch		1–1.5	1–1.5	1–1.5	

8.3 The Issue of Dose Exposure

The major criticism to CTC, in particular if to be used for screening, is represented by the exposure of patients to a potentially high radiation. Reasons are different: (1) routine use of double scanning, prone and supine, mandatory for technical reasons, but doubling the dose to the patient (Chen et al. 1999); (2) geometric efficiency of the detectors, definitely worse on 4- and 8-rows scanners compared with new 16-rows and above (Giacomuzzi et al. 2001); (3) use of thin collimation (now even submillimetric, 0.5/0.6 mm), offering advantages in terms of spatial resolution, but at the expenses of an increase in mA value and consequently effective dose exposure (Luz et al. 2007).

Since the beginning of CTC, dose exposure has been a debated issue, with the results that many researchers have developed low-dose scanning techniques also on SSCT equipments (Hara et al. 1997).

CTC offers a great opportunity to optimize low-dose protocols, because of the high intrinsic contrast of the structures under evaluation: colonic wall, with a soft tissue density (30–50 HU) and endoluminal air (−500 HU and lower). This is similar to lung scan where low mA techniques have been implemented since many years. The reduction of dose exposure has an obvious consequence in the increase in image noise, but, thanks to the high intrinsic contrast, without losing accuracy in lesion identification (Fig. 8.3) (van Gelder et al. 2002; Iannaccone et al. 2003; Iannaccone et al. 2005; Cohnen et al. 2004). However, if this is true for colonic lesions, the same concept

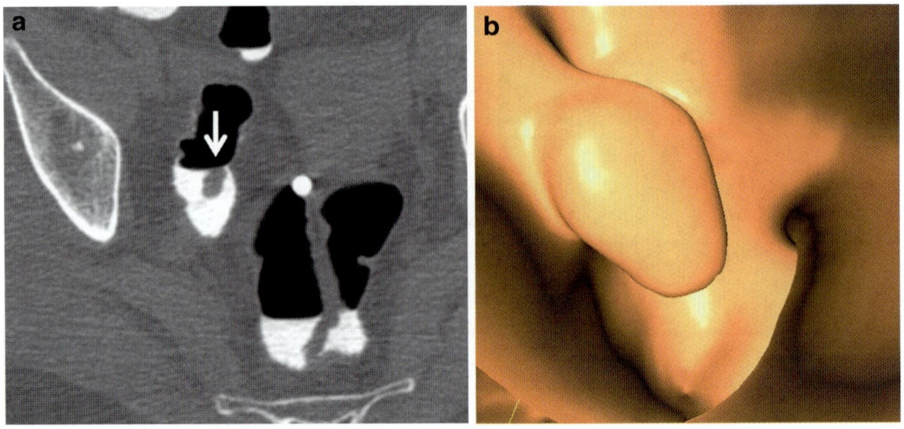

Fig. 8.3. Low-dose (100 mAs) axial scan (**a**) of a polyp (*arrow*) of the sigmoid colon, submerged by tagging agent. Virtual endoscopic view (**b**) of the same polyp following electronic cleansing

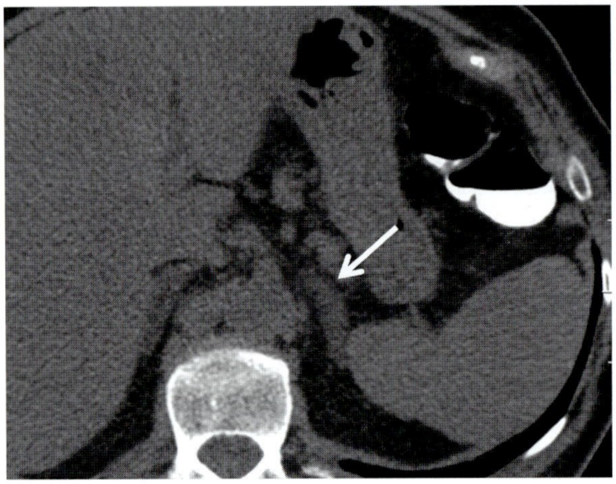

Fig. 8.4. Eighty mAs image, abdominal window. Despite the low-dose protocol, a left adrenal adenoma (*arrow*) is perfectly depicted

cannot be applied to extra-colonic findings, and particularly to parenchymatous organs (liver, spleen, pancreas, kidneys). In fact, a low-dose scanning protocol does not allow optimal characterization of hepatic or renal lesions; even simple characterization of cysts may be affected by the image noise, although major findings can still be detected (Fig. 8.4) (Kalra et al. 2002). Thus, it is clear that whenever intravenous injection of contrast medium is required, a full dose protocol similar to routine CT of the abdomen and pelvis, should be used (see Table 8.1).

8.3.1
Optimization of Low-Dose Protocol

The optimization of low-dose scanning protocol needs the modification of scanning parameters and also the use of automatic dose modulation systems.

Main technical parameters related to radiation exposure are: milliampere/s (mAs), kilovolt peak (kVp), and pitch.

8.3.1.1
mAs and kVp

The major factor affecting a low-dose scanning protocol is mAs value, having an inverse linear correlation with noise: the lower the mAs value, the lower the dose and the higher the intrinsic noise within the image. The interest of researchers in the past few years was to understand the lower limit of mAs, without affecting the sensitivity of CTC for the detection of small polyps. The conclusions of the studies were as follows: (1) decrease of mAs is associated with increase of image noise and progressive consequent degradation of image quality, also in three-dimensional reconstructions (van Gelder et al. 2002); (2) studies conducted both *in vivo* and *in vitro* have shown that mAs can be lowered to a value of 10 or even less with no decrease in sensitivity for polyps >5 mm (Fig. 8.5) (Hara et al. 1997; Iannaccone et al. 2003; Iannaccone et al. 2005; Cohnen et al. 2004; Florie et al. 2007; van Gelder et al. 2004); (3) ultra low-dose protocols (<50 mAs) do not allow an adequate evaluation of extra-colonic findings and suffer of severe limitations in obese patients (Fig. 8.6) (Huda et al. 2000).

Considering dose exposure, low-dose protocols using 30–80 mAs are associated with a radiation exposure, including both prone and supine scans, of about 2.5 mSv in men and about 2.9 mSv in women, when using 30 mAs, and about 5.7 mSv in men and about 6.4 mSv in woman, when using 80 mAs (Luz et al. 2007). For ultra low-dose protocols, at 10 mAs, radiation exposure is about 1.8 mSv in men and about 2.4 mSv in women (Iannaccone et al. 2003, 2005; Cohnen et al.

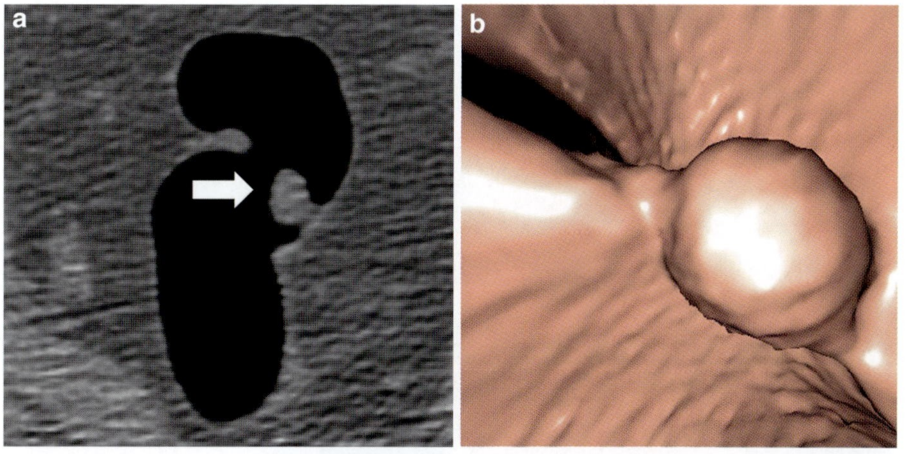

Fig. 8.5. Ultra low-dose (10 mAs) scan of a sessile polyp of the sigmoid colon. Despite the ultra low-dose and the high intrinsic noise degrading the overall image quality (see the streak artifacts within the fat tissue and the relative inhomogeneity of the soft tissue density of the polyp), optimal visualization of the polyp (*arrow*) is achieved on both axial image (**a**) and endoluminal view (**b**)

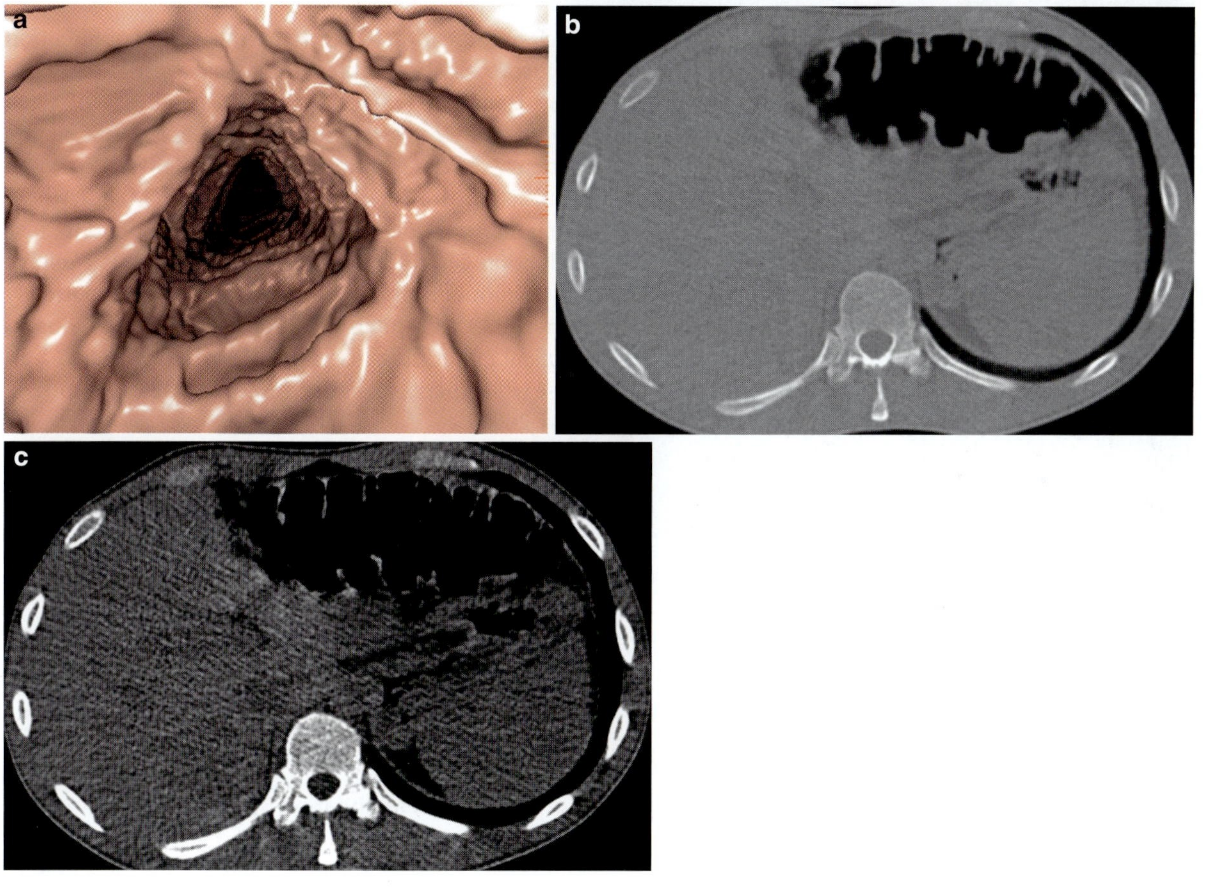

Fig. 8.6. Ultra low-dose (10 mAs) scan of familiar polyposis. Endoluminal view (**a**) showing multiple tiny sessile polyps in the transverse colon. On the axial image visualized with colon window (**b**), the colonic lumen is clearly analyzable. On the abdominal window (**c**), the extreme noise of an ultra low-dose scan is evident, preventing any evaluation about extra-colonic organs and in particular liver and spleen

2004). These values are substantially lower compared with those reported in previous publications, not only for SSCT and MDCT, but also in comparison with barium enema (5–7 mSv) (Kemerink et al. 2001).

Another technical parameter strictly related to dose exposure is kiloVolt peak (kVp). Compared with mAs, having a direct linear inverse relation with dose exposure, kVp has an exponential dependence: it means

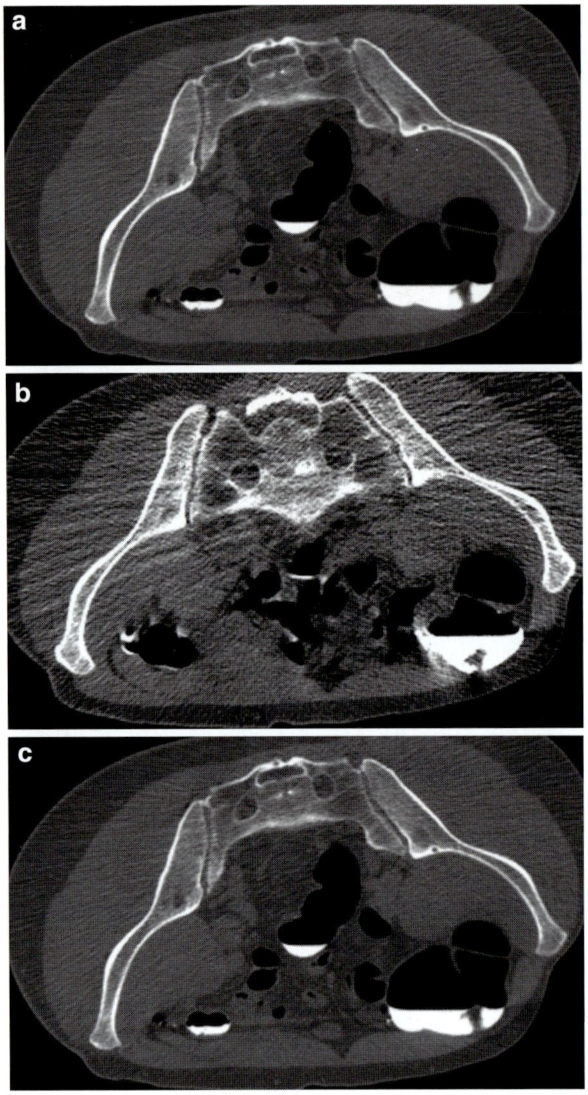

Fig. 8.7. Modifications of image quality induced by the selection of different kVp values, at the same mAs (100 mAs). Using the standard value (120 kVp) (**a**) image quality is excellent, considering the reduced mAs. Using 80 kVp (**b**), noise is severely increased, as observed by beam hardening artifacts, but intrinsic contrast is increased, with fecal residues tagged with iodine being more hyperdense. At 140 kVp (**c**), noise is slightly reduced, together with intrinsic contrast within the image

that small variations may profoundly affect radiation exposure and inversely noise. However, changes in kVp result in a modification of the energy of photon beam as well: the higher the kVp the more penetrating the photons, with the result of higher energy delivered to detectors. Such modifications influence image noise, contrast resolution, and dose delivered to the patient, but also density values of different structures. In fact, the more penetrating the photon beam (it means the higher the kVp value), the lower is the density of the structures, with a consequent reduction in contrast resolution. On the contrary, the lower the kVp, the higher is the contrast, especially for high-density structures (i.e., barium, iodine) (Huda et al. 2000) (Fig. 8.7). Because of the profound influence on absorbed radiations as well as the quality of radiation which modifies intrinsic contrast in the image, it is better to keep kVp at a fixed value, that is 120 in normal-size individuals and 140 in obese patients (see Table 8.1) (Taylor et al. 2007).

8.3.1.2
Pitch

Pitch modification to minimize the impact of radiation exposure has been extensively used with SSCT scanning protocols (Hara et al. 2001): increase of pitch would reduce proportionally dose exposure, at the expenses of degradation of image quality (Whiting et al. 2000). More complex is the issue on MDCT, where pitch increase does not necessarily correspond to dose reduction. This is due to some automatic tools available on certain equipments that are able to automatically adapt mAs with pitch variation. In such cases, a paradoxical effect may occur with a possible increase in dose when increasing pitch value (Theocharopoulos et al. 2006).

Anyway, as a general guideline, it is advisable to avoid using pitch value <1, not justified by any necessary increase in image quality (as in cardiac CT, for example) and try to select values between 1 and 1.5 (Luz et al. 2007; Laghi et al. 2003; Wessling et al. 2003; Rottgen et al. 2003; Luz et al. 2004; Tolan et al. 2007). The exact pitch value depends on the available equipment.

8.3.1.3
Automatic Dose Modulation Systems

Automatic dose modulation systems are tools able to modify the tube current (mA) during the scan as a function of the anatomic region under evaluation, trying to keep the dose as lower as possible and the image quality as higher as possible (McCollough et al. 2006). They are not a new technology, since they were initially implemented on SSCT scanners (Kalender et al. 1999), but recently they have been upgraded, being able to simultaneously combine angular and longitudinal (*x-*, *y-*, and *z-axis*) tube current modulation: it means a variation of the tube current not only during gantry rotation, but also along the *z-axis* of the patient (i.e., from the anteroposterior direction to the lateral direction, and from the shoulders to the abdomen) (Mastora et al. 2001).

Automatic dose modulation systems used with MDCT, however, should be considered as a secondary tool of radiation dose reduction because they save between 19 and 27% of the radiation dose on the patient, regardless of initial mAs preset (Tack et al. 2003). However, initial decreases of mAs presets by the physician should be considered the primary tool for radiation dose reduction. And in fact in the single study available on this topic in CTC, it was possible to reduce the radiation dose to 2.38 mSv by using an automated dose modulation technique working on the three axes with an X-ray beam collimation of 16×0.75 mm at a pitch factor of 1, 120 kV, and the simultaneous use of 40 mAs (Graser et al. 2006).

8.3.2 Other Considerations

The matter of radiation exposure related to the increased number of CT examinations worldwide, in particular with the advent of MDCT technology, is deeply experienced by public opinion, media, as well as radiologists. Alarming conclusions about the potential number of radiation-induced cancers derive from published papers based on physics theories whose data are extrapolated using a mathematical model from those obtained at the time of atomic explosions during the World War II (Brenner and Hall 2007). And this is because if the carcinogenic effect of high and intermediate ionizing radiation (>100 mSv) are well known (Preston et al. 2003), with regard to weak doses, as those used in diagnostic radiology the effects, if any, are so weak that it would be very difficult if not impossible to identify them during epidemiological studies (Brenner et al. 2003). This would require an international study involving tens of thousands of people, supposing that it would be possible to monitor such a population throughout their entire lives. In fact, for example, if a sample size of 1,000 persons were needed to quantify the effect of a 1.0-Sv dose, 100,000 persons would be needed to quantify the effect of a 100-mSv dose and 10 million persons for a 10-mSv dose (Verdun et al. 2008). Today, it is not possible to come to a conclusion as the existence, or not, of a dose threshold below which there would be no effect related to the exposure to ionizing radiation. For the purpose of managing risks and protection, there is an international consensus to consider, out of prudence, that any exposure to ionizing radiation at any level can possibly result in an effect, even weak, across a population group. For exposures to weak doses, where a true risk has been neither proven nor disproven, the probability of developing stochastic effects is, by agreement, considered as being proportional with the dose received. The quantification of the relation between the dose and the effect is, in this context, established by extrapolating from what has been observed with higher doses. This is the so-called *linear-non-threshold (LNT)* model (NCRP 2001). However, other models do exist considering the results of LNT overestimated (*Adaptive response* model) or underestimated (*Bystander Effect Sensitive Subpopulation* model) and other more hypothesizing the existence of a threshold value (between 3 and 10 mSv) below which the dose does not increase the probability of a cancer (Huang et al. 2007).

Besides the dispute on physics theories, since CTC is now considered as a possible screening option (Levin et al. 2008), dose exposure should be minimized so that an appropriate benefit–risk ratio is maintained (Nicholson et al. 2005; Brenner and Georgsson 2005). Data from a European survey conducted in 2002 (van Gelder et al. 2002) among centers using 4-row MDCTs, median effective dose per CTC examination was about 8.8 mSv. Using the LNT model, it turns into a potential risk of inducing cancer in 50-year-old individuals of around 0.02%. In a different study (Brenner and Georgsson 2005), considering as effective mean dose a value between 7.6 and 13.2 mSv, variable as a function of the equipment being the same the scanning parameters, the estimated radiation-associated absolute lifetime risk for colon cancer induction was 0.044% for a CTC scan at age 50 and 0.022% for a scan at age 70. This risk can be further reduced by a factor of 5 (and perhaps as much as a factor of 10) if specific low-dose protocols are implemented. And in a very recent survey, it was shown that currently, in 34 institutions around the world, the median effective dose of CTC for screening protocols (5.6 mSv) is 38% lower than that for protocols in daily practice (9.1 mSv) (Liedenbaum et al. 2008).

The first consideration, based on these data, is that even if the cancer risk associated with the radiation exposure from CTC is not zero, it is much smaller than the CRC-related risk of 6% and the related mortality of 3% (Brenner and Georgsson 2005).

The second consideration deals with the amount of radiation any single individual is exposed during

Table 8.2. Reference average values of radiation exposure

	mSv
Background dose caused by natural radiation exposure	2.4 (Liedenbaum et al. 2008)
CTC (≤10 mAs)	1.4–1.8♂; 2.0–2.4♀ (van Gelder et al. 2002; Iannaccone et al. 2003; Cohnen et al. 2004)
CTC (30 mAs)	2.5♂; 2.9♀ (Luz et al. 2007; Hara et al. 1997; van Gelder et al. 2002; Florie et al. 2007)
CTC (80 mAs)	5.7♂; 6.4♀ (Luz et al. 2007; van Gelder et al. 2002; Florie et al. 2007)
Barium enema	5–7 (Kemerink et al. 2001)
Round-trip flight, Paris–Tokio	0.18 (Thorne 2003)
Annual exposure airline cabin crew	2–5 (Bottollier-Depois et al. 2007)
Lifelong exposure airline pilots	~80 (Bottollier-Depois et al. 2007)

his life (Table 8.2). In fact, it consists of a natural background radiation of around 2.4 mSv/year (Thorne 2003) plus the effect of other activities, for example airplane flights. As an example, an intercontinental roundtrip flight between Paris and Tokio corresponds to around 0.18 mSv (Bottollier-Depois et al. 2007). And the impact of flights is particularly evident in a category of workers, i.e., airline crews, whose annual radiation exposure, apart from the background, is between 2 and 5 mSv/year with a lifelong exposure of around 80 mSv. Because of the radiation exposure, several epidemiological studies have been conducted on this population group showing that "*among airline cabin crew in Europe, there was no increase in mortality that could be attributed to cosmic radiation or other occupational exposures to any substantial extent*" (Zeeb et al. 2003). These results are an indirect demonstration of the low impact of radiation exposure of a CTC examination on the possible induction of a cancer.

In conclusion, CTC should be performed using MDCT scanners (the use of SSCT is no longer recommended) optimizing the choice of scanning parameters. Thin collimation and reconstruction index are necessary to obtain high accuracy for lesion detection. A careful use of mAs is mandatory to minimize the impact of radiation exposure, especially important in the case of screening examinations: in fact, despite the fact that the risk associated with a radiologic examination is rather low compared with the natural risk, it should be weighed against the benefits for patients. It means that justification and optimization of a procedure are absolutely essential. In symptomatic patients, with the need of injection of contrast medium, a standard dose protocol for abdominal MDCT should be implemented in the supine scan.

References

Vining DJ, Gelfand DW, Bechtold RE et al (1994) Technical feasibility of colon imaging with helical CT and virtual reality. Am J Roentgenol 62(Suppl):104

Taylor SA, Laghi A, Lefere P, Halligan S, Stoker J (2007) European Society of Gastrointestinal and Abdominal Radiology (ESGAR): consensus statement on CT colonography. Eur Radiol 17:575–579

Saini S (2004) Multi-detector row CT: principles and practice for abdominal applications. Radiology 233:323–327

Laghi A, Iannaccone R, Panebianco V et al (2001) Multislice CT colonography: technical developments. Semin Ultrasound CT MR 22:425–431

Cody DD, Mahesh M (2007) Technologic advances in multidetector CT with a focus on cardiac imaging. Radiographics 27:1829–1837

Luz O, Buchgeister M, Klabunde M et al (2007) Evaluation of dose exposure in 64-slice CT colonography. Eur Radiol 17:2616–2621

Hamberg LM, Rhea JT, Hunter GJ et al (2003) Multi-detector row CT: radiation dose characteristics. Radiology 226: 762–772

Rogalla P, Meiri N (2001) CT colonography: data acquisition and patient preparation techniques. Semin Ultrasound CT MR 22:405–412

Mc Collough CH (2002) Optimization of multidetector array CT acquisition parameters for CT colonography. Abdom Imaging 27:253–259

Power NP, Pryor AM (2002) Optimization of scanning parameters for CT colonography. Br J Radiol 75:401–408

Laghi A, Iannaccone R, Mangiapane F et al (2003) Experimental colonic phantom for the evaluation of the optimal scanning technique for CT colonography using a multidetector spiral CT equipment. Eur Radiol 13:459–466

Wessling J, Fischbach R, Meier N et al (2003) CT colonography: protocol optimization with multi detector row CT – study in an anthropomorphic colon phantom. Radiology 228: 753–759

Taylor SA, Halligan S, Bartram I et al (2003) Multi-detector row CT colonography: effect of collimation, pitch, and orientation on polyp detection in a human colectomy specimen. Radiology 229:109–118

Kim SH, Lee JM, Shin CI et al (2008) Effects of spatial resolution and tube current on computer-aided detection of polyps on CT colonographic images: phantom study. Radiology 248:492–503
Rottgen R, Schroder RJ, Lorenz M et al (2003) CT-colonography with the 16-slice CT for the diagnostic evaluation of colorectal neoplasms and inflammatory colon diseases. Rofo 175:1384–1391
Luz O, Schaefer J, Heuschmid M et al (2004) Evaluation of different 16-row CT colonography protocols using a procine model. Rofo 176:1493–1500
Tolan DJ, Armstrong EM, Burling D et al (2007) Optimization of CT colonography technique: a practical guide. Clin Radiol 62:819–827
Chen SC, Lu DSK, Hecht JR et al (1999) CT colonography: value of scanning in both the supine and prone positions. Am J Roentgenol 172:595–599
Giacomuzzi SM, Torbica P, Rieger M et al (2001) Radiation exposure in single slice and multi-slice spiral CT (a phantom study). Rofo 173:643–649
Hara AK, Johnson CD, Reed JE et al (1997) Reducing data size and radiation dose for CT colonography. Am J Roentgenol 168:1181–1184
Van Gelder RE, Venema HW, Serlie IW et al (2002) CT colonography at different radiation dose levels: feasibility of dose reduction. Radiology 224:25–33
Iannaccone R, Laghi A, Catalano C et al (2003) Performance of lower dose multi-detector row helical CT colonography compared with conventional colonoscopy in the detection of colorectal lesions. Radiology 229:775–781
Iannaccone R, Catalano C, Mangiapane F et al (2005) Colorectal polyps: detection with low-dose multi-detector row helical CT colonography versus two sequential colonoscopies. Radiology 237:927–937
Cohnen M, Vogt C, Beck A et al (2004) Feasibility of MDCT Colonography in ultra-low-dose technique in the detection of colorectal lesions: comparison with high-resolution video colonoscopy. Am J Roentgenol 183:1355–1359
Kalra MK, Prasad S, Saini S et al (2002) Clinical comparison of standard-dose and 50% reduced-dose adominal CT: effect on image quality. Am J Roentgenol 179:1101–1106
Florie J, van Gelder RE, Schutter MP et al (2007) Feasibility study of computed tomography colonography using limited bowel preparation at normal and low-dose levels study. Eur Radiol 17:3112–3122
van Gelder RE, Venema HW, Florie J et al (2004) CT colonography: feasibility of substantial dose reduction–comparison of medium to very low doses in identical patients. Radiology 232:611–620
Huda W, Scalzetti EM, Galina L et al (2000) Technique factors and image quality as functions of patient weight at abdominal CT. Radiology 217:430–435
Kemerink GJ, Bortslap AC, Frantzen MJ et al (2001) Patients and occupational dosimetry in double contrast barium enema examinations. Br J Radiol 74:420–428
Hara AK, Johnson CD, MacCarty RL et al (2001) CT colonography: single- versus multi-detector row imaging. Radiology 219:461–465
Whiting BR, Mc Farland EG, Brink JA et al (2000) Influence of image acquisition parameters on CT artefacts and polyp depiction in spiral CT colonography: in vitro evaluation. Radiology 217:165–172
Theocharopoulos N, Perisinakis K, Damilakis J et al (2006) Dosimetric characteristics of a 16-slice computed tomography scanner. Eur Radiol 16:2575–2585
McCollough CH, Bruesewitz MR, Kofler JM (2006) CT dose reduction and dose management tools: overview of available options. Radiographics 26:503–512
Kalender WA, Wolf H, Suess C et al (1999) Dose reduction in CT by on-line tube current control: principles and validation on phantoms and cadavers. Eur Radiol 9:323–328
Mastora I, Remy-Jardin M, Suess C et al (2001) Dose reduction in spiral CT angiography of thoracic outlet syndrome by anatomically adapted tube current modulation. Eur Radiol 11:590–596
Tack D, De Maertelaer V, Gevenois PA (2003) Dose reduction in multidetector CT using attenuation-based online tube current modulation. Am J Roentgenol 181:331–334
Graser A, Wintersperger BJ, Suess C et al (2006) Dose reduction and image quality in MDCT colonography using tube current modulation. Am J Roentgenol 187:695–701
Brenner DJ, Hall EJ (2007) Computed tomography – an increasing source of radiation exposure. N Engl J Med 357:2277–2284
Preston DL, Shimizu Y, Pierce DA et al (2003) Studies of mortality of atomic bomb survivors. Report 13: solid cancer and noncancer disease mortality: 1950–1997. Radiat Res 160:381–407
Brenner DJ, Doll R, Goodhead DT et al (2003) Cancer risks attributable to low doses of ionizing radiation: assessing what we really know. Proc Natl Acad Sci U S A 100: 13761–13766
Verdun FR, Bochud F, Gudinchet F et al (2008) Radiation risk: what you should know to tell your patient. Radiographics 28:1807–1816
NCRP (2001) Evaluation of the linear-nonthreshold dose-response model for ionizing radiation, report no.136. National Council on Radiation Protection and Measurements, Bethesda, MD
Huang L, Kim PM, Nickoloff JA et al (2007) Targeted and nontargeted effects of low-dose ionizing radiation on delayed genomic instability in human cells. Cancer Res 67: 1099–1104
Levin B, Lieberman DA, McFarland B et al (2008) Screening and surveillance for the early detection of colorectal cancer and adenomatous polyps, 2008: a joint guideline from the American Cancer Society, the US Multi-Society Task Force on Colorectal Cancer, and the American College of Radiology. CA Cancer J Clin 58:130–160
Nicholson FB, Barro JL, Bartram CI et al (2005) The role of CT colonography in colorectal cancer screening. Am J Gastroenterol 100:2315–2323
Brenner DJ, Georgsson MA (2005) Mass screening with CT colonography: should the radiation exposure be of concern? Gastroenterology 129:328–337
Liedenbaum MH, Venema HW, Stoker J (2008) Radiation dose in CT colonography-trends in time and differences between daily practice and screening protocols. Eur Radiol 18:2222–2230
Thorne MC (2003) Background radiation: natural and man-made. J Radiol Prot 23:29–42
Bottollier-Depois JF, Blanchard P, Clairand I et al (2007) An operational approach for aircraft crew dosimetry: the Sievert system. Radiat Prot Dosimetry 125:421–424
Zeeb H, Blettner M, Langner I et al (2003) Mortality from cancer and other causes among airline cabin attendants in Europe: a collaborative cohort study in eight countries. Am J Epidemiol 158:35–46

How to Interpret CTC Data: Evaluation of the Different Lesion Morphologies

Beth G. McFarland

CONTENTS

Beth G. McFarland
Center for Diagnostic Imaging, Chesterfield, MO 63017, USA

9.1 Introduction

A climatic new era of data validation has been reached for CTC screening in both asymptomatic cohorts and patients at increased risk (Johnson et al. 2008; Graser et al. 2009; Regge 2009; Kim et al. 2007; Pickhardt et al. 2003). In 2008 the American Cancer Society released a joint guideline with the US Multisociety colorectal task force and the American College of Radiology recommending CTC, along with other proven modalities, for colorectal screening (Levin et al. 2008). Thus, the pathway to broader community implementation of CTC for screening has began to evolve in the United States and worldwide (Thomas et al. 2008). Concordant with the continued technological evolution and increased translation into screening cohorts, there is a need to reinforce how to most effectively interpret the data.

Important differences in acquisition methods have varied in stool tagging and low-dose techniques, while image display techniques have ranged from primary detection with 2D multiplanar reformation (2D MPR) to 3D endoscopic fly-through techniques. Although differences exist, there are key issues of image display techniques which are important to understand for data interpretation.

This chapter focuses on (1) current mainstream image display techniques for data interpretation, (2) four basic steps to detect and characterize lesions, (3) influence of tagging on image interpretation, (4) major categories of colorectal lesion morphologies, and (5) issues of standardization of reporting clinically significant colorectal findings in CTC.

9.2 Current Mainstream Image Display Techniques

After the initial years of use of 2D MPR as a primary review with 3D to solve problems, the success of the study of Pickhardt et al. in (2003), aided by improved computer graphics, demonstrated that 3D as a primary review could be used effectively as a primary review. Although a few still debate whether 2D versus 3D is better, most agree that an understanding of how to cohesively apply each of these techniques in the appropriate setting is optimal.

How are we now to approach data interpretation? Currently, the answer probably is a seamless interaction between 2D MPR and 3D endoscopic fly-through techniques, which may vary across patients or within specific colonic segments of a patient. The 3D fly-through as a primary review uses 3D to detect, with 2D MPR to help characterize. Conversely, the technique of 2D MPR as a primary review uses 2D to detect, with 3D MPR to help characterize. In addition to these techniques, the 3D transparency view allows an overall view of the colonic anatomy, simulating the visualization from a barium enema. Recent improvements have led to the increasing use of the 3D flattened view, which permits an open view of the colon, like reading a paper. However, image distortion around areas of tortuosity still exists. In order to best apply these techniques, it is important to understand the uses, advantages, and disadvantages.

Appropriate training is important to acquire the new skills of these techniques. Currently, both academic and commercial programs for reader training are widely available in the United States and Europe. An essential component of training is for each trainee to have hands-on, interactive training, using an independent workstation with dedicated 3D CT colonography software. A recently developed clinical service may benefit initially from double reading of cases among trained colleagues.

9.2.1 2D Multiplanar Reformation

Primary 2D MPR review for lesion detection can provide a time-efficient evaluation of the colon, exploiting a cross sectional field of view for improved orientation of the colonic segments. This visualization is based on a real-time sectoring through the colonic subsegments in cine mode, in a continuous direction typically from the rectum to the cecum. Two window levels settings are typically utilized. The polyp window (width 1500, level 200) imparts the high-contrast interface to detect intraluminal colorectal polypoid lesions. The soft tissue window setting (width 400, level 10) is critical to evaluate more advanced wall lesions, discern the high density of false positives or the fat density of lipomas, and to evaluate the extra-colonic findings. In some areas of retained tagged fluid, a modified setting may be needed to better see within the dense fluid level (window 1000, level 200).

To use 2D MPR as a primary review, it can be helpful to initially perform a 1 min coronal cine of both the prone and supine data sets to get a "lay of the land." This allows the reader to determine the degree of tortuosity and the colonic course, as well as the image quality of colonic distention and fluid/stool retention. The data set with the best image quality can be chosen to evaluate first. Typically, as each lesion is detected, characterization of the lesion on the other 2D MPR views and 3D views can be made between prone and supine data sets. Images of true positive lesions are taken and an internet report of findings for future dictation can be initiated. This type of organization of effort, involving lesion detection and characterization, followed by image capture of important findings, along the continuous retrograde path of the colon from rectum to cecum, allows an efficient and thorough evaluation of the colonic surface area. If interrupted by another task, the colon segment reached can be recorded and then evaluation can be reinitiated at this segment, once the interpretation can be resumed. After finishing the first data set (typically supine) with characterization of each lesion detected, the other data set (typically prone) can be briefly viewed with an axial cine to potentially see any additional findings. Using embedded arrows for lesions already detected allows one not to waste time reevaluating the same lesions between data sets.

What are the advantages and disadvantages of 2D MPR? The use of 2D MPR offers several important advantages. First, there is the direct display of the source attenuation data of a focal lesion to determine density. Specifically, the density of a focal lesion, such as fat in a lipoma or high density or focal pockets of air in stool, provides important characteristics to confirm false positive lesions. This can be especially helpful in patients with significant retained densely tagged stool, which make the 3D primary review tedious. Another advantage of 2D MPR is the ability to visualize the location of a lesion from an extraluminal viewpoint, rather than the immersed endoscopic view of 3D fly-through. This can be helpful to confirm whether a lesion is in the same segment between prone and supine data sets (especially helpful in tortuous colons), as well as whether the lesion is dependent or nondependent within a given segment. If a lesion shifts in position to different segments or changes to a dependent position on both prone and supine views without a visualized stalk, the concern for a false positive (e.g., retained stool) increases. Another advantage is that 2D MPR can be a time-efficient evaluation of the colonic findings, since a thorough cine of both data sets is done once, compared to the need of forward and retrograde 3D fly-through views in both prone and supine data sets. Subtle mural lesions can often best be seen in the MPR soft tissue window settings, with higher contrast to the surrounding mesenteric fat compared to the polyp settings. The disadvantages of 2D MPR as a primary review may be decreased sensitivity, compared to the increased surface area visualization of 3D fly-through. Although this has not been directly confirmed in validation studies, the improved results of 3D as a primary review in the Pickhardt et al. study are compelling. Reader fatigue also can be greater with 2D MPR, given the potentially more subtle and briefer visualization of lesions during the cine method of sectoring through the data.

9.2.2 3D Endoscopic Fly-Through

The use of 3D fly-through as a primary review provides a continuous fly-through of the colon, using the endoscopic field of view. The exciting advances of this technique have become more generalizable across 3D workstations. One feature which has been supported is the use of field of views greater than 90° (typically 110–120°) to improve surface area visualization, although mild image distortion can still be present.

To use 3D as a primary review, endoscopic fly-through in antegrade and retrograde paths for both supine and prone data sets are typically done. Some advocates of 3D however state that if excellent visualization with no lesions found is present after forward and backward fly-through paths of the supine data set, only a retrograde fly-through is needed in the prone data set (e.g., eliminates antegrade fly-through in the second data set). Similar to 2D MPR, use of embedded arrows bookmarked in focal findings as they are evaluated decreases any time inefficiencies in the inadvertent reevaluation of the same findings in a later flight path or MPR review. A critical point is the need to also sector through the axial MPR data in soft tissue settings (done at the start or end of review) to exclude a flat lesion or advanced mural lesion. Circumferential narrowing or partial wall involvement of the colon in advanced cancers or flat lesions can be seen in the 3D endoscopic view; however, in some cases these changes can be better seen in the extraluminal viewpoint of 2D MPR using the soft tissue settings. Thus the 3D and 2D views are very complementary for detection of these advanced lesions.

What are the advantages and disadvantages of 3D endoscopic fly-through techniques? A strong advantage is the increased surface area visualization, which continues to be aided by improved navigational tools. In nontortuous segments of colon, there is a longer period of visualization of a focal colorectal lesion over the course of the fly-through, compared to the brief visualization seen while sectoring through a sub segment of the colon using 2D MPR cine techniques. This advantage, however, is diminished in marked areas of tortuosity or areas of collapse. Focal polypoid lesions can also be more visibly apparent within the colon lumen, compared to 2D, and thus can be easier to see in 3D fly-through. Both the potential advantages of longer visualization and increased ease of visualization of a lesion can lead to greater detection rates with less reader fatigue. The disadvantages of 3D endoscopic fly-through can include longer length of evaluation to complete review of the antegrade and retrograde paths. Retained focal stool can increase false positive rates since stool can appear similar to true polyps in 3D. Correlation of findings in 3D with the 2D data sets to exclude dense stool or air greatly improves diagnostic accuracy. In tortuous colons, surface areas visualization around the inner curve of a turn can be initially missed. However, some software programs display areas of nonvisualized regions for the reader to evaluate after the flight path is completed. For 3D to improve lesion detection rates with increased surface area visualization, false positive rates must be minimized with further characterization of findings with 2D correlation.

In summary, use of 2D MPR and 3D display techniques optimally are best used with seamless integration to exploit their inherent advantages and diminish their disadvantages. Even if 3D fly-through techniques are used as the primary review, the use of 2D MPR as a primary review may still be needed in specific segments or subsegments not amendable to 3D. Specifically, areas best evaluated with 2D MPR primarily may include areas of marked muscular hypertrophy from diverticulosis, sharp hairpin turns, colonic collapse, or marked fluid retention. In these areas, the 3D fly-through may be suspended, with transition to 2D MPR through a given region. In addition, in areas where multiple focal findings are being detected in 3D raising the concern for stool retention, evaluation in 2D MPR may allow a more efficient overall characterization. Thus, given the differences in image quality and anatomy which vary within or between patients, complementary use of 2D or 3D can be selectively utilized for improved visualization.

9.2.3 3D Transparency View (Edge-Enhanced View)

In addition to the primary modes of interpretation, the 3D transparency view provides an effective visualization to display the overall colonic anatomy and to demarcate where focal findings are. Although this view is not helpful in making the diagnosis, its role to summarize the findings in a consistent and accurate way is important for current management and future surveillance of lesions. Similar to the barium enema in appearance, this view can give an effective roadmap for the gastroenterologist or surgeon. Even in cases with no lesions, standard AP and bilateral oblique views can be helpful for future reference.

9.2.4 Future Advances of Image Display Techniques

Other 3D image display techniques are growing in their use. One example is the virtual dissection view, which straightens the colon along its central axis and then unfolds it. This open view can be completely flat like reading a page from a book, or be partially flattened. The ease of use in evaluating the surface area is an advantage, with each focal finding then registered back to the source axial, MPR, and 3D endoscopic views. The disadvantage can be image distortion which occurs in areas of marked tortuosity of the colon.

How we interpret virtual colonography currently will probably change dramatically in the next 5–10 years. Important influences will be the further refinement of computer-aided diagnosis and molecular imaging. Computer-aided diagnostic algorithms in CTC are being actively explored in academic and commercial efforts. If sensitivity can be achieved across the complexity of colorectal morphologies, without a compromise of specificity, remarkable efficiency of the data evaluation will be achieved. It will be interesting to evaluate whether CAD is used optimally as a primary read or a secondary read. As molecular imaging techniques continue to evaluate functional information at cellular and molecular levels, colorectal applications may shift to other modalities, such as MR and optical imaging. Certainly, the success of molecular imaging could lead to a phenomenal break-through of detection of clinically significant lesions in the polyp-carcinoma pathological continuum, along with focused therapy.

9.3 Four Basic Steps to Detect/Characterize Focal Lesions

There are four basic steps using 2D and/or 3D techniques to detect and characterize a focal colorectal lesion (Fig. 9.1).

First, *lesion morphology* is evaluated. A true polyp typically is smoothly marginated, in contrast to the potentially angulated margins that can be seen with retained stool. In 3D, evaluation of the morphology of the focal lesion in relationship to surrounding folds is very useful. Namely, the common dilemma of discernment of a thickened fold (or confluence of a compound fold) from a polyp on a fold can usually be best discerned in the 3D view. In 2D, complementary use of axial, sagittal, and coronal MPR can be helpful to evaluate morphology of a lesion.

Second, the *density* of a lesion is an important and easy step to delineate. To efficiently confirm that a lesion is soft-tissue density suggests a polyp and allows the evaluation to continue. However, to confirm that a focal finding has high density (tagged stool or retained pills), fat density (lipoma), or internal focal pockets of air (stool) allows the exclusion of this lesion as a true polyp, and no further evaluation is needed. The 2D axial view provides the true source attenuation data, typically viewed in a soft-tissue density setting (width 100, level 10). Some vendors provide an opacity map of the lesion within the 3D endoscopic view, which helps display the profile of density differences across the lesion.

Fig. 9.1. Four basic steps to characterize a polyp (*arrow*)-*morphology, density, location, measurement*: (**a**) 3D endoscopic view demonstrates typical morphology of a smoothly marginated polyp, (**b**) supine 2D axial MPR (1,500 W, –200L) shows corresponding morphology of polyp, (**c**) 2D axial MPR (400W, 10 L) shows soft tissue density of polyp, (**d**) prone 2D axial MPR shows similar location of polyp along anterior wall of cecum, with polyp submerged in tagged fluid, (**e**) 3D edge enhanced view serves as an anatomic roadmap to demarcate location of cecal polyp, (**f**) 3D endoscopic view demonstrates polyp measurement along long axis of polyp

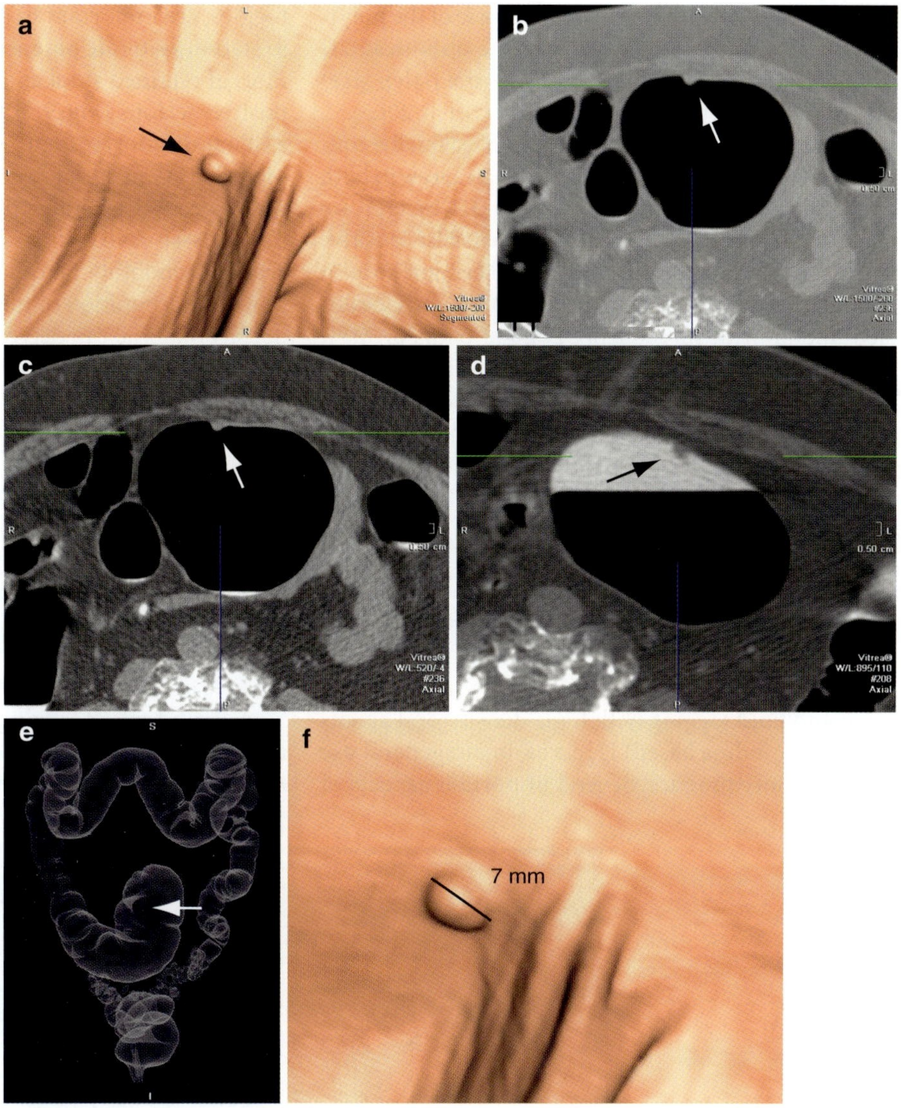

Third, confirmation of a lesion's *anatomic location* on the corresponding prone or supine data set is needed. Since the confirmation of the anatomic location of a potential polyp can be the most consuming step, this is typically done only after the first two steps suggest a probable polyp to increase time efficiency. Increasing use of automated registration of supine and prone data sets is becoming technically feasible in the 3D endoscopic views and has proved to be a great time saver. However, when automatic registration fails due to the wide in vivo range in position of a focal finding between prone and supine positions, 2D MPR (coronal often) or the 3D transparency views with their extracolonic field of view most efficiently are used to localize the anatomic position of specific lesion in the colon. Confirmation of the same location within a colonic segment on both prone and supine data sets (when image quality permits) greatly increases confidence to confirm the presence of a true positive lesion. A few exceptions should be noted. Namely, with pedunculated lesions on a long stalk, the polyp head can shift from one colonic segment to an adjacent segment, such as from the descending colon to sigmoid colon. Also, along the redundancy of the colonic mesentery, a lesion can appear to drop dependently between positions, when in fact it has remained constant but the entire mesentery has flipped (Laks et al. 2004).

Fourth, *lesion measurement* is important to do consistently and accurately. As the C-RADS structured reporting guideline describes, a polyp should be measured as the longest diameter along the polyp head, excluding the stalk if present. A sessile polyp should be measured along its long axis at the base of the polyp. The use of 3D endoscopic views or the optimized 2D MPR (MPR view which best elongates the polyp size) are ideal for measurement (Pickhardt et al. 2005).

For reporting, when a focal lesion is finally confirmed, it is *bookmarked* typically with an arrow in both data sets and representative 2D and 3D images are taken for the final report. Ideally, even false positive findings can be marked in a designated fashion, so as to not spend any additional time on a previously evaluated finding with subsequent 3D flight paths or MPR reviews. For the trained reader, the organized method to mark lesions during review of both prone and supine data sets as the case is read is essential to optimize time-efficiency and completeness of the data interpretation.

9.4 Influence of Stool and Fluid Tagging on Image Interpretation

Stool and fluid tagging with high-density oral agents (barium or iodine based) is increasing in general use in community practice. Several important aspects of tagging are important to understand for image interpretation, with the potential to decrease false positive rates of retained stool and increase sensitivity of true positive lesions (Fig. 9.2).

First, the most recognized use of tagging is to impart high-density material selectivity to retained stool from oral ingestion of either barium and/or iodine based products, so as to decrease false positive rates. Namely, retained smoothly margined stool can mimic polyps; however recognition of the tagging of stool with high-density material can decrease false positives. Two caveats need to be recognized. One caveat is that not all retained stool gets densely tagged, demonstrating partial or no tagging. An example is retained stool within densely tagged fluid, with the focal stool remaining relatively nontagged within the fluid, but usually dropping dependently between positions. Another caveat is that not all densely tagged focal findings represent stool; however, no true positive lesions of clinical significant are densely tagged. One example is ingested pills which can range from being high in density in the absence of tagging to being low in density.

A second role of tagging is to increase the conspicuity of submerged polyps to decrease false negative rates. As Fig. 9.2b shows, the submerged soft tissue density of

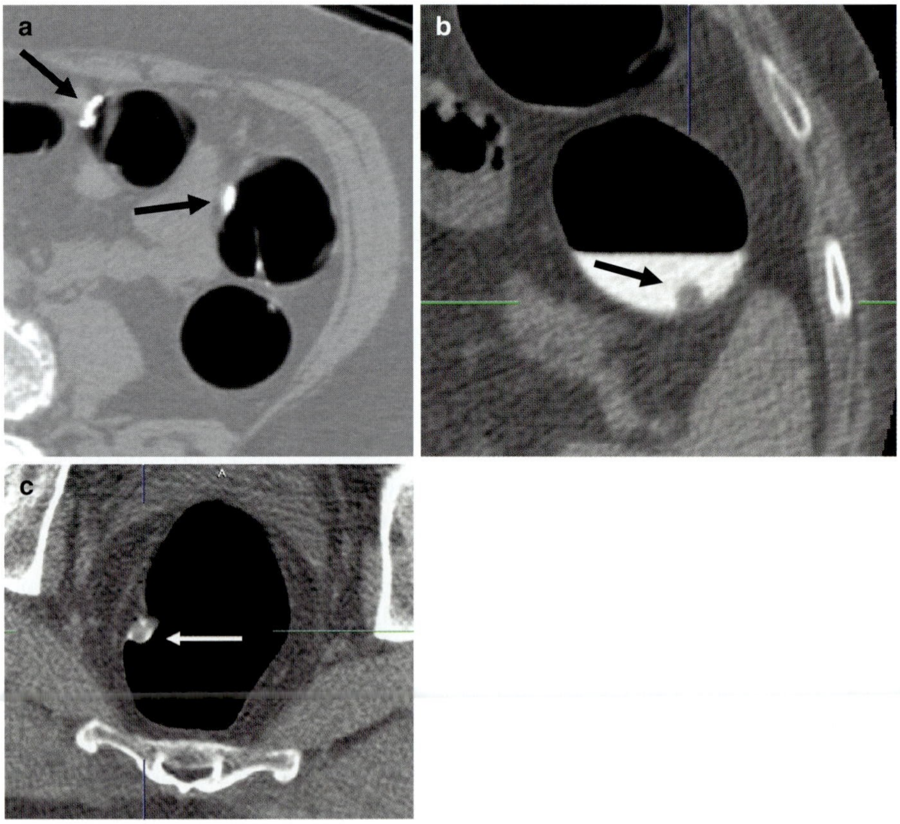

Fig. 9.2. Three basic uses of stool and fluid tagging: (**a**) Dense tagging of retained stool (*arrows*) can decrease false positives, but is most useful in the 2D views. (**b**) Tagged fluid can improve detection of submerged true polyp (*arrow*). (**c**) Linear or globular coating can occur along surface of a true polyp (*arrow*)

a polyp is sharply contrasted by the surrounding densely tagged fluid to improve detection. By using the different MPR views, the attachment of the polyp to the wall can help confirm this is a true polyp finding.

Third, it is important to recognize that polyps can have partial coating with tagged agents, which can either appear as dense linear coating or conglomerate droplets along the polyp surface. O'Connor et al. evaluated a subanalysis of 216 screening patients and found that 46% of 312 polyps demonstrated some adherent contrast coating the surface of polyps from the tagging agents (O'Connor et al. 2006).

9.5 Major Categories of Colorectal Lesion Morphologies

There are common types of colorectal morphologies evaluated in CT colonography. These include the focal polypoid lesion, pedunculated lesion, flat or sessile lesion, and advanced mural lesions. This section describes these morphologies and their corresponding false positive counterparts. The differential application of 2D and 3D image displays to assess these morphologies is also reinforced.

9.5.1 Focal Polypoid Lesions (r/o Stool)

One of the most common colorectal morphologies is the focal polypoid lesion. This is also the most common morphology of the false positive lesion of retained stool. Thus discernment between a focal polyp and stool are critical. Key features include the following:

The morphology of a focal polyp is typically smoothly marginated and round (Fig. 9.1). Although stool can also be similar in morphology, margins which are more geometrical or angular are highly suggestive of stool (Fig. 9.3). A polypoid lesion is typically of soft- tissue density. In contrast, lesions which are high in density are highly specific of stool or other false positive findings, such as retained pills. Stool can also be of low attenuation or opaque; however, this can overlap with the partial volume effects of smaller polyps, depending on the collimation used.

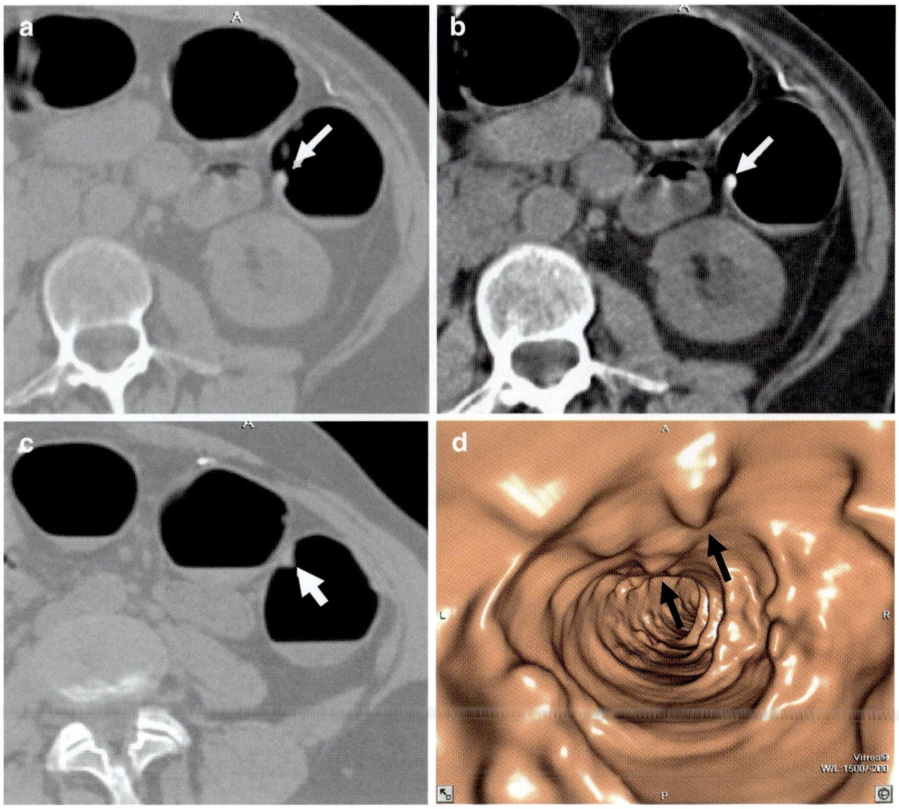

Fig. 9.3. Typical features of false positive retained stool (*arrows*), with angular or geometric margins and high density: (**a**) Axial 2D MPR (W 1,500, L –200) shows focal polypoid lesion, compared to (**b**) axial 2D MPR (W 400, L 10) in soft tissue settings better demonstrates high density of stool, (**c**) Axial 2D MPR shows angular margins of retained stool, (**d**) 3D perspective volume rendered view demonstrates multiple false positive lesions, many with angular margins

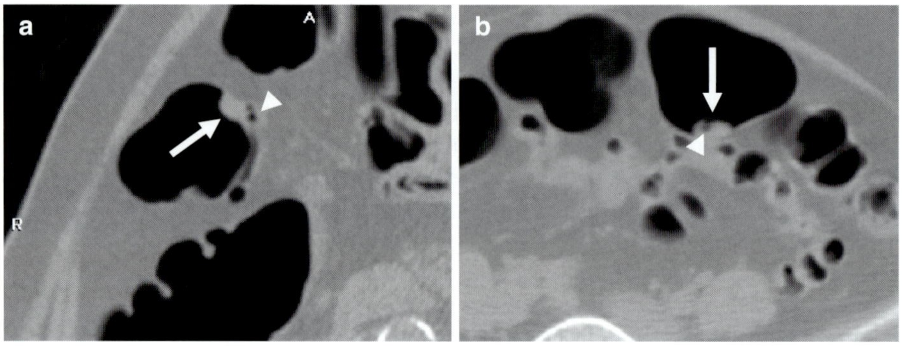

Fig. 9.4. Polypoid lesions with focal pockets of air seen in true polyp vs. stool: (**a**) True positive polyp (*arrow*) with air around edges of lesion (*arrowheads*), where lesion abuts the wall, (**b**) false positive of stool (*arrow*) with central pockets of air (*arrowheads*)

A focal polyp can have air around the edges, if it is coated next to the wall; however, central focal pockets of air within a lesion is diagnostic of stool (Fig. 9.4). Shift versus constancy of location of a focal finding relative to the colon wall is important. A polypoid lesion will stay fixed in the same position relative to the wall between prone and supine images. In contrast, the finding of stool which drops dependently is highly characteristic. There are exceptions to this. A sigmoid polyp may appear to shift dependently on prone and supine images, but actually the redundancy of the sigmoid mesentery is what shifts (Laks et al. 2004). Stool can be adherent to the wall, which has been described with the phospha-soda preps. Also, a pedunculated polyp which does not demonstrate its stalk can appear to drop dependently. Finally, if intravenous contrast is used, differences in enhancement can be seen. Polyps potentially can enhance, whereas stool will not enhance. As diagnostic CT is exploited to stage the liver along with evaluation of the colorectal lesions, the increasing use of IV contrast may lead to better understanding of the enhancement characteristics of polyps.

Both 2D and 3D techniques help to evaluate these characteristics. The morphologic features of round or smooth versus angular or geometric margins are best seen with 3D endoscopic views. Inherent density, location, focal pockets of air, and the degree of enhancement are best evaluated with 2D MPR. As stool tagging continues to be developed, the ability to see high density within residual stool further aids differentiation of polyp from stool.

9.5.2 Pedunculated Lesions

The pedunculated lesion, comprised of a round polyp head with a linear stalk, is a very distinguishable lesion. The challenge is how different these lesions can appear between prone and supine data sets (Fig. 9.5). On one data set, the polyp head can be suspended dependently from the stalk, whereas on the corresponding data set, both polyp head and stalk can lie dependently together along the wall. If the stalk is long enough, lesions on the border between two segments can lie in different adjacent segments between prone and supine views. Also of importance is the variability in lesion measurement with such morphological differences between views. A consistent reporting style is to measure the polyp head, with exclusion of the stalk. Thus, choosing the image where the polyp head and stalk are best discerned provides the more accurate and reproducible measurement (Fig. 9.5b).

In general, 3D endoscopic views can provide improved visualization of these morphological features. One exception would be the visualization of the highly characteristic stalk of a pendunculated lesion in a segment with marked muscular hypertrophy of diverticulosis. In this setting, 2D MPR may offer an advantage, due to the impaired endoscopic visualization within the thickened folds (Fig. 9.6).

9.5.3 Sessile/Flat Lesions (r/o Thick or Confluent Folds)

These lesions currently can be challenging to detect and differentiate from globally thickened folds (Fig. 9.7). One important issue is the variability in definition of the terms. "Sessile" is generally defined as a lesion with a polyp base that is twice as long as the polyp height. Thus, a one centimeter high lesion with a two centimeter base could be defined as sessile. This is very different than a "flat" lesion which is generally defined as a lesion measuring one to three millimeters in height. Unfortunately, the literature is

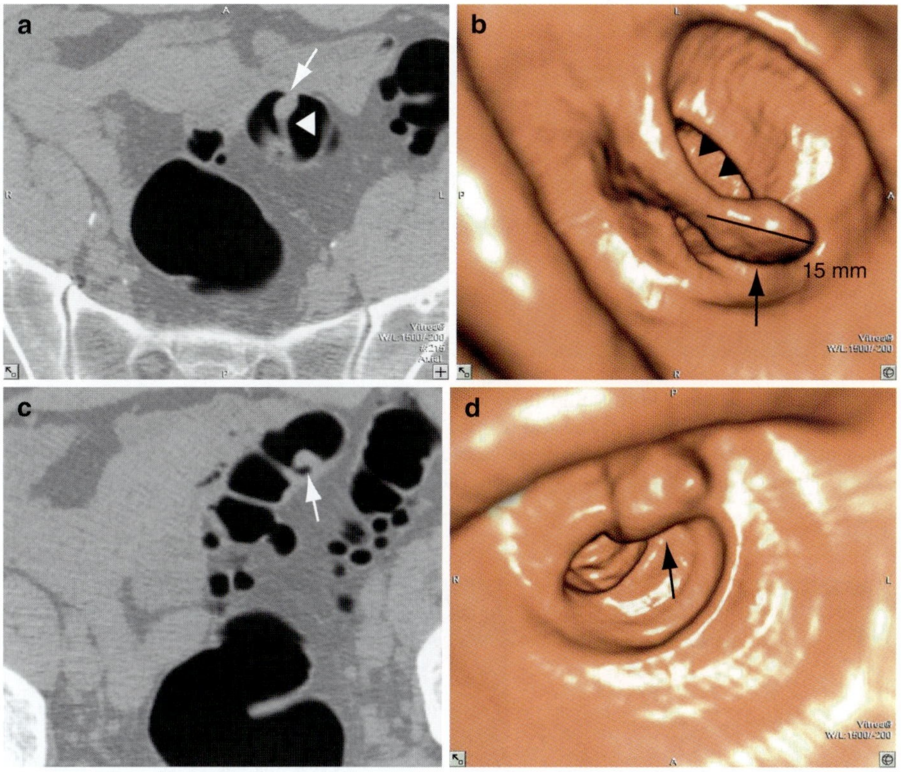

Fig. 9.5. Typical features of a pedunculated polyp in sigmoid colon, demonstrating polyp head (*arrow*) and characteristic stalk (*arrowheads*), with marked changes between positions: (**a**) Axial 2D MPR and (**b**) 3D volume rendered view in supine position demonstrates polyp head (*arrow*) and stalk (*arrowheads*). Accurate measurement of long axis of polyp head, excluding the stalk, is shown. (**c**) Axial 2D MPR and (**d**) 3D volume rendered view in prone position shows remarkable shift in position and change in morphology

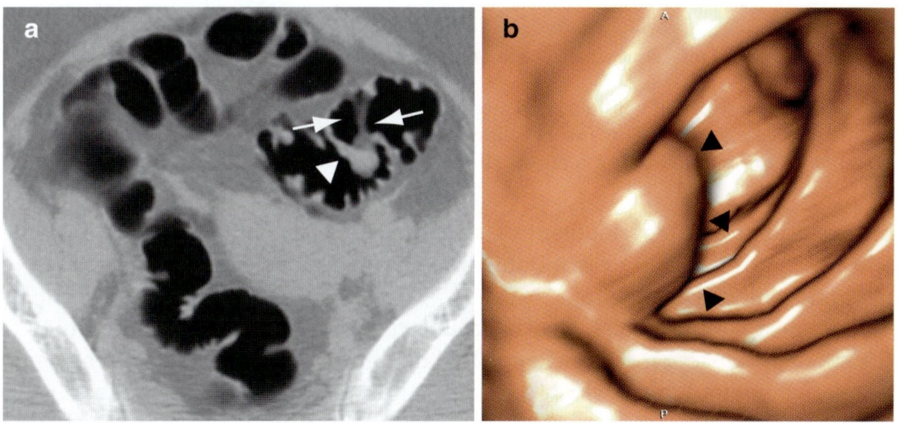

Fig. 9.6. Pedunculated lesion in area of luminal narrowing and marked diverticulosis: (**a**) Axial 2D MPR view best visualizes the characteristic stalk (*arrows*) from the polyp head (*arrowheads*), compared to (**b**). 3D volume rendered view, with polyp head shown (*arrowheads*), but stalk obscured by muscular hypertrophy and luminal narrowing

inconsistent with these definitions, and reported sensitivities have varied. Fidler et al. reported a sensitivity range of 15–65% to detect 22 sessile polyps (size range of 0.4–3.5 cm) in a cohort of 547 patients (Fidler et al. 2002). Pickhardt et al. reported a sensitivity of 80% (47/59 polyps) to detect sessile lesions (defined as lesions with a base greater than height) in the cohort of 1233 screening patients (Pickhardt et al. 2004). Recently, Soetikno et al. reported the prevalence of nonpolypoid colorectal neoplasia in a mixed cohort of 1819 veterans, using the subgroups defined as superficially elevated, flat and depressed (Soetikno et al. 2008). In this cohort, the prevalence of nonpolypoid neoplasia was 9.35% overall and 5.84% among screening patients. Although there is still active debate about the associated risk of cancer

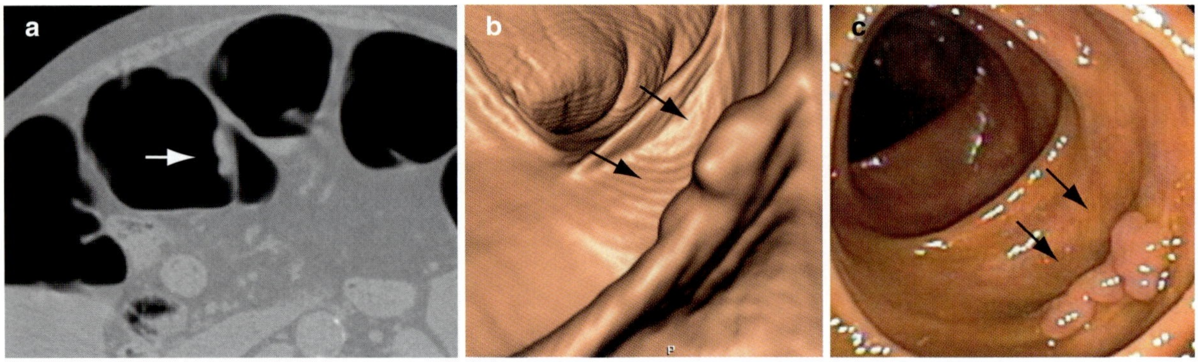

Fig. 9.7. Sessile lesion along a fold (*arrows*): (**a**) Axial 2D MPR shows focal nodularity of a sessile lesion along the mid point of a fold, (**b**) 3D endoscopic view best demonstrates overall morphology of the sessile lesion relative to the entire fold, (**c**) Corresponding endoscopic view from optical colonoscopy nicely correlates with 3D view (copyright given by *Clinics in Colon and Rectal Surgery*, for Thomas et al. 2008)

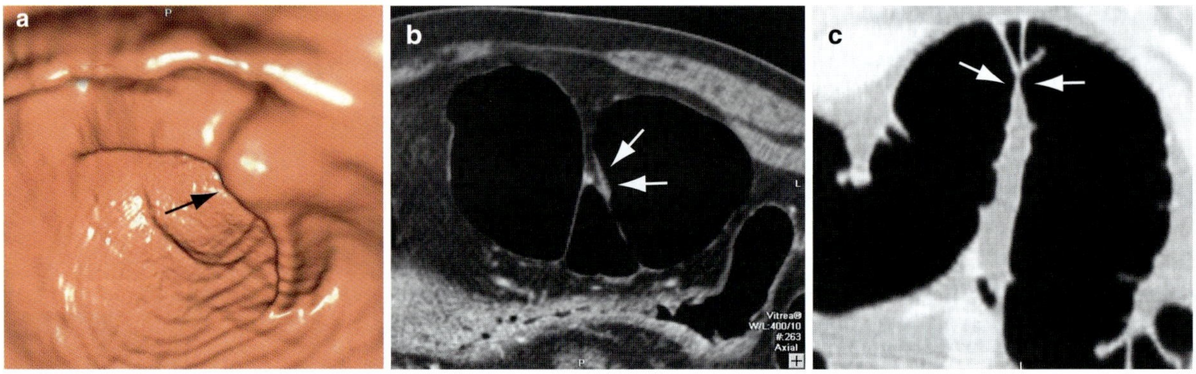

Fig. 9.8. False positive of confluence of a compound fold at flexure mimicking a flat lesion: (**a**) 3D volume rendered view raises concern for a flat lesion (*arrow*), (**b**) Axial 2D MPR in soft tissue settings also demonstrates flat morphology (*arrow*), (**c**) Sagittal 2D MPR best demonstrates confluence of compound folds

in these subgroups, development of a more consistent lexicon of terms to describe this range of morphologies will be very helpful.

The most common false positive counterpart to the flat or sessile lesion is a thickened fold or confluence of compound folds, which are common at the flexures (Fig. 9.8). For these types of challenging lesions, both 2D MPR (in soft tissue window-level settings) and 3D views are complementary. Both techniques should be explored to best detect and characterize these lesions.

9.5.4 Advanced Mural Lesions (r/o Collapse)

CT colonography has reliably shown high sensitivity in detecting advanced mural lesions (Fig. 9.9). A potential challenge in CT colonography is the discernment between an advanced mural lesion of advanced cancer from an area of focal collapse with relative wall thickening (often seen at points of flexures, tortuosity, or muscular hypertrophy). At CT colonography, an advanced cancer will tend to stay fixed between prone and supine imaging, whereas an area of collapse can change in distention between positions. A cancer will typically have irregularity of the soft-tissue rind along the wall, whereas focal collapse or muscular hypertrophy will be more smooth and symmetric (Fig. 9.10). If intravenous contrast is given, a cancer may have more irregular enhancement, whereas focal collapse of normal colon will enhance symmetrically.

The importance of 2D MPR with soft-tissue settings (window 400, level 10) needs to be emphasized with these types of lesions. Whether this is subtle

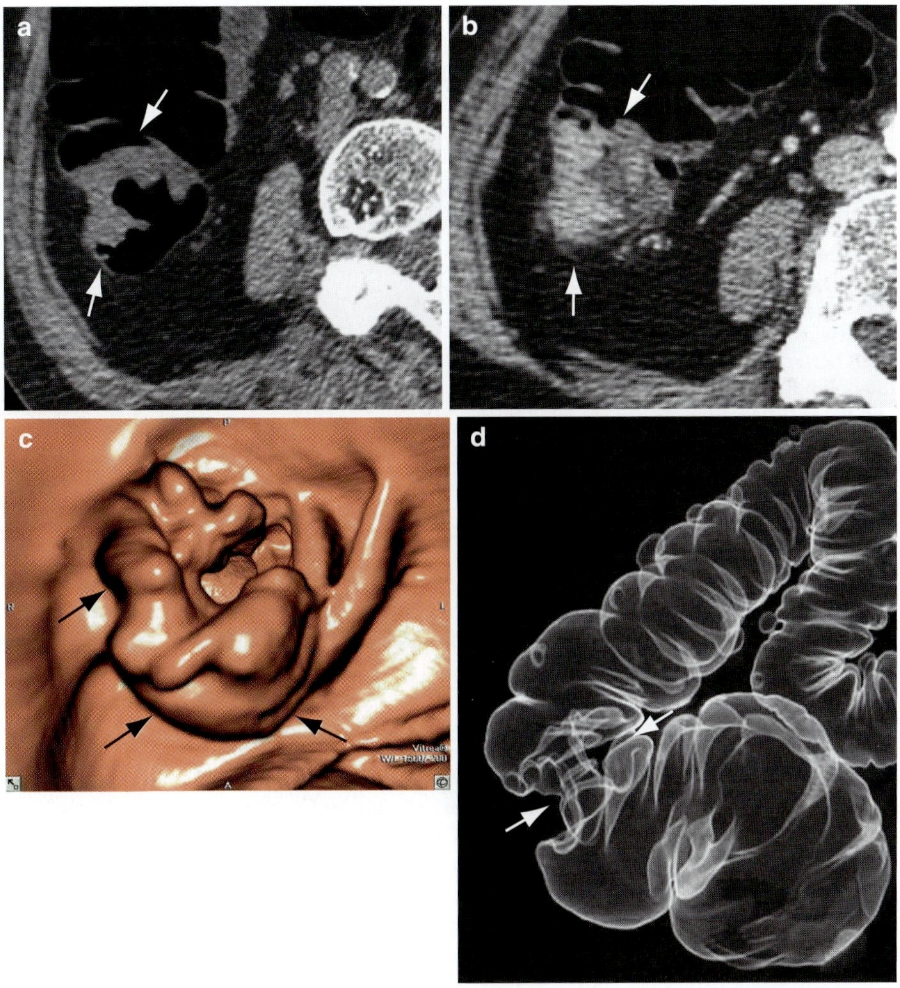

Fig. 9.9. Advanced mural lesion (*arrows*): (**a**) Prone noncontrast axial 2D MPR demonstrates advanced mural lesion, (**b**) Supine contrast enhanced axial 2D MPR shows enhancing mass immersed in fluid, (**c**) 3D volume rendered intraluminal view of cancer, (**d**) 3D transparency view shows classic apple-core lesion

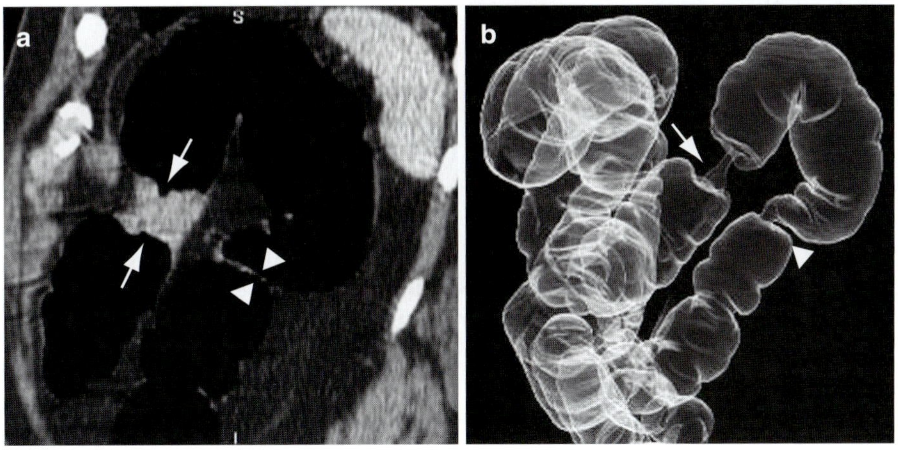

Fig. 9.10. Advanced mural lesion (*arrows*) vs. collapse (*arrowheads*): (**a**) Sagittal 2D MPR view shows mural thickening of advanced cancer vs. area of luminal collapse without mural thickening, (**b**) 3D edge enhanced view also demonstrates these two areas

mural thickening or advanced, the 2D MPR views give valuable information of the mural relationships, which extend beyond the "lumenography" of the 3D fly-through (Fig. 9.11). In addition, the 3D transparency view, which simulates the barium enema, can be a powerful view to display the lesion for others to appreciate the length and location of the cancer.

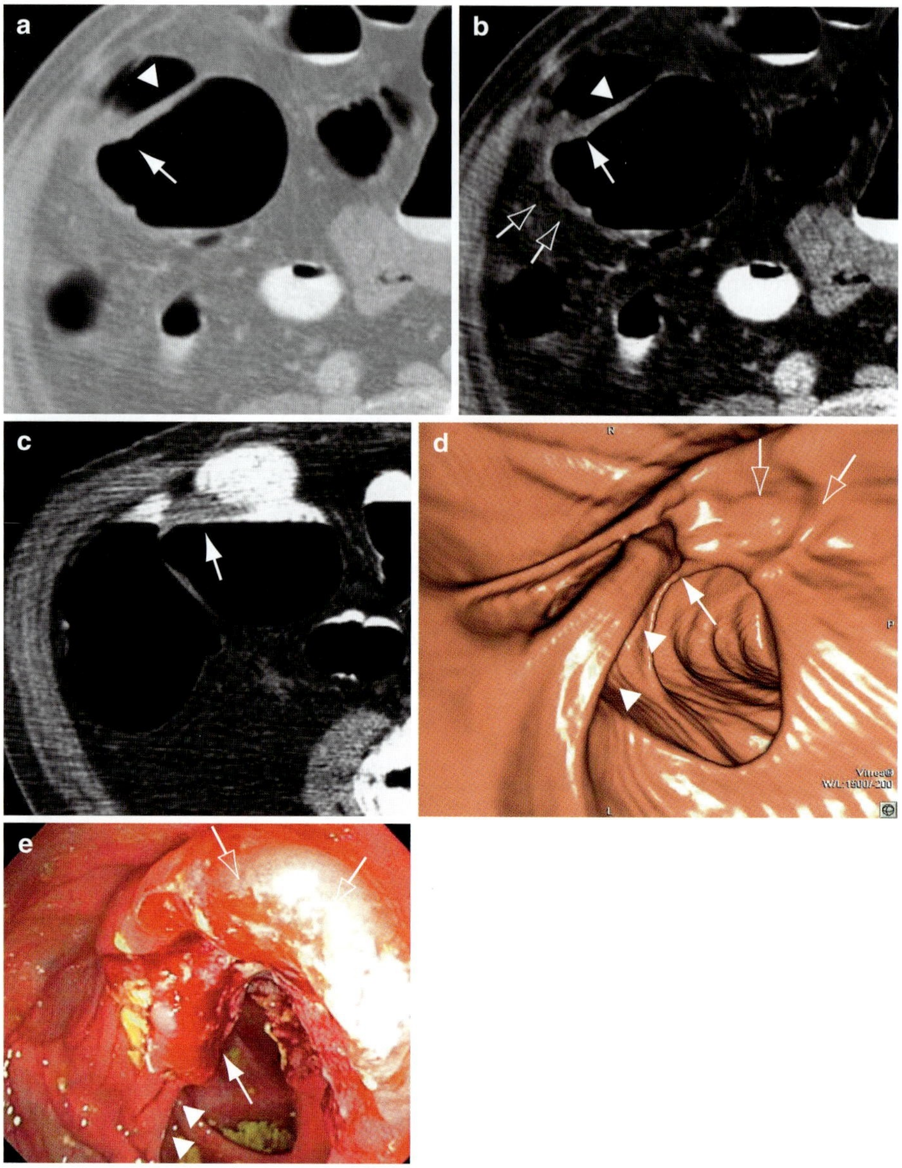

Fig. 9.11. Advanced mural lesion with polypoid head (*white arrow*), stalk (*white arrowheads*) and infiltrative T3 mural components, (*open arrows*) best seen in soft tissue MPR views: (**a**) Supine axial 2D MPR (W 1,500, L –200) does not demonstrate lesion as well, compared to (**b**) Supine axial 2D MPR in soft tissue settings (W 400, L 20) better demonstrates the polypoid component and flat soft tissue mural infiltration, (**c**) Prone axial 2D MPR shows immersed polypoid lesion (*arrows*) with a narrower soft tissue window setting (W 900, L 300), (**d**) Optimized 3D view shows polypoid and infiltrative mural component, which nicely correlates to (**e**) Corresponding view at optical colonoscopy

9.6 Standardization of Reporting of Clinically Significant Colorectal Findings and Quality Assurance

The Virtual Colonoscopy Working Group, represented by an organized group of CTC investigators at the International Virtual Colonoscopy annual meeting, published a consensus statement in 2005 regarding the development of a reporting structure of colorectal and extra-colonic findings (Zalis et al. 2005). This reporting structure, named "C-RADS" helps to lay the groundwork for structured reporting of lesion morphology, size, and location, along with preliminary recommendations of lesion surveillance. Although this effort now needs to be refined with multidisciplinary consensus, it represents an important step toward more consistent and reproducible reporting at CT colonography.

C-RADS describes the use of three morphologies of lesions: sessile (broad based lesion whose width is greater than its vertical height), pedunculated (polyp with a separate stalk), and flat (polyp with vertical height less than 3 mm). Lesion measurement is critical for clinical management and can vary between readers if defined criteria are not used. C-RADS defines the measurement of a polypoid lesion to be the maximal long axis of the polyp head, with exclusion of the stalk, if present. For sessile lesions, the maximal length along the base of the polyp should be used. Both optimized 2D MPR and 3D techniques have been advocated for measurement, both of which certainly are felt to exceed the accuracy of axial measurements. Lesion location refers to the standardized colonic segments of rectum, sigmoid, descending, transverse, ascending, and cecum.

Recommendations of lesion management based on size criteria continue to be debated (Levin et al. 2008; Thomas et al. 2008; Van Dam et al. 2004). The recent consensus 2008 guidelines by the American Cancer Society, US Multisociety Colorectal Task Force (comprised of the three major gastroenterology societies) and American College of Radiology, recommends that all patients with polyps 6 mm or greater in size should be offered polypectomy (Levin et al. 2008), recognizing that management may need to be individually tailored, based on clinical context. Specifically, some patients with 6–9 mm polyps may be more suited for short-term surveillance, based on comorbidity, age, or other risk factors. Further multidisciplinary consensus and on-going research will now be needed to refine these recommendations.

Finally, C-RADS discusses the reporting of extra-colonic findings. To achieve cost effectiveness, the judicious reporting of extra-colonic findings to minimize unnecessary additional imaging tests will be critical. Significant extra-colonic findings, such as abdominal aortic aneurysms, solid renal or liver masses, adenopathy, and lung nodules (greater than 1 cm) are emphasized. Less significant findings, such as small liver and renal cystic lesions (common findings which are often difficult to characterize without contrast), and gallstones hopefully will be under-reported. Further definition of how to categorize and follow these findings will be important.

Similar to the initiative for measuring quality of colonoscopy (Lieberman 2006), quality metrics for CTC are also being developed. In 2008, the ACR began development of individual and practice-based quality metrics for CTC, including low-dose CT technique, bowel preparation, adequacy of insufflation, and outcomes measures of positive predictive value of clinically significant polyps, incidence of perforations and reporting of significant extracolonic findings. These metrics began a pilot phase in late 2008 using the National Radiology Data Registry (NRDR), which is an active ACR national data warehouse. In time, these data may help provide a pay for performance model for CTC to promote quality of performing and interpreting the examination.

In summary, the increasing use of C-RADS since its introduction in 2005 continues to improve standardization as the technique migrates out into more general use in screening cohorts. Multidisciplinary consensus of radiologists, gastroenterologists, internists, surgeons, pathologists, and epidemiologists will hopefully continue to define and standardize clinical issues of importance. At the core of these issues will be definition of what constitutes a clinically significant lesion, with appropriate surveillance based on the clinical context. As standardization is refined during ongoing evolution of the technique, an active process of quality assurance will be essential for broader community implementation.

References

Johnson CD, Chen MH, Toledano AY et al (2008) Accuracy of CT colonography for detection of large adenomas and cancers. NEJM 359:1207–1217

Graser A, Stieber P, Nagel D et al (2009) Comparison of CT colonography, colonoscopy, sigmoidoscopy and fecal occult blood tests for the detection of advanced adenoma in an average risk population. Gut 58:241–248

Regge D, Laudi C, Galatola G, et al (2009) Accuracy of CT colonography in subjects at increased risk of colorectal carcinoma: a multi-center trial of 1,000 patients. JAMA 301:2453–2461.

Kim DH, Pickhardt PJ, Taylor AJ et al (2007) CT colonography versus colonoscopy for the detection of advanced neoplasia. N Engl J Med 357:1403–1412

Pickhardt PJ, Choi JR, Hwang I, Butler JA, Puckett ML, Hildebrandt HA et al (2003) Computed tomographic virtual colonoscopy to screen for colorectal neoplasia in asymptomatic adults. N Eng J Med 349:2191–2200

Levin B, Lieberman DA, McFarland B, Smith RA, Brooks D, Andrews KS et al (2008) Screening and Surveillance for the early detection of colorectal cancer and adenomatous polyps 2008: a joint guideline from the American Cancer Society, the US Multi-society task force on colorectal cancer, and the American College of Radiology. CA Cancer J Clin 58:130–160

Thomas J, Carenza J, McFarland E (2008) Computed tomographic colonography (virtual colonoscopy): climax of a new era of validation and transition into community practice. Clin Colon Rectal Surg 21:220–232

Laks S, Macari M, Bini EJ (2004) Positional change in colon polyps at CT colonography. Radiology 231:761–766

Pickhardt PJ, Lee AD, McFarland EG, Taylor AJ (2005) Linear polyp measurement at CT colonography: in vitro and in vivo comparison of two-dimensional and three-dimensional displays. Radiology 236:872–878

O'Connor SD, Summer RM, Choi JR, Pickhardt PJ (2006) Oral contrast adherence to polyps on CT colonography. J Comput Assit Tomogr 30:51–57

Fidler JL, Johnson CD, MacCarty RL, Welch TJ, Hara AK, Harmsen WS (2002) Detection of flat lesions in the colon with CT colonography. Abdom Imaging 27:292–300

Pickhardt PJ, Nugent PA, Choi JR, Schindler WR (2004) Flat colorectal lesions in asymptmatic adults: implications for screening with CT virtual colonoscopy. AJR 183: 1343–1347

Soetikno RM, Kaltenbach T, Rouse RV, Park W, Maheshwari A, Sato T et al (2008) Prevalence of nonpolypoid (flat and depressed) colorectal neoplasia in asymptomatic and symptomatic adults. JAMA 299:1027–1035

Zalis ME, Barish MA, Choi JR, Dachman AH, Fenlon HM, Ferrucci JT, Glick SN, Laghi A, Macari M, McFarland EG, Morrin MM, Pickhardt PJ, Soto J, Yee J (2005) CT colonography reporting and data system: a consensus proposal. Radiology 236:3–9

Van Dam J, Cotton P, Johnson CD, McFarland BG, Pineau BC, Provenzale D, Ransohoff D, Rex D, Rockey D, Wootton T (2004) AGA future trends report: CT colonography. Gastroenterology 127:970–984

Lieberman D (2006) A call to action–measuring the quality of colonoscopy. N Engl J Med 355:2588–2589

How to Avoid Pitfalls in Imaging:

Causes and Solutions to Overcome False-Negatives and False-Positives

Stefaan Gryspeerdt and Philippe Lefere

CONTENTS

Stefaan Gryspeerdt, MD
Philippe Lefere, MD
Department of Radiology, Stedelijk Ziekenhuis, Bruggesteenweg, 90, 8800, Roeselare, Belgium

10.1 Introduction

A major requisite, prior to the use of computed tomography-colonography (CTC) as a screening tool, has been to achieve an accuracy level comparative to that of conventional colonoscopy. Until now, a wide range of sensitivities has been reported (Fletcher et al. 2005), even for the largest lesions (>9 mm): Johnson et al. (2003) reported a major inter-observer variability, with sensitivity ranges of only 32–73%, whereas Pockhardt et al. (2003) reported excellent sensitivities of 93.8%. This wide range of reported sensitivities is one of the major reasons for gastrointestinal endoscopists not to advocate the technique as a screening tool yet (Hwang and Wong 2005; Pickhardt 2005).

In-depth analysis of the different results has shown numerous possible causes for the reported differences in accuracy, including a learning curve, influencing sensitivity (Spinzi et al. 2001), as well as specificity (Gluecker et al. 2002). This learning curve includes the whole process of CTC: patient preparation, scanning technique (including patient positioning, colon insufflation, and scanning parameters), and image manipulation and interpretation (Taylor et al. 2004).

Each step in the process of a CTC examination has its own potential dangers of hindering a final correct diagnosis.

In this chapter, different causes of false-positive and false-negative diagnosis are reviewed, and the possible solutions to overcome these problems are proposed.

In the first part, false-positive diagnosis will be reviewed, and in the second part, false-negative diagnosis will be reviewed.

The figures represent a pictorial review of the different pitfalls, with lessons to overcome those pitfalls, marked in italics in the figure legend.

10.2 False-Negative Diagnosis

Overall, false-negative diagnosis can be related to errors in characterization, failure to detect the lesions, or both (Fidler et al. 2004; Nio et al. 2007).

10.2.1 Failure to Detect the Lesion

10.2.1.1 Preparation-Related False-Negative Diagnosis

There are two main bowel preparations available: cathartics, such as magnesium citrate and phospho-soda, and gut lavage solutions, such as polyethylene glycol (PEG).

PEG is known as a "wet prep", leaving a clean colon filled with residual fluid. Residual fluid does not hinder colonoscopic evaluation because of the ability of the colonoscopist to aspirate the residual fluid. In CTC, however, PEG results in fluid-filled segments, impeding full mucosal visibility, resulting in false-negative diagnosis.

Prone or supine imaging might overcome this problem in some way (Fig. 10.1), but is still insufficient to guarantee a complete colon evaluation (Gryspeerdt et al. 2002).

Fluid tagging has been proposed to overcome the problem of drowned segments: the fluid can be tagged either by barium, iodinated contrast material, or a combination (Lefere et al. 2002; Zalis et al. 2003; Pickhardt et al. 2003). As a result, the polyp can be detected as a hypodense structure in the tagged, hyperdense fluid levels (Fig. 10.2). Additionally, there is the possibility of electronic cleansing, removing the tagged fluid level, resulting in complete mucosal visibility (Zalis et al. 2003; Pickhardt et al. 2003).

Preparation without cathartic cleansing, the so-called "dry preparation", is currently being evaluated as the ultimate reduced preparation, further improving patient compliance, and almost eliminating residual fluid (Bielen et al. 2003; Callstrom et al. 2001; Lefere et al. 2004; McFarland and Zalis 2004; Pickhardt et al. 2003; Zalis et al. 2003).

10.2.1.2 Technical Artifacts

A major technical artifact is caused by suboptimal distended or even undistended segments, possibly hiding the polyps.

Spasmolytic agents can be used to improve colonic distention.

There are two main spasmolytic agents: glucagon, a single-chain polypeptide hormone that increases the blood glucose and relaxes the smooth muscle of the gastrointestinal tract; and buthylhioscin (Buscopan®), used in Europe and Asia to induce bowel hypotonia.

The rationale to use spasmolytic agents is a possible improved colonic distention and reduced procedural pain.

Goei et al. (1995) found Buscopan® to be more effective in distending the colon than glucagon, which is in conjunction with the findings of both Yee et al. (1999) and Morrin et al. (2002), who found that colonic distention was not improved after glucagon administration. Therefore, the use of glucagon has been currently abandoned.

Bruzzi et al. (2003) found that Buscopan® should not be used routinely, but observed that it is useful in patients with diverticular disease. Taylor et al. (2003a–d), on the other hand, found that the effect of

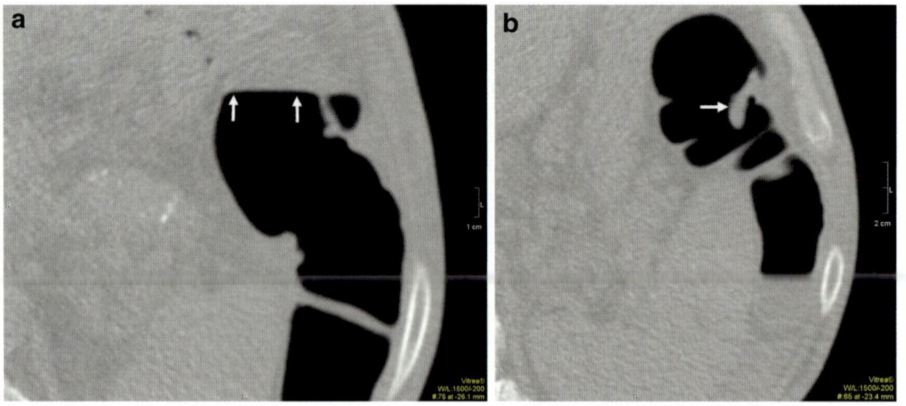

Fig. 10.1. False-negative diagnosis due to a non-tagged, fluid-drowned segment. (**a**) Prone image shows a fluid level (*arrows*), impeding visualization of a stalked polyp. (**b**) The stalked polyp is clearly seen on the supine image (*arrow*). *Lesson: Prone/supine imaging is useful to prevent false-negative diagnosis in case of fluid-filled segments*

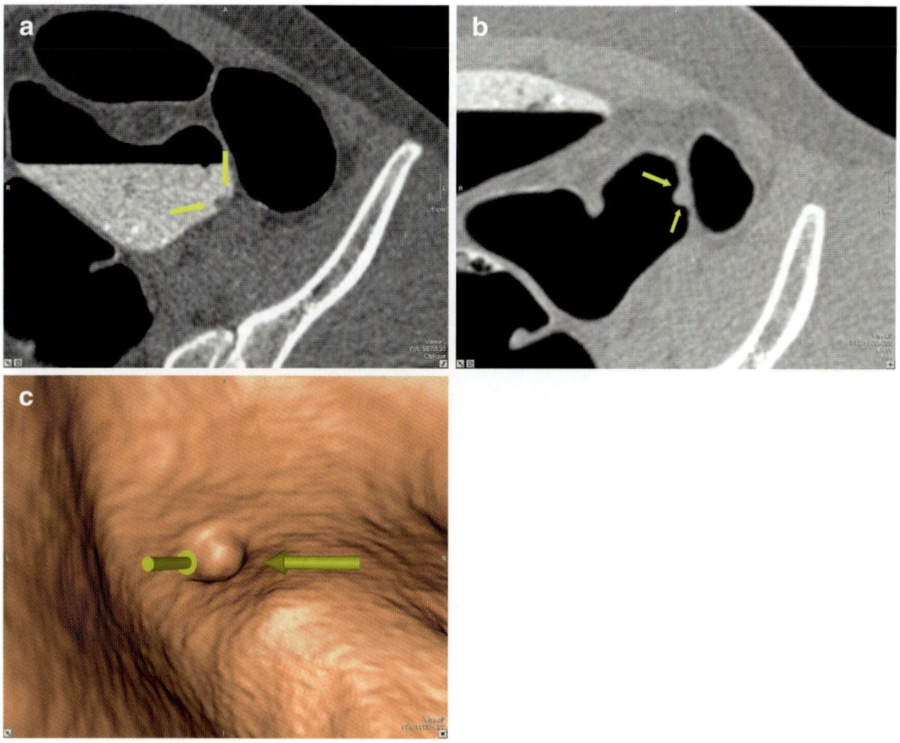

Fig. 10.2. True positive diagnosis in a tagged, fluid-drowned segment. (**a**) Supine image shows a hypodense structure in a tagged, hyperdense fluid level (*arrows*), suspicious for a sessile polyp. The presence of a 5-mm sessile polyp (*arrows*) is confirmed on (**b**) prone and (**c**) endoluminal 3D image. *Lesson: Fluid tagging can be used to overcome the problem of drowned segments: polyps can be detected as a hypodense structure in a tagged, hyperdense fluid level*

Buscopan® also extends to those without diverticular disease.

Orally administered Buscopan® has also proven useful during barium enema (Bova et al. 1999).

In our institution, we routinely use Buscopan®: 10 mL diluted in 100 mL of 0.9% sodium chloride and administered intravenously at a rate of 10 mL/min.

The reason is the subjective impression of reduced procedural pain, and the fact that procedural spasm can mimic tumor (see later) or impede adequate evaluation.

A persistent spasm can be differentiated from tumoral lesions by its smooth contours and the absence of surrounding lymph nodes. In some instances, additional inflation might be necessary to solve the problem (see Sect. 10.2.2.2).

The problem of segmental collapse can also be solved by prone/supine imaging (Fig. 10.3).

10.2.1.3 Normal Anatomy: Blind Spots and Areas of Danger

Normal anatomy may cause false-negative diagnosis because normal anatomical structures can hide polyps, for example, causing blind spots (Mang et al. 2007): thickened semilunar folds typically hide polyps in either antegrade or retrograde three-dimensional (3D) evaluation (Fig. 10.4). The same holds true for complex folds at the hepatic or splenic flexure, possibly hiding small polyps, impossible to detect using standard antegrade and retrograde 3D views. To overcome the problems of inadequate visualization of the colonic lumen, different 3D reconstruction methods have been developed, improving the detection of polyps on 3D endoscopic views such as virtual colonic dissection or unfolded cube (Hoppe et al. 2004; Vos et al. 2003; Luo et al. 2004). Each of these different viewing modes aims to display the whole colonic lumen at one view, obviating the need of turning the virtual camera in different angles.

The cecum, hepatic flexure, transverse colon, splenic flexure, and sigmoid colon, should be considered as "areas of danger" because of the convoluted and mobile nature.

The mobile nature of these segments mimics the positional change of lesions, possibly causing erroneous diagnosis of "mobile" residual stool (Fig. 10.5) (Park et al. 2005).

Although the rectum is straight and not mobile, one has to take care of not missing rectal lesions. False-negative diagnosis of rectal lesions may be caused by "reader's fatigue" if one starts at the cecal level, or by rectal balloon catheter that hides the rectal lesions (Pickhardt and Choi 2005) (Fig. 10.6).

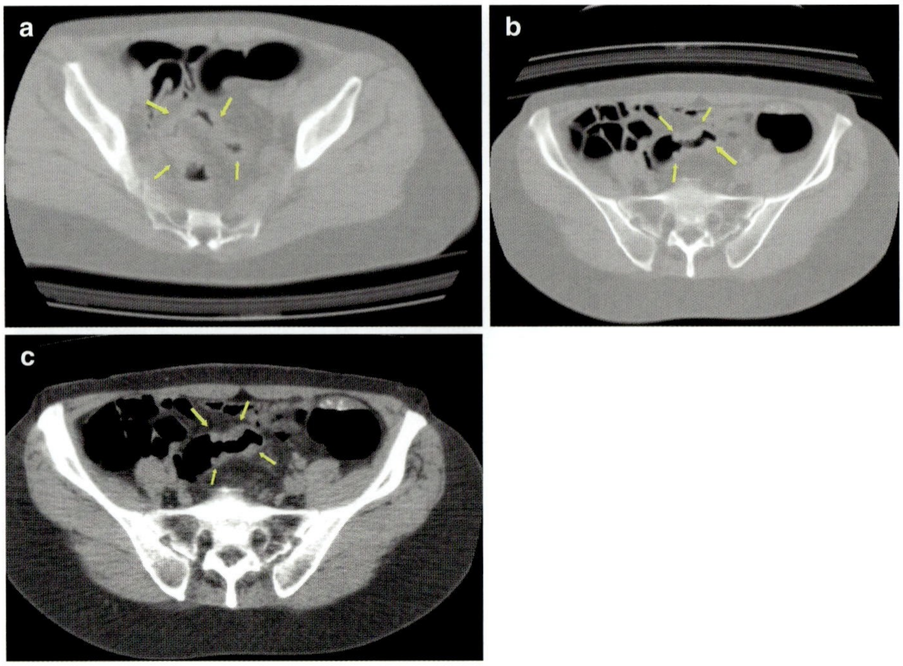

Fig. 10.3. False-negative diagnosis due to incomplete distension. (**a**) Supine image shows a suboptimal distended sigmoid (*arrows*). (**b**) Prone image shows a good distension of the sigmoid, revealing the presence of a tumoral lesion (*arrows*). (**c**) The tumoral lesion is better appreciated using abdominal window settings (*arrows*), compared with intermediate window settings (*arrows* in (**b**)). *Lesson: Optimal distension is a prerequisite to detect colonic lesions. Optimal distension can be achieved by dual positioning and routine use of buthylhioscine (Buscopan®)*

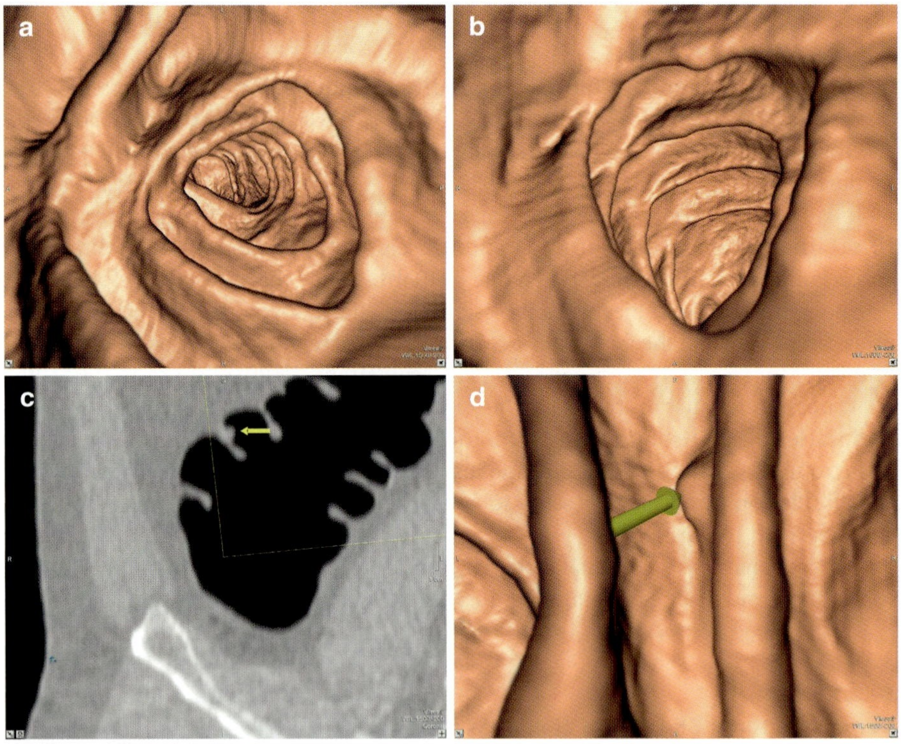

Fig. 10.4. False-negative diagnosis due to blind spots: small sessile lesions, located between haustral folds. (**a**) Antegrade and (**b**) retrograde endoluminal views show normal haustral folds in the ascending colon. (**c**) Corresponding coronal MPR image shows a small sessile lesion, located between two haustral folds (*arrow*). (**d**) Lateral endoluminal 3D image reveals the polyp, located between haustral folds (*arrow*). *Lesson: Primary 3D read should include different viewing angles, by turning the virtual camera, using dedicated software, or offering different 3D reconstruction methods, thus showing the whole colonic wall*

The ileocecal valve is an important "mimicker" of pathology (see later), but one has to keep in mind that the ileocecal valve might hide the polyps (Figs. 10.7 and 10.8), or can even be cancerous (Fig. 10.9). Cancers of the ileocecal valve should not be mistaken for lipomatous or papillary transformations. Different window settings are helpful in revealing the cancerous nature of the lesions.

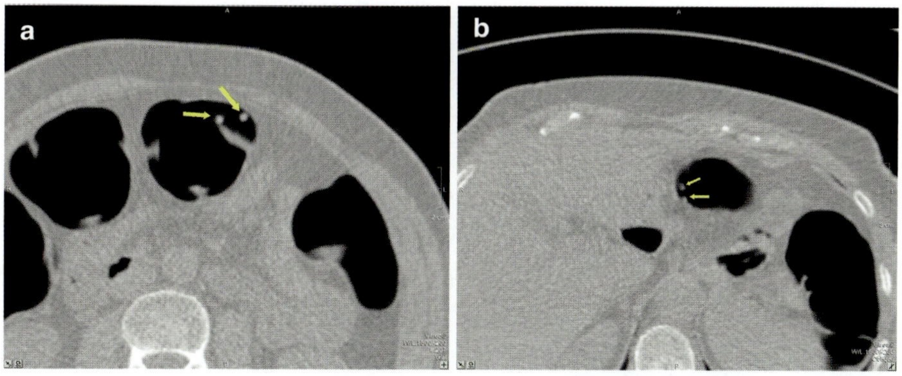

Fig. 10.5. False-negative diagnosis: polyps simulating fecal residue in mobile segments. Differential diagnosis of mobile stool or small sessile lesions in a mobile transverse colon. (**a**) Supine scan shows two lesions in the transverse colon (*arrows*). (**b**) Prone scan shows the lesions in the transverse colon in an apparent different position (*arrows*). Conventional colonoscopy revealed the presence of two small sessile polyps. *Lesson: Polyps, located in mobile colonic segments such as the transverse colon can cause erroneous diagnosis of "mobile" residual stool*

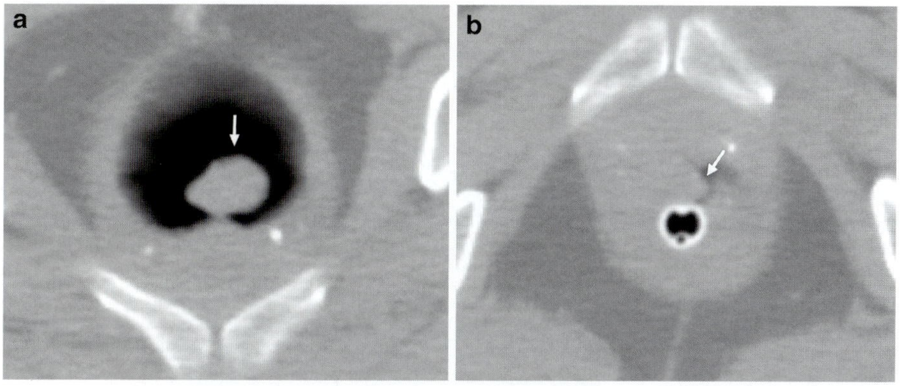

Fig. 10.6. False-negative diagnosis: rectal balloon catheter hiding rectal polyp. (**a**) Prone scan after removing the rectal balloon clearly shows a large stalked polyp (*arrow*). (**b**) The polyp is hidden by the rectal balloon on supine image (*arrow*). *Lesson: Thick rectal balloon catheters can hide rectal lesions. Therefore, remove rectal balloon catheter on prone scan*

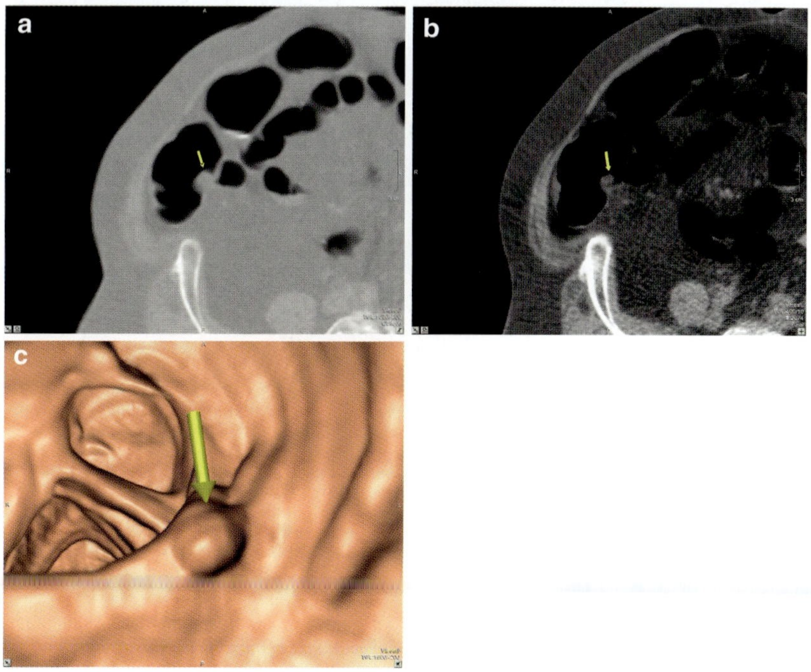

Fig. 10.7. False-negative diagnosis: differentiate small sessile polyps located on the ileocecal valve from normal variations of the ileocecal valve. Although the ileocecal valve is an important "mimicker" of pathology, one has to keep in mind that polyps can arise *on* the ileocecal valve (*arrows* in **a**–**c**). (**a**) Evaluation in "intermediate" window setting, as well as (**b**) "abdominal window setting", combined with (**c**) 3D endoluminal view, are helpful to differentiate polyps from tumoral (see Fig. 10.9) or lipomatous transformation of the ileocecal valve (see Fig. 10.26). *Lesson: For the evaluation of the pathology of the ileocecal valve, always use different window settings, in combination with endoluminal 3D evaluation*

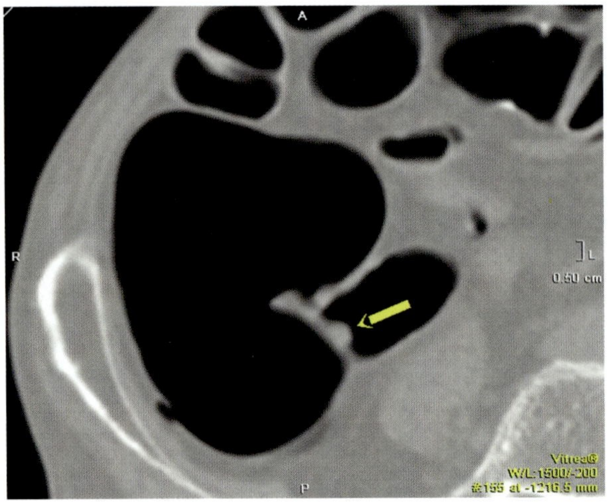

Fig. 10.8. Small sessile polyp located in the ileocecal valve. Although most polyps are located on the ileocecal valve, polyps can also arise in the ileocecal valve (*arrow*)

10.2.1.4
Diverticular Disease

In the case of diverticular disease, prominent semi-circular folds, luminal narrowing, and distortion impede good visualization of the colonic surface, resulting in difficult detection of polypoid lesions. In fact, as optimal detection of polyps is only achieved in well-distended segments of the colon, special care has to be taken when examining the involved segments with shortened haustrations and increased luminal tortuosity. To avoid interpreting a polyp as a thickened fold, or vice versa, it is important to examine each semicircular fold by scrolling back and forth through the axial images. Imaging in both abdominal and lung window settings is mandatory to detect focal-wall thickenings and luminal filling defects, respectively (Lefere et al. 2003). Frequent comparison between two-dimensional (2D) and 3D images is recommended (McFarland 2002) (Fig. 10.10).

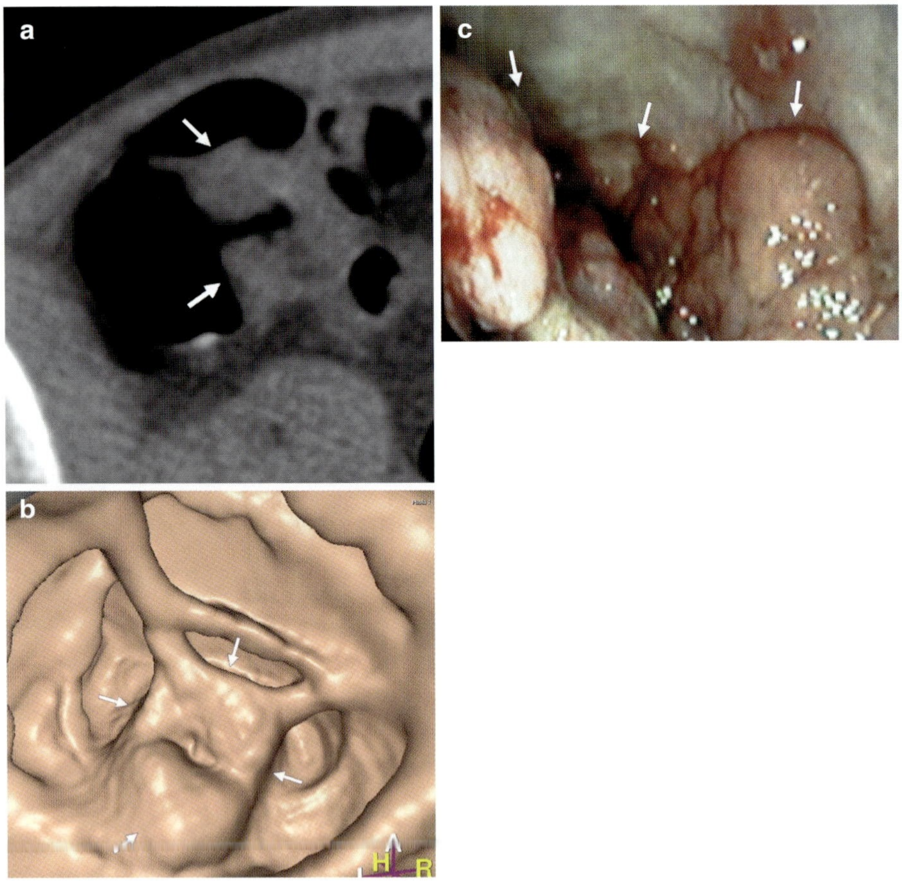

Fig. 10.9. False-negative diagnosis: patient with Crohns' disease: tumoral transformation of the ileocecal valve to be differentiated from lipomatous transformation of the valve. (**a**) Axial 2D image shows a dense, extremely enlarged ileocecal valve on abdominal window settings (thus excluding the possibility of lipomatous transformation) (*arrows*). (**b**) A hypertrofic ileocecal valve is also seen on endoluminal 3D images (*arrows*). (**c**) Corresponding conventional colonoscopic image shows tumoral transformation of the ileocecal valve (*arrows*). *Lesson: In case of an extremely enlarged and dense ileocecal valve, keep in mind the possibility of tumoral transformation, to be differentiated from papillary transformation or lipomatous infiltration of the ileocecal valve (Fig. 10.27). Abdominal window settings are helpful in excluding the possibility of lipomatous transformation of the ileocecal valve*

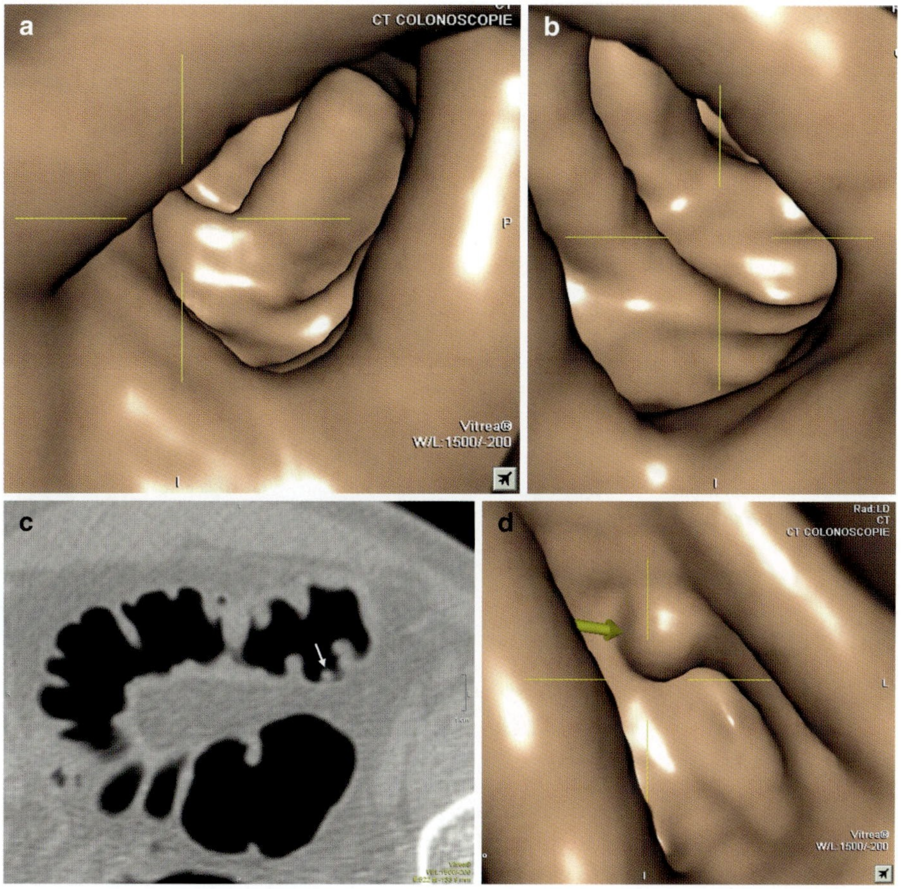

Fig. 10.10. False-negative diagnosis: thickened folds in diverticular disease, hiding a small sessile polyp. Diverticular disease is characterized by thickened semilunar folds. The luminal narrowing and the thickened semilunar folds make primary 3D evaluation extremely difficult. There is a normal antegrade (**a**) and retrograde view (**b**) of the narrow lumen with thickened folds in a patient with diverticular disease. (**c**) Corresponding axial 2D image shows a small polyp, interspaced between two thickened semilunar folds (*arrow*). (**d**) Tailored endoluminal 3D image shows the small polyps (*arrow*) interspaced between thickened haustral folds. *Lesson: In case of diverticular disease, frequent comparison between 2D and 3D images is necessary, to avoid missing small polyps interspaced between thickened haustral folds*

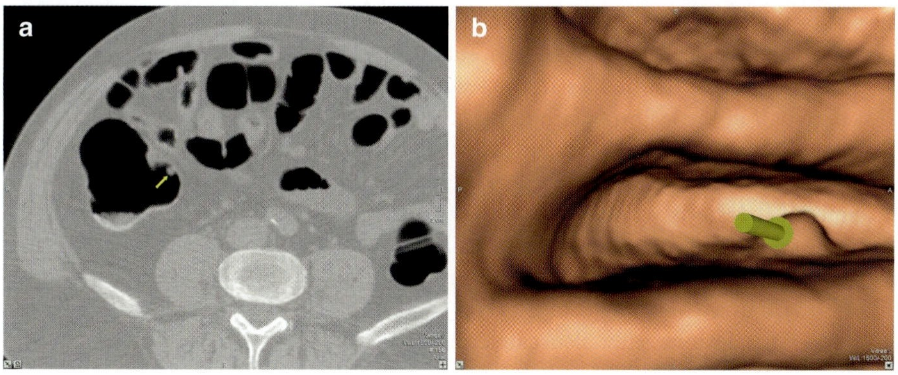

Fig. 10.11. Sessile polyp located between a haustral fold. (**a**) Polyps located *between* normal haustral folds are easy to detect on axial 2D image (*arrow*), and (**b**) corresponding endoluminal 3D image (*arrow*)

10.2.1.5 Sessile Polyps

Although sessile polyps have a high conspicuity if located between folds (Fig. 10.11), the lesions may remain undetected if they are located on a semilunar fold (Fig. 10.12).

A thickened fold in an otherwise well-distended colon might therefore point to the correct diagnosis of a sessile polyp on a haustral fold (Fidler et al. 2004) (see also Fig. 10.18).

10.2.1.6 Small Lesions and Small Flat Lesions

Park et al. (2005) found that for the lesions that were not detected for reasons not apparent on retrospective

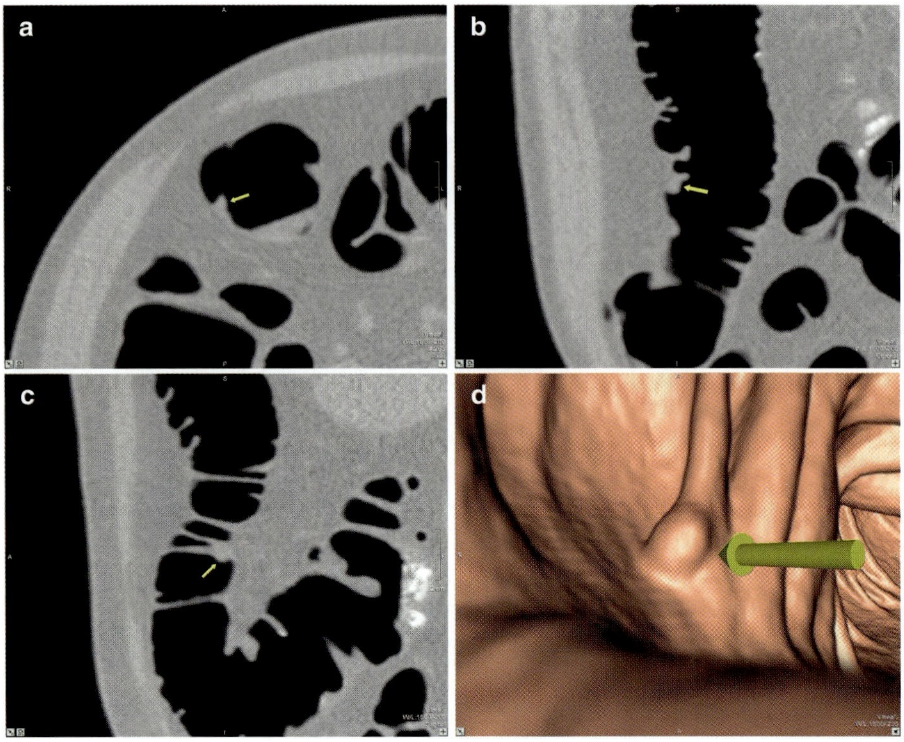

Fig. 10.12. False-negative diagnosis: sessile polyp located on a haustral fold. (**a**) Polyps located on a haustral fold are difficult to detect on axial 2D images (*arrow*). (**b**) Sagittal and (**c**) coronal 2D images show a thickened haustral fold in an otherwise well-distended segment. (**d**) Corresponding endoluminal 3D image clearly shows a polyp on a haustral fold (*arrow*). *Lesson: A thickened haustral fold in an otherwise well-distended segment is suspicious for a polyp on a haustral fold*

analysis, the size of the lesion was the only significant factor associated with lesion detectibility. Lesions of 5 mm or smaller are more difficult to visualize than those that are 6 mm or larger. Up to 50% or more of lesions smaller than 5 mm are, however, non-adenomatous, and the necessity to detect those lesions is therefore questionable (Macari et al. 2004; Pickhardt et al. 2004a, b).

Flat lesions are defined as lesions with a height less than half of the lesion's diameter (Dachman and Zalis 2004). This definition includes a wide range of flat lesions, including small as well as large lesions.

Small flat lesions will be missed, even on retrospective analysis, for the same reason as in the case of small sessile lesions: small lesions are just more difficult to visualize (Macari et al. 2003) (Fig. 10.13).

Larger flat lesions may also cause false-negative diagnosis because of failure to correctly characterize the lesion (see Sect. 10.1.2.2).

10.2.2 Failure to Characterize the Lesions

10.2.2.1 Annular Structuring Lesions

Annular structuring lesions may be misinterpreted as either spasm (Figs. 10.14 and 10.15) or residual fecal material. The use of fecal tagging with an oral contrast agent (Thomeer et al. 2003; Zalis et al. 2003; Pickhardt et al. 2005) seems to help in avoiding interpretive errors caused by residual fecal material.

10.2.2.2 Larger Flat Lesions

Flat lesions can be divided into flat adenomas, flat depressed adenomas, plaque-like carcinomas, and carpet lesions (Galdino and Yee 2003).

As discussed, small flat lesions are difficult to detect for the same reason as small sessile lesions: detection is hampered by resolution.

Larger flat lesions, however, are also difficult to detect and characterize because of several reasons.

First, there is the problem of insufficient awareness and familiarity with those lesions: surveillance programs, based on the known adenoma–carcinoma sequence, have mainly focused on identifying sessile pedunculated polyps. This explains why flat lesions are frequently characterized in normal folds. As a rule, a thickened fold in an otherwise well-distended colon should raise the question of whether or not this lesion could represent a flat lesion.

Second, the plaque-like morphology is likely to be mistaken for residual fecal material (Park et al. 2005):

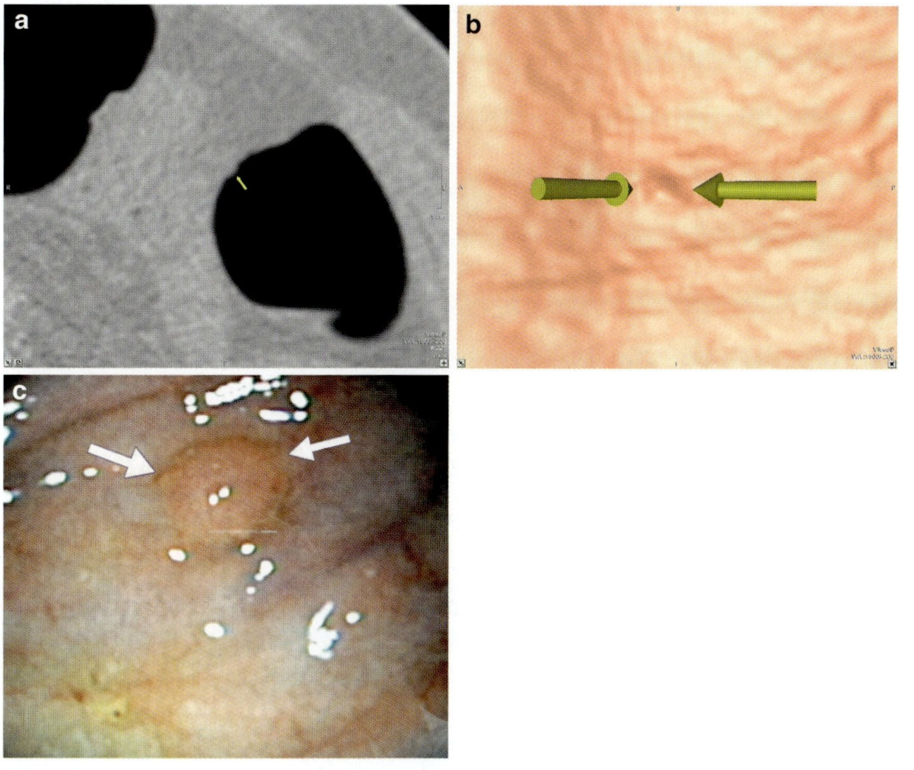

Fig. 10.13. False-negative diagnosis: small (<5 mm) sessile lesion. (**a**) Shows a small sessile 3-mm polyp, prospectively missed. Retrospectively, the lesion was identified on axial (*arrow*) and (**b**) endoluminal 3D image (*arrows*). (**c**) Corresponding conventional colonoscopic image shows a small polyp, representing a hyperplastic polyp on pathological examination (*arrows*). *Lesson: Small polyps (<5 mm) are difficult to detect. However, up to 50% of those lesions are non-adenomatous, and the necessity to detect those lesions is therefore questionable*

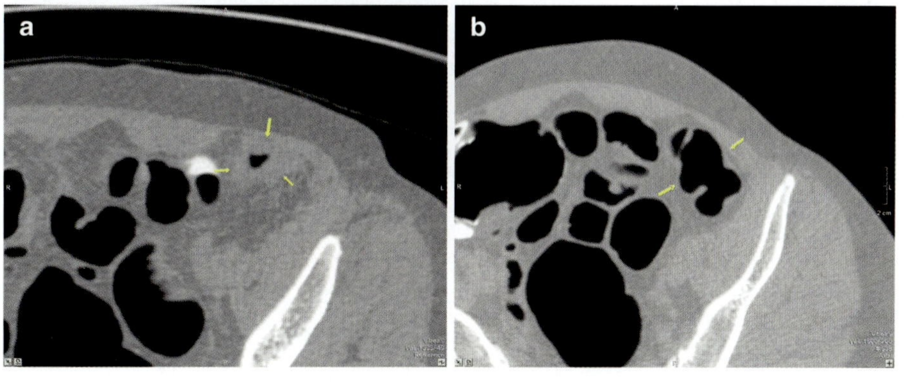

Fig. 10.14. False-positive diagnosis: spasm mimicking annular structuring lesion. Spasm can closely resemble annular structuring lesions (see Fig. 10.15). The *arrows* in (**a**) point towards a non-distended sigmoid region in prone position, (**b**) corresponding supine image shows a normal sigmoid

the use of oral contrast media may therefore help in detecting flat lesions. Third, the size and morphology of the lesions explain the necessity of different window settings (Dachman et al. 2004; Fidler et al. 2002; Park et al. 2007): detection of flat lesions is improved by using abdominal window settings, rather than the routinely used intermediate window settings. The necessity to change window settings also explains the low conspicuity of flat lesions, even the larger ones.

Reviewing the literature shows three different morphological characteristics for flat lesions:

plaque-shaped mucosal elevations with or without central depression, thickened haustral folds, nodular mucosal surfaces (Park et al. 2007) (Figs. 10.16–10.18).

Optimal bowel preparation and distention are therefore prerequisites to detect flat lesions.

Flat adenomas measuring 6 mm or greater are, however, uncommon in a typical Western screening population, and advanced neoplasms are rare. Flat lesions should therefore not be considered a significant drawback for virtual colonoscopy screening (Pickhardt et al. 2004a, b).

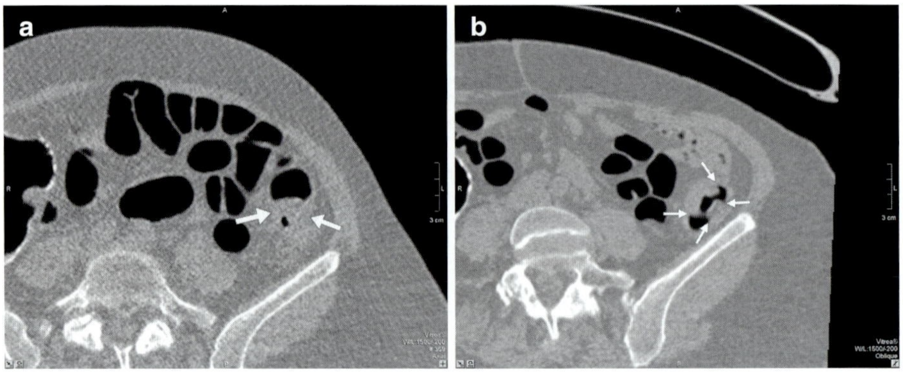

Fig. 10.15. False-negative diagnosis: failure to characterize lesions: annular structuring lesions compared with spasm. The *arrows* in (**a**) point toward a non-distended sigmoid region in supine position. (**b**) Corresponding prone images show a persistent wall thickening with shoulder forming (*arrows*). Conventional colonoscopy showed a tumoral lesion. *Lesson: Annular structuring lesions can closely resemble spasm. Dual positioning is mandatory to avoid those pitfalls (compare Figs. 10.14 and 10.15)*

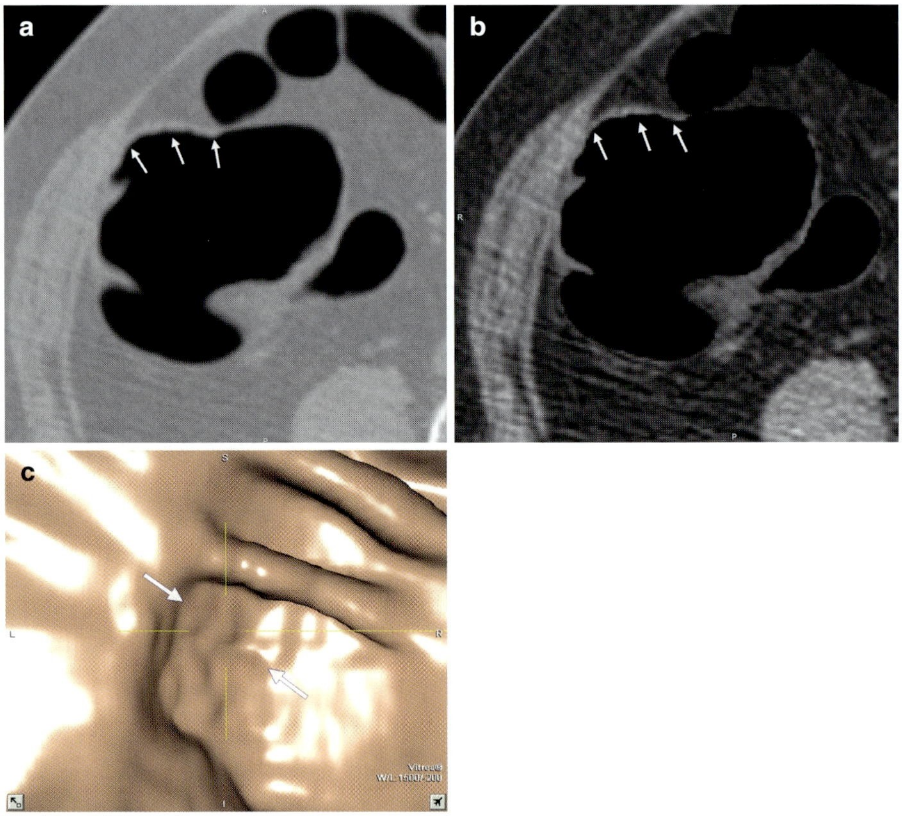

Fig. 10.16. False-negative diagnosis: failure to characterize lesions: Flat lesions. (**a–c**) Flat lesion in the cecum at the level of the ileocecal valve with nodular mucosal surface. (**a**) Axial image at the level of the ileocecal valve shows subtle wall thickening on intermediate window settings (*arrows*), better appreciated on (**b**) abdominal window settings (*arrows*). (**c**) 3D endo-view image shows subtle wall thickening (*arrows*). Pathology showed a tubular adenoma. *Lesson: Flat lesions have been defined as lesions with a height less than half the lesion diameter. This nature makes them difficult to recognize. As in this patient, changing the window settings is helpful in diagnosing these lesions*

10.2.2.3
Small Sessile Polyps

Small sessile polyps frequently represent hyperplastic polyps. Hyperplastic lesions tend to flatten out in well-distended segments, explaining the fact that those lesions might only be visible in somewhat underdistended segments. In that way, those lesions are frequently only recognized on either prone or supine position, and can therefore be mistaken as residual stool.

Hyperplastic lesions, however, are not to be considered precancerous, and should therefore be considered as "leave-alone" lesions. Misinterpreting those lesions as residual stool is therefore rather beneficial for the

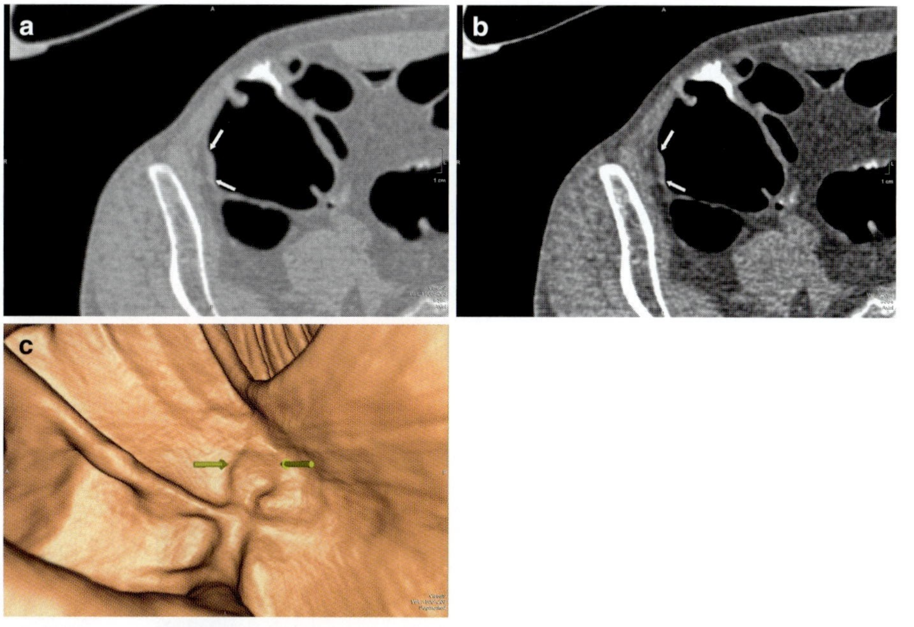

Fig. 10.17. Flat lesion appearing as plaque-shaped mucosal elevation without central depression. (**a**, **b**) 2D axial image at intermediate window settings shows a slightly elevated lesion (*arrows*), more apparently appreciated on abdominal window settings (*arrows* in (**b**)). (**c**) 3D endo-view image shows the slightly elevated lesion, without central depression (*arrows*). Diagnosis: flat adenoma with moderate-grade dysplasia

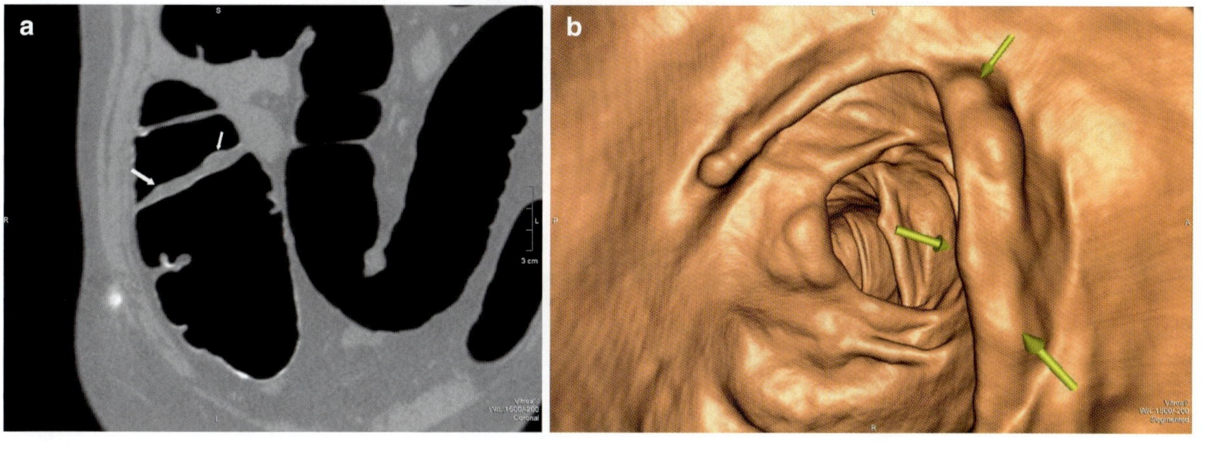

Fig. 10.18. Flat lesion appearing as thickened hasutral fold. (**a**) Coronal image shows a thickened haustral fold in the right hemicolon (*arrows*). (**b**) 3D endo-view image shows lesion that presents as nodular thickening of haustral fold (*arrows*). Diagnosis: flat adenoma with low-grade dysplasia. Courtesy: Cremers, MMC, Eindhoven, The Netherlands

patients, avoiding unnecessary conventional colonoscopy (Pickhardt et al. 2004a) (Fig. 10.19).

10.2.2.4 Sessile Cancers

Sessile cancers, if detected, may remain unrecognized due to the fact that the lesions are characterized as normal fold; correlating axial 3D images with endoluminal views is helpful in this respect (Fig. 10.20).

Sessile cancers may also be mistaken for residual stool because of marked surface irregularity, usually attributed to residual stool (Gluecker et al. 2004).

10.2.2.5 Pedunculated Lesions

Pedunculated lesions may remain undetected because of mischaracterization as fecal residues or even residual fluid.

Mischaracterization as fecal residues is caused by the fact that there are three observations that are made to distinguish stool from polyps: presence of gas, morphology (polyps and small cancers have rounded and lobulated smooth borders), and mobility. Especially the mobility of the lesions is used in favor of residual stool, analogous to the findings on double-contrast barium enema (Laks et al. 2004).

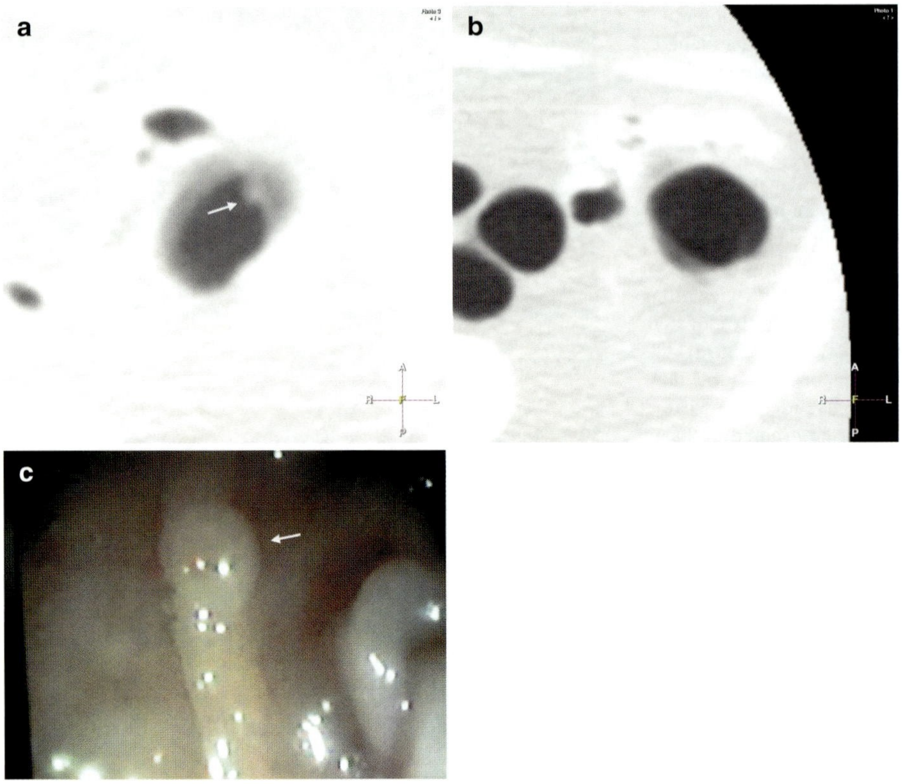

Fig. 10.19. False-negative diagnosis: failure to characterize lesions: hyperplastic lesions. (**a**) Axial, supine 2D image shows a small polyp-like lesion (*arrow*) in a suboptimal distended segment. (**b**) Corresponding prone scan shows a better distended descending colon, and does not show the lesion anymore. Differential diagnosis was made between hyperplastic polyp and fecal residue. (**c**) Corresponding conventional colonoscopy revealed a small hyperplastic polyp. *Lesson: Hyperplastic lesions tend to flatten out in well-distended segments, impeding visualization in prone or supine position. Therefore, they are frequently misinterpreted as mobile fecal residue*

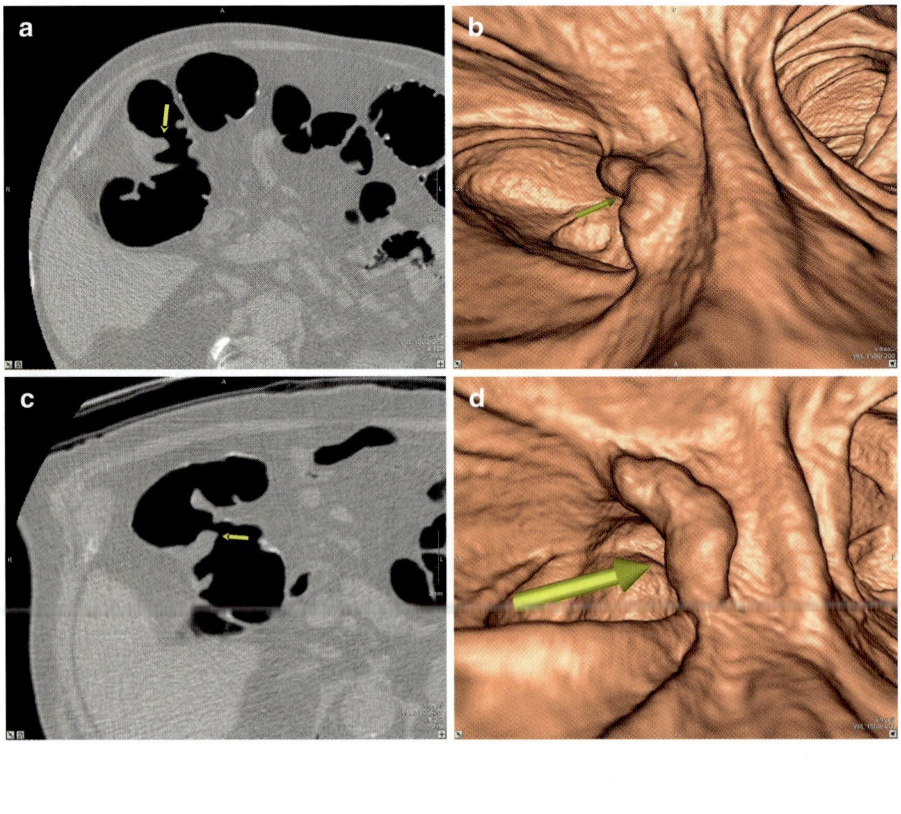

Fig. 10.20. False-negative diagnosis: failure to characterize the lesions: sessile cancer. (**a**, **c**) show a broad-based thickened haustral fold on supine (*arrows* in (**a**)) and prone image (*arrows* in (**c**)) at the hepatic flexure. Differential diagnosis: complex haustral fold, normal thickened fold or sessile cancer. Corresponding endoluminal 3D images (**b**, **d**) showed distorted and thickened haustral fold on supine (*arrow* in (**b**)) as well as prone scan (arrow in (**d**)). Conventional colonoscopy showed a flat sessile cancer. *Lesson: Endoluminal 3D images are useful to differentiate normal thickened folds from sessile cancers (compare with Fig. 10.32)*

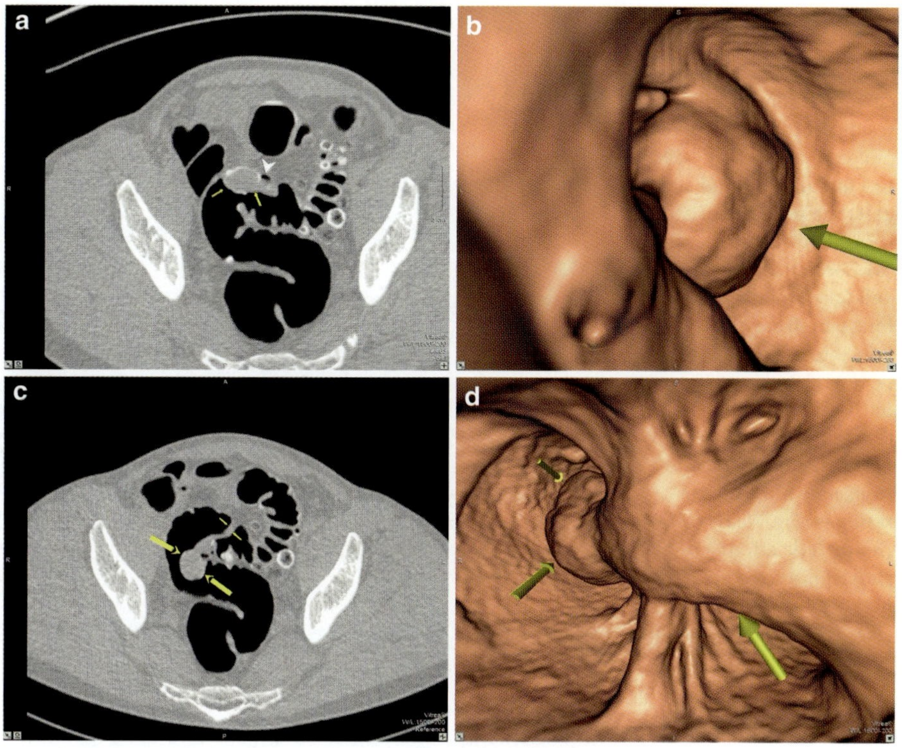

Fig. 10.21. False-negative diagnosis: failure to characterize the lesions – pedunculated lesions mimicking residual stool. (**a**) Prone image shows a nodular mass (*arrows*), with air included in the mass (*arrowhead*). (**b**) Corresponding endoluminal 3D image shows a nodular lesion (*arrow*). (**c**) Supine image shows that the lesion is highly mobile (*large arrows*), and suggests the presence of a stalk (*small arrows*). (**d**) The supine-endoluminal image clearly shows a pedunculated lesion (*arrows*)

Pedunculated polyps, however, change in position between prone and supine images, and may moreover include gas between the stalk and the bowel wall, mimicking residual stool (Fig. 10.21). A pedunculated polyp can also mimic residual fluid (Fig. 10.22).

10.3 False-Positive Diagnosis

10.3.1 Preparation-Related False-Positive Findings

One of the major reasons why virtual colonoscopy is attractive to the patients is its ability to evaluate the colon without the need of an intensive colon-cleansing regimen. Different reduced preparations have been evaluated: reduced amount of PEG in combination with bisacodyl, magnesium carbonate with citric acid (Citramag®, Pharmaserve LTD, Manchester), a combination of sodium picosulfate with magnesium citrate (Picolax®, Ferring Pharmaceuticals Ltd, Berkshire), magnesium citrate combined with bisacodyl tablets and suppository (Losoprep®, EZ-EM , Westbury, NY), and fleet phosphosoda (Yee 2002; Taylor et al. 2003a–d; Gryspeerdt et al. 2002; Macari et al. 2001).

Compared with the standard colon-cleansing regimens, each of these reduced preparations showed fewer side effects and disturbances in the patient's daily life, while inviting improved patient compliance.

The driest preparations (Picolax®) (Taylor et al. 2003a–d), Losoprep® (Lefere et al. 2002) and fleet phosphosoda (Macari et al. 2001); however, are associated with more retained residue, with subsequent increased risk of false-positive findings. False-positive findings are mainly related to small fecal residue: larger residues will shift between prone and supine imaging, while smaller residues stick to the wall.

Therefore, there is the need for fecal tagging: fecal tagging reduces false-positive diagnosis (Lefere et al. 2002; Gryspeerdt et al. 2002) (Figs. 10.23–10.25).

10.3.2 Technical Artifacts Causing False-Positive Findings

10.3.2.1 Breathing Artifacts

Most published studies using single-slice CT have used a collimation of 3–5 mm and a pitch of 1–2, resulting in breathhold times ranging from 35 to 50 s.

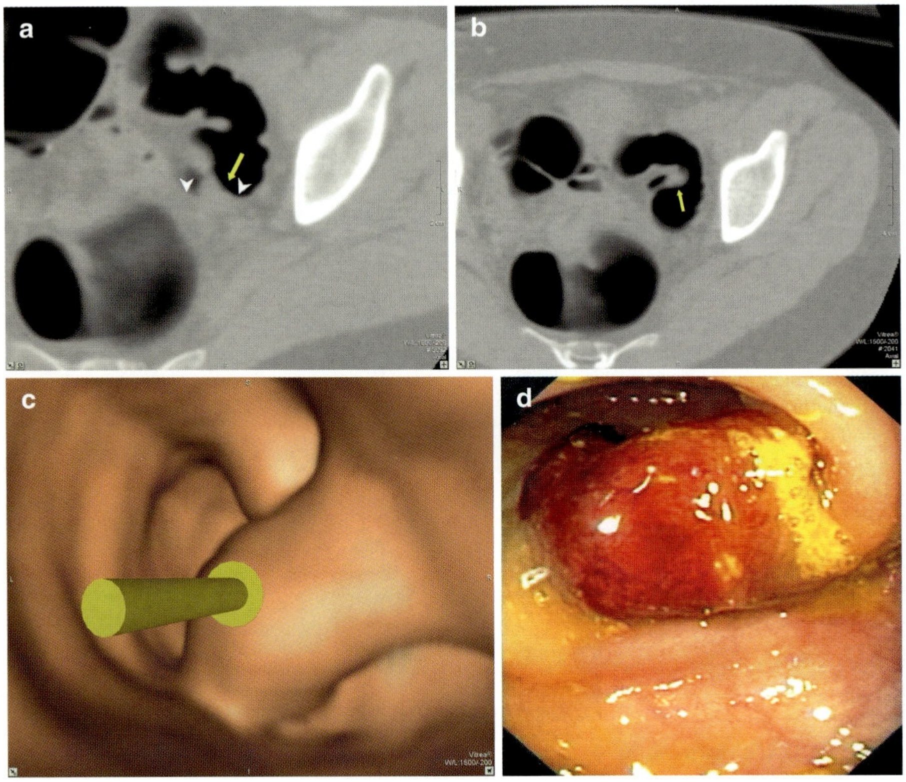

Fig. 10.22. False negative diagnosis: failure to characterize the lesions – pedunculated lesions mimicking residual fluid. (**a**) Supine image shows a thick haustral fold (*arrow*) and suggests the presence of a fluid level (*arrowheads*). (**b**) Corresponding axial and (**c**) endoluminal 3D image in prone position shows the stalk of a pedunculated lesion (*arrows* in (**b–d**)), proven on (**d**) conventional colonoscopy. *Lesson: Pedunculated lesions may mimic fecal residues (Fig. 10.21) (they can include air, due to their stalked nature, and are highly mobile) or fluid levels (Fig. 10.22). Identifying the stalk on 3D endoluminal images points to the diagnosis of a pedunculated lesion*

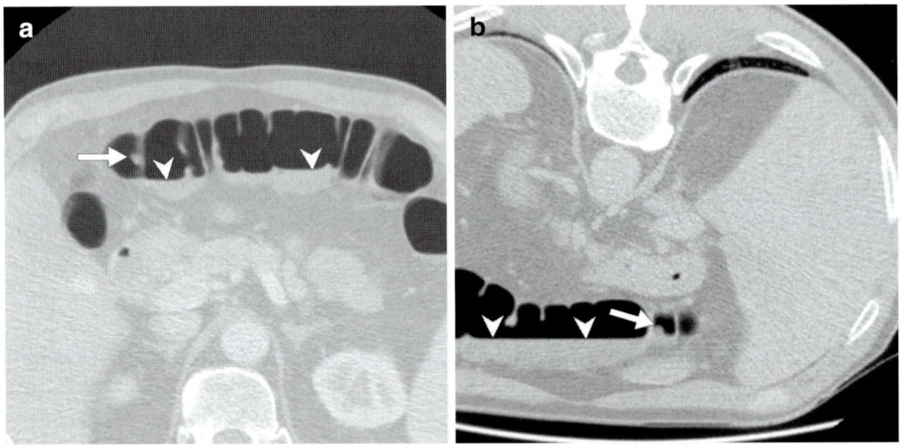

Fig. 10.23. False-positive diagnosis: adherent fecal residue. Fecal tagging facilitated differential diagnosis between fecal residue and polyp. Standard colonoscopic cleansing: false-positive diagnosis of polyp due to adherent fecal residue. (**a**) Supine and (**b**) prone images in a patient with incomplete visualization of the cecum due to redundancy, suggested the presence of a 10-mm polypoid lesion in the transverse colon (*arrow* in (**a**, **b**)). As the transverse colon was reached on repeated conventional colonoscopy, and no lesion was detected, this lesion was interpreted as false-positive due to adherent fecal residue. *Arrowheads* in (**a**, **b**) non-tagged fluid levels, adherent to standard colonoscopic preparation

Such long breathhold periods are prone to breathing artifacts, simulating polyps. The introduction of multislice CT technology now permits thinner collimation (1–2.5 mm) and reduced breathhold time (15–20 s) (Embleton et al. 2003; Taylor et al. 2003a–d). These reduced breathhold times virtually eliminate severe artifacts. If the patients are still unable to maintain a breathhold time, then the left decubitus scanning has

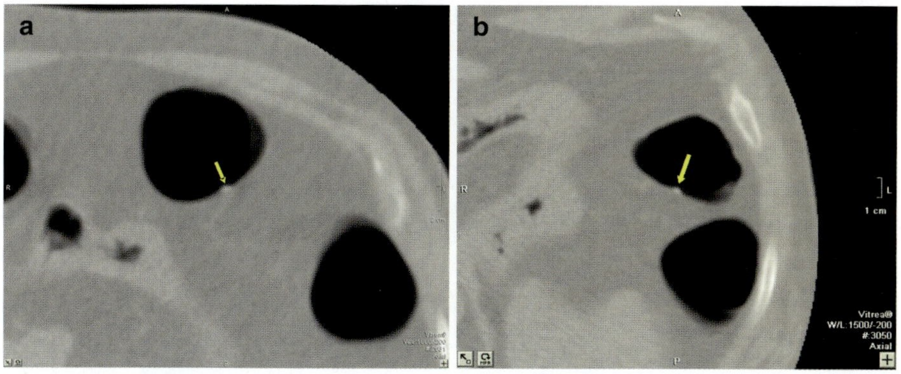

Fig. 10.24. False-positive diagnosis: adherent fecal residue. Fecal tagging facilitated differential diagnosis between fecal residue and polyp. Reduced preparation with fecal tagging using barium as the sole tagging agent: There is a 4-mm lesion on (**a**) supine (*arrow*) and (**b**) prone (*arrow*) image. The lesion is hyperdense, pointing toward a tagged fecal residue. Conventional colonoscopy did not show any lesions in this patient

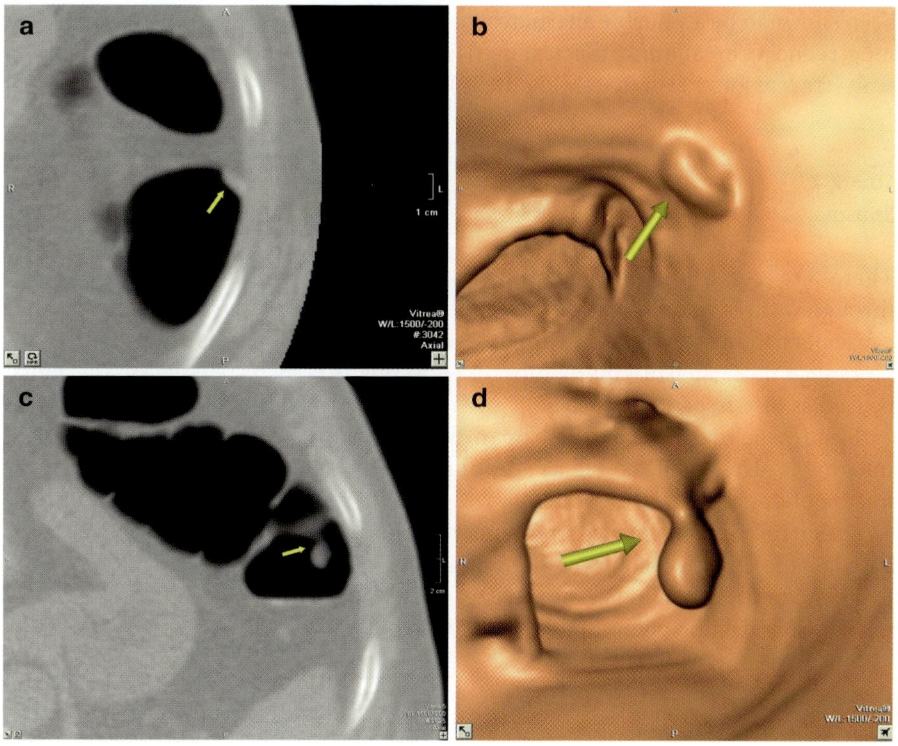

Fig. 10.25. False-positive diagnosis: adherent fecal residue. Fecal tagging facilitated differential diagnosis between fecal residue and polyp. Reduced preparation with fecal tagging using barium as the sole tagging agent: (**a**) axial and (**b**) endoluminal 3D image in prone position. There is a 6-mm non-tagged lesion at the splenic flexure (*arrow* in (**a**, **b**)). The non-tagged nature suggests the presence of a polyp. (**c**) Corresponding axial and (**d**) endoluminal 3D image in supine position: the non-tagged lesion, seen on prone image, corresponds to a pedunculated polyp (*arrow* in (**c**, **d**)). *Lesson: fecal tagging reduces false-positive findings due to adherent fecal residue, improves conspicuity of polyps, and reduces false positives, as the tagged or non-tagged nature of the lesions allows easy differentiation between polyps and fecal residues*

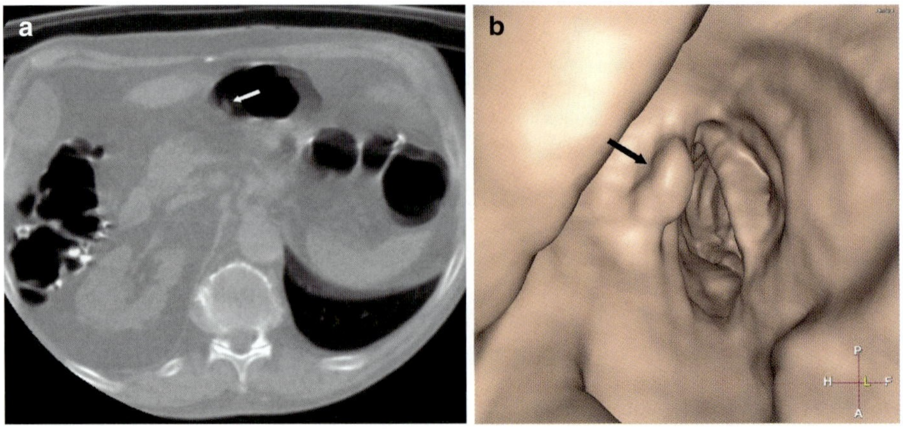

Fig. 10.26. False-positive diagnosis: pseudopolyp due to breathing artifacts. (**a**) Axial 2D image obtained in a 66-year-old patient in prone position shows breathing artifacts (*arrow*). (**b**) Corresponding endoluminal 3D image shows pseudopolypoid appearance of the colonic wall, caused by breathing artifact (*arrow*). *Lesson: In patients who are extremely short of breath, especially prone scanning can be hampered by breathing artifacts, causing pseudo-polypoid appearance on endoluminal 3D images. Left/decubitus scanning instead of prone scanning can be used as an alternative*

been shown to be a valuable alternative to prone scanning, reducing breathing artifacts if used as the second scan (Gryspeerdt et al. 2004) (Fig. 10.26).

10.3.2.2 Spasm

There are seven different sphincters distributed throughout the colon. Each of these sphincters can cause persistent spasms, mimicking tumoral disease. To reduce those spasms, buthylhioscin (Buscopan®) is used as discussed previously.

Besides the routine use of Buscopan, dual position imaging is also useful, as well as additional inflation in case of doubt (Fig. 10.27).

Spasm can be differentiated from tumoral pathology, based on the smooth contours of the spasms, in contrast to the circumferential tumors. The presence of surrounding lymph nodes also points toward tumoral pathology.

10.3.3 Pitfalls Related to Normal Anatomy and Non-Tumoral Lesions

10.3.3.1 Ileocecal Valve

The ileocecal valve is located between the large and small bowel, and consists of two segments, the upper and lower lips. The ileocecal valve can appear as a thin slit-like structure, large intraluminal mass, or being almost invisible. There are three different endoscopic appearances: the labial type, with a slit-like appearance, the papillary type, with a dome shaped appearance, and lipomatous type, with deposits of fat within the lips.

Most visible valves are of the labial type (78%), 21% is of the papillary type, and 3% is lipomatous.

Lipomatous and papillary ileocecal valves can mimic neoplasms, and should be differentiated from polyps on the ileocecal valves (Fig. 10.28).

Prolapsing ileocecal valves appear prominent, irrespective of the labial or papillary morphology, and may mimic polyps (Fig. 10.29) (Iafrate et al. 2007, Regge et al. 2005).

10.3.3.2 Extrinsic Impression

Any organ or structure outside the colon can cause external impression. They compress the colon and may appear as focal neoplasms on 3D endoluminal images. We have noted impressions from the spleen, liver, other bowel loops, spine, psoas muscle, aorta and iliac arteries, as well as uterine fibroids (Fig. 10.30) (Macari and Megibow 2001).

10.3.3.3 Complex or Thickened Folds

Complex or thickened folds are typically encountered at the splenic and hepatic flexures. Axial CT images might raise the possibility of intraluminal soft-tissue

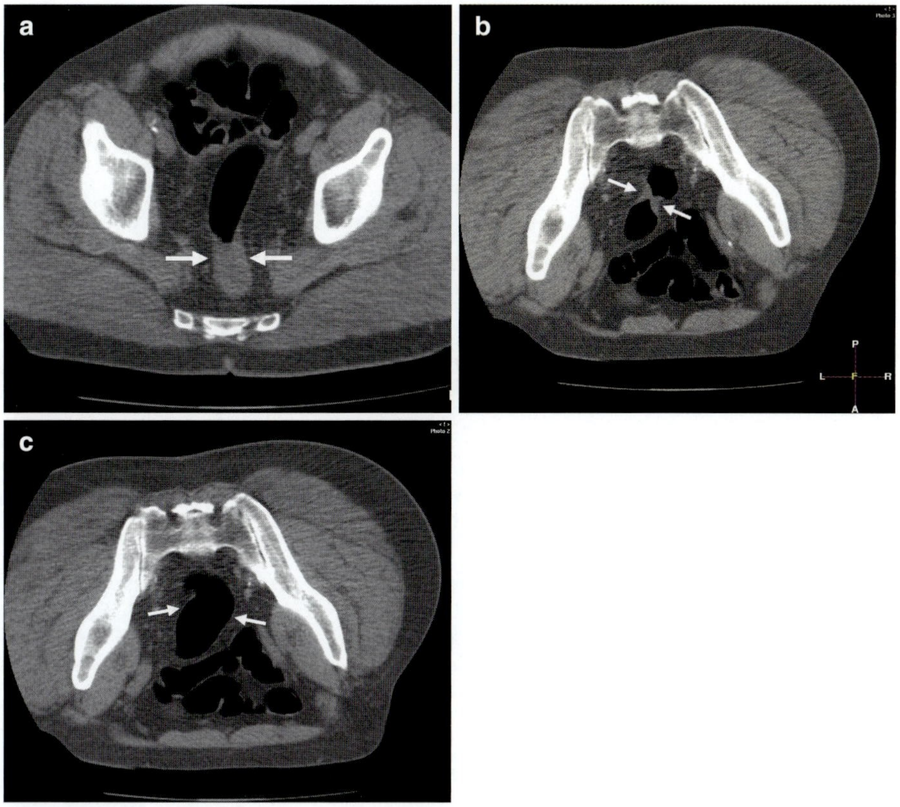

Fig. 10.27. False-positive diagnosis: spasm of the Ring of Rossi mimicking tumoral disease. (**a**) Supine and (**b**) prone scanning images show persistent incomplete distention of the sigmoid (*arrows* in (**a**, **b**)). Differential diagnosis was made between spasm of the Ring of Rossi and tumoral disease. The soft contours of the lesions suggested a persistent spasm. Additional inflation was performed and subsequent re-evaluation showed normal sigmoid. (**c**) Diagnosis of spasm of the Ring of Rossi was made. *Lesson: Persistent spasms of colonic sphincters can mimic tumoral disease. Administration of Buthylhioscin (Buscopan®) or additional inflation helps to relieve the spasm. Morphological characteristics, helpful in differential diagnosis, are the smooth contours and absence of lymph nodes in case of spasm*

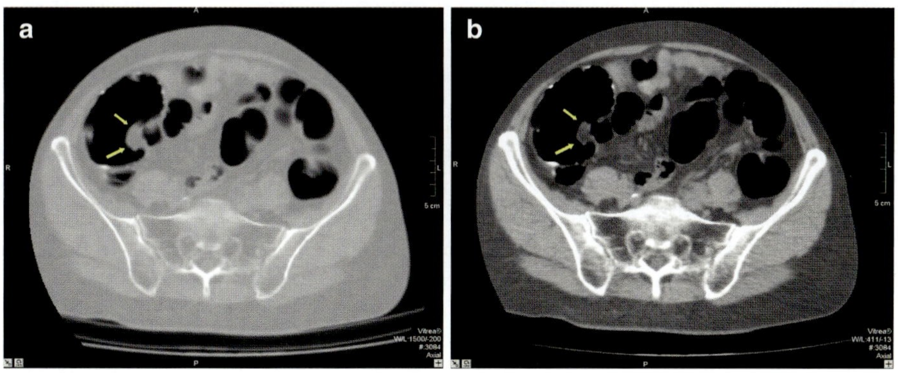

Fig. 10.28. False-positive diagnosis: lipomatous transformation of the ileocecal valve. (**a**) Supine image in intermediate window settings shows a hypertrophic nodular ileocecal valve. Differential diagnosis: tumor – lipomatous or papillary transformation of the ileocecal valve. (**b**) Same image as (**a**): abdominal window setting clearly shows the lipomatous transformation of the ileocecal valve. *Lesson: Lipomatous transformation is a "pseudotumoral" alteration of the ileocecal valve. Use different window settings to reveal the lipomatous nature of the valve. Compare with Figs. 10.7–10.9*

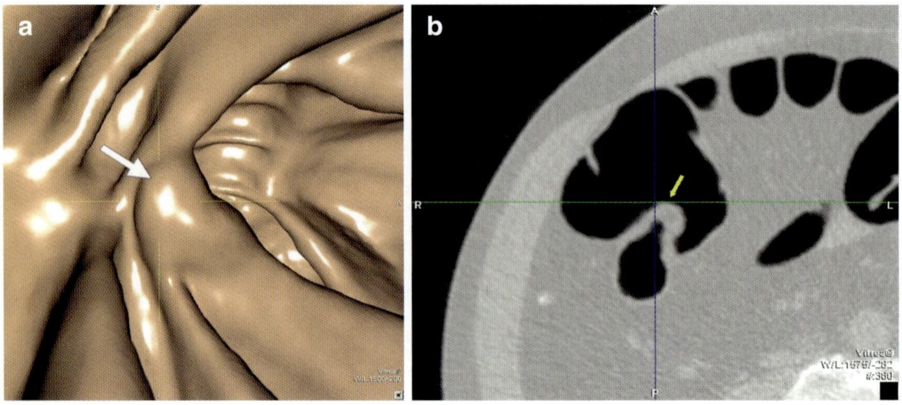

Fig. 10.29. False-positive diagnosis: prolapsing ileocecal valve. (**a**) Endoluminal 3D image shows a nodular appearance of the ileocecal valve (*arrow*). (**b**) Corresponding axial image shows that the polypoid appearance is caused by a prolapsing ileocecal valve. *Lesson: A prolapsing ileocecal valve mimics polypoid pathology on endoluminal 3D image. In comparison, axial 2D correctly points to the diagnosis*

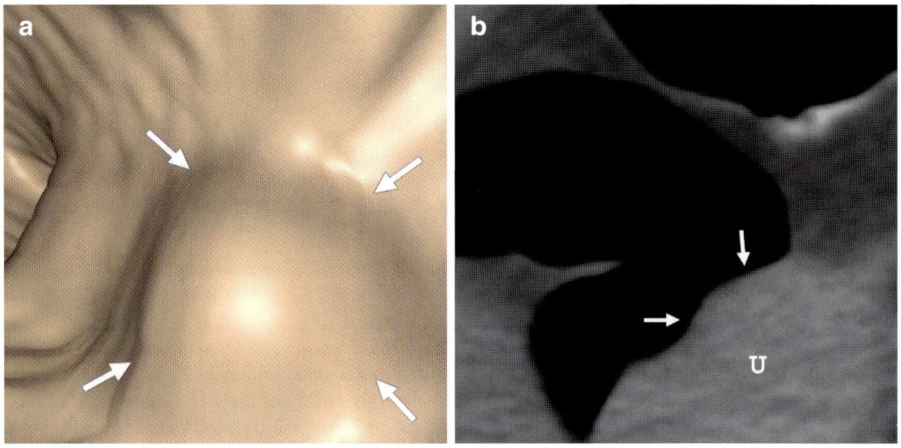

Fig. 10.30. False-positive diagnosis: external impression. (**a**) Endoluminal 3D image shows a smoothly delineated nodule in the sigmoid (*arrows*). (**b**) Corresponding axial image shows the nodule is caused by extrinsic uterine impression (*arrows*; *U* uterus). *Lesson: Any organ or structure outside the colon can cause external compression. On endoluminal view, these extrinsic impressions simulate tumoral or polypoid disease. Careful correlation of endoluminal 3D image with axial images points toward the diagnosis of external impression*

masses or tumoral thickened folds. Endoluminal views are frequently helpful in identifying the mass as a complex pattern of normal haustral folds. Endoluminal imaging is also extremely helpful in showing the smooth contours of complex normal folds, as opposed to the irregularity caused by tumoral pathology (compare Fig. 10.31 with Fig. 10.20).

10.3.3.4 Submucosal Non-Tumoral Lesions

Lipomas are rare, but well-recognized "tumors" of the colon. They are more common in the right colon than the left colon. They arise from the submucosa, and may protrude into the lumen as either polypoid or nodular tumor-like lesions. Diagnosis of their lipomatous nature can be easily be made by viewing the "tumor" in abdominal window settings. (Pickhardt 2004) (Fig. 10.32).

Colonic varices are a complication of portal hypertension, and can be seen in the anorectal region, as well as throughout the whole colon. Varices are typically smoothly delineated linear lesions. Identification of afferent venous structures points toward the diagnosis (Fig. 10.33).

Hemorrhoids can be tiny, or extremely large, mimicking tumoral pathology. They typically appear

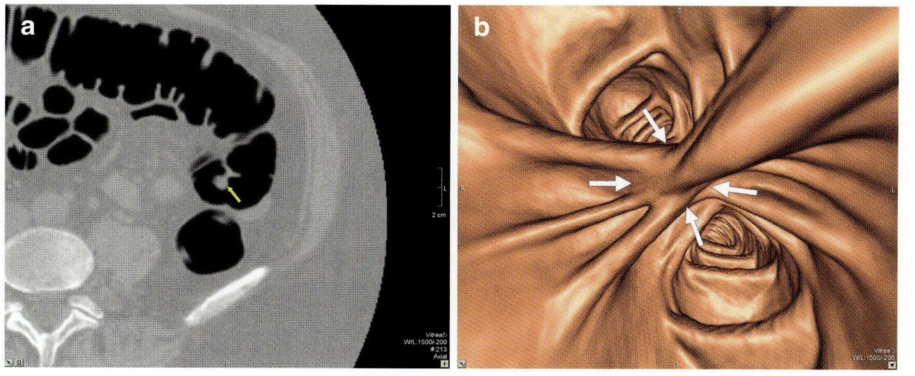

Fig. 10.31. False-positive diagnosis: complex folds. (**a**) Axial image shows the splenic flexure, with a thickened nodular-like fold (*arrow*). (**b**) Corresponding endoluminal 3D image clearly shows that the thickened nodular appearance can be explained by the complexity of the folds at the splenic flexure. *Lesson: Complex or thickened folds are typically encountered at the splenic and hepatic flexures, and should be differentiated from sessile cancers or polyps. Endoluminal 3D images are extremely helpful for differential diagnosis. Compare with Fig. 10.18*

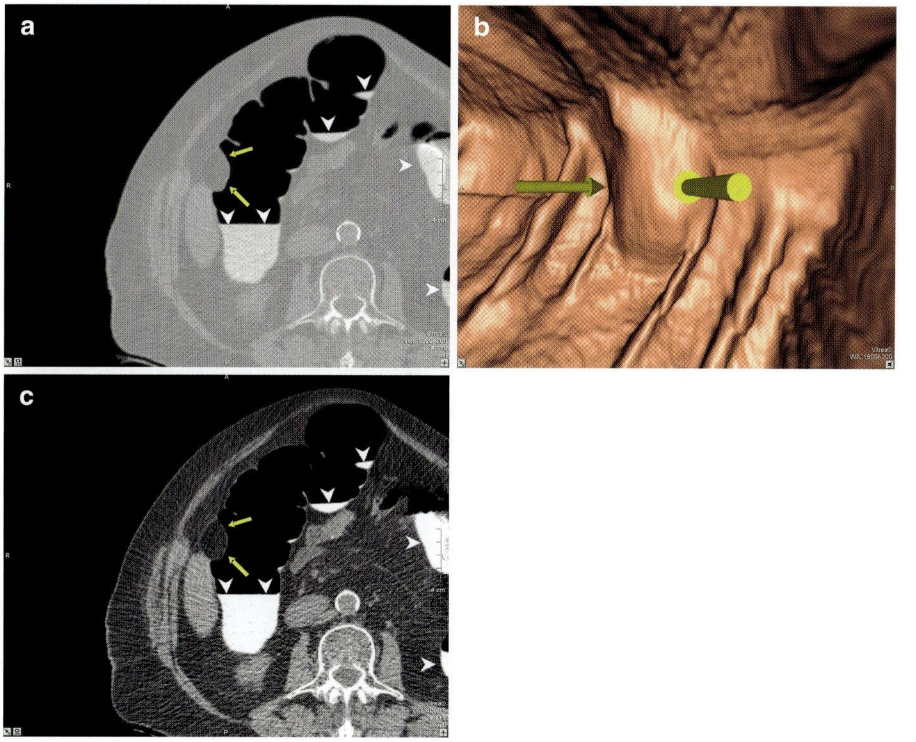

Fig. 10.32. False-positive diagnosis: lipoma. Axial image (**a**; intermediate window settings) and (**b**) endoluminal 3D image show a nodular distortion of the colonic wall at the hepatic flexure (*arrows* in (**a**, **b**)). (**c**) Corresponding axial image using abdominal window settings shows the lipomatous nature of this lesion. Diagnosis: lipoma. Note: *arrowheads* point toward tagged fluid levels. *Lesson: Lipomas are submucosal lesions that are to be considered as "leave-alone" lesions. Correct diagnosis can easily be made by viewing the "tumor" in abdominal window settings*

as linear, smoothly delineated mucosal irregularities proximal to the anorectal margin (Fig. 10.34).

Cystic pneumomatosis of the colon is a rare disease, characterized by tiny air-filled cysts. It may be related to a large variety of diseases like ischemia or infection of the colon, or idiopathic (Sala et al. 2005). Pickhardt reported asymptomatic right-sided colonic pneumatosis as a rare self-limited condition associated with carbon dioxide delivered at CTC (Pickhardt et al. 2008) (Fig. 10.35).

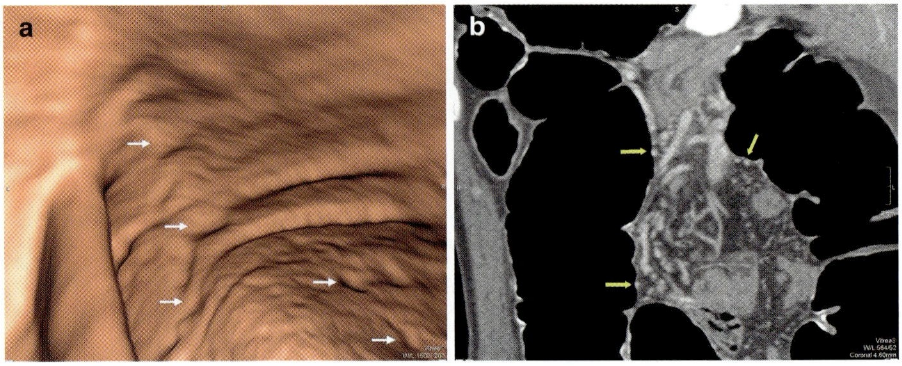

Fig. 10.33. False-positive diagnosis: submucosal vascular lesions. (**a**) Endoluminal 3D image in a patient with severe portal hypertension shows multiple tiny polyp-like lesions, distributed throughout the colon (*arrows*). (**b**) Corresponding contrast-enhanced coronal reformatted MPR image shows multiple submucosal veins, explaining the polyp-like lesions on endoluminal 3D images (*arrows*). *Lesson: In patients with known portal hypertension, consider possible submucosal colonic varices, explaining multiple tiny nodular lesions on endoluminal 3D imaging. Identification of afferent venous structures points toward the diagnosis*

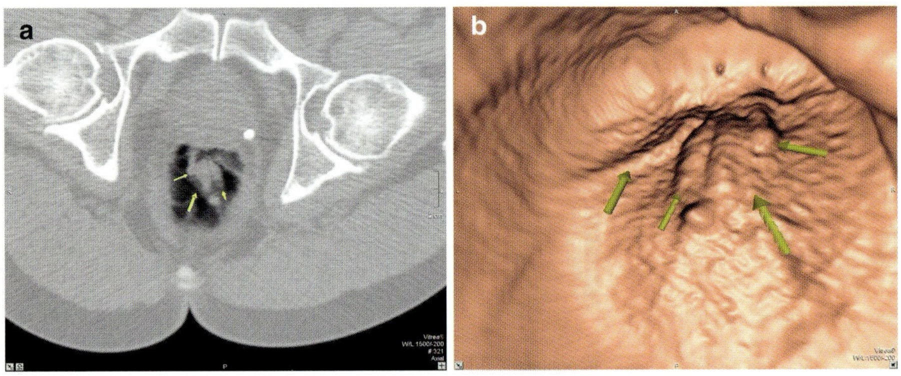

Fig. 10.34. False-positive diagnosis: internal hemorrhoids. (**a**) Axial image shows irregular, linear structures at the anorectal region (*arrows*). (**b**) Corresponding endoluminal 3D image shows linear, smoothly delineated structures at the anorectal junction (*arrows*). Diagnosis: internal hemorrhoids

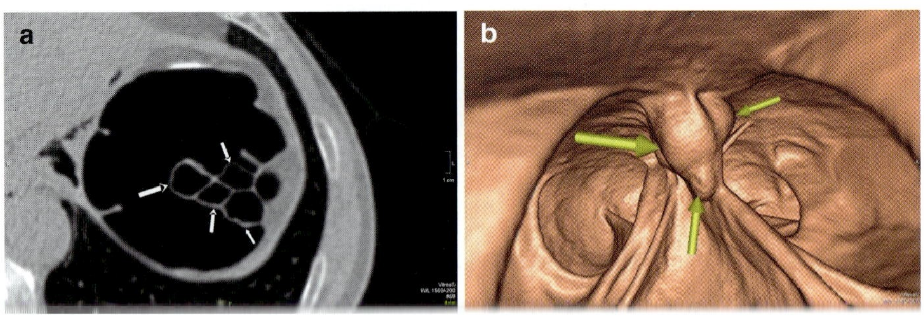

Fig. 10.35. False-positive diagnosis: pneumatosis coli. (**a**) Axial image using lung window settings clearly shows multiple rounded well-defined intramural air collections in the wall of the distended colon at the splenic flexure (*arrows*). (**b**) Corresponding endoluminal 3D image shows multiple polypoid lesions (*arrows*). Diagnosis: accidentally discovered pneumatosis coli. Courtesy: Ranschaert, Jeroen Bosch Ziekenhuis, Hertogenbosch, The Netherlands

10.3.3.5
Appendiceal Orifice

The normal appearance of appendiceal orifice is a slit-like orifice (Fig. 10.36). The appendiceal orifice can however also protrude, simulating polypoid disease (Fig. 10.37). In case of previous appendectomy, the appendiceal stump can also simulate polypoid disease. The anatomical location, clearly illustrated on coronal or sagittal reformats, points to the diagnosis (Taylor et al. 2003a–d).

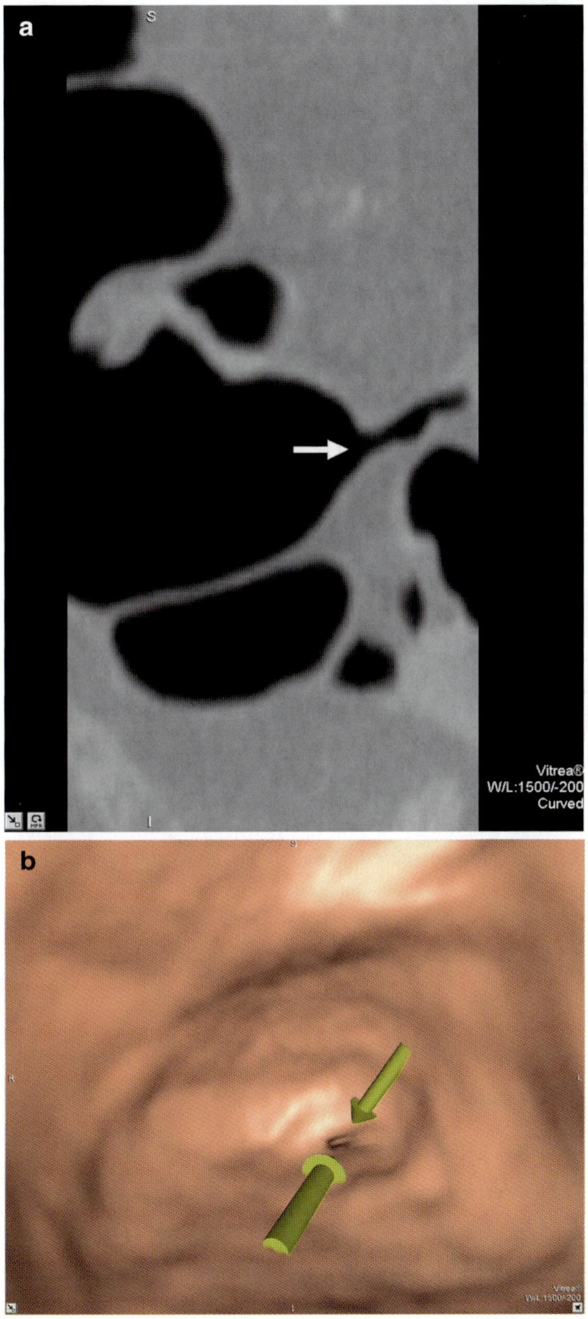

Fig. 10.36. Normal appendiceal orifice. (**a**, **b**) Curved reformatted MPR image shows normal appendiceal orifice (*arrow* in (**a**)), appearing as a slit-like orifice on endoluminal 3D images (*arrows* in (**b**))

10.3.3.6
Scar After Polypectomy

After polypectomy, the colonic wall remains edematous, simulating flat or polypoid lesions on virtual

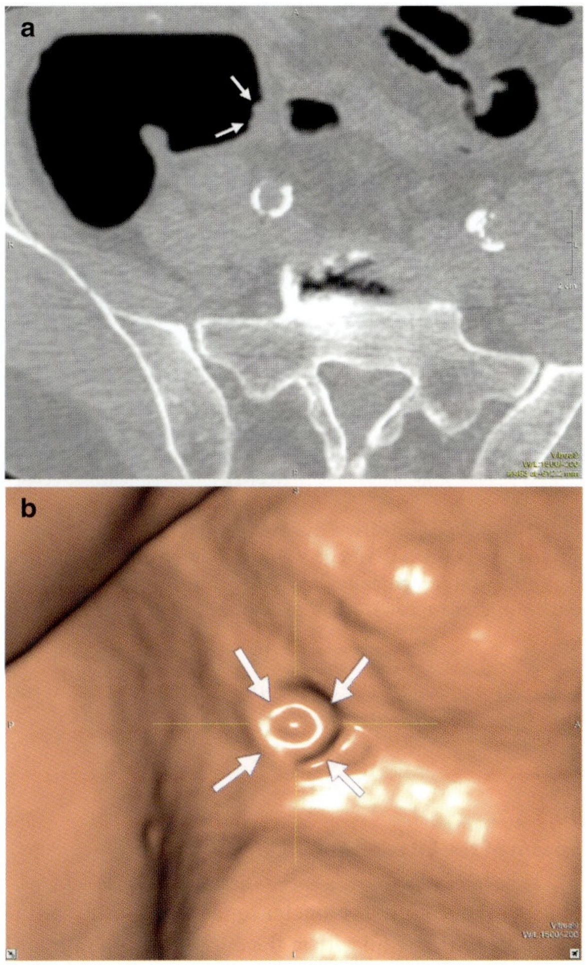

Fig. 10.37. Prolapsing appendiceal orifice, causing false-positive diagnosis. (**a**) Axial image at the level of the appendiceal orifice shows a nodular-like lesion (*arrows*). (**b**) Corresponding endoluminal 3D image shows a prolapsing appendiceal orifice (*arrows*). *Lesson: Before making the diagnosis of a polyp in the cecum, closely correlate the lesion with the anatomical landmarks to exclude prolapsing appendiceal orifice or ileal prolapse (Figs. 10.27 and 10.35)*

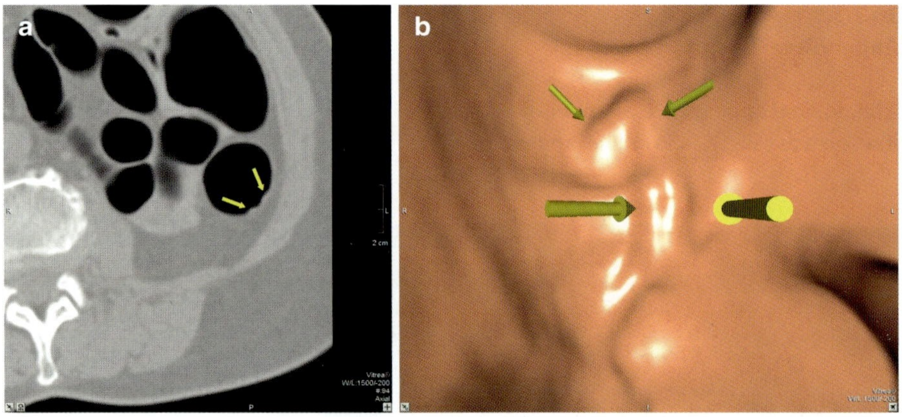

Fig. 10.38. False-positive diagnosis: scar after polypectomy. (**a**) Axial image shows a focal mucosal thickening in the descending colon (*arrows*). (**b**) Corresponding endoluminal 3D image confirms the presence of a mucosal lesion, suggesting a flat lesion (*arrows*). This patient had a polypectomy 3 days prior to the examination. Diagnosis: Scar after polypectomy. *Lesson: The mucosa appears edematous and prominent after polypectomy, closely resembling flat lesions*

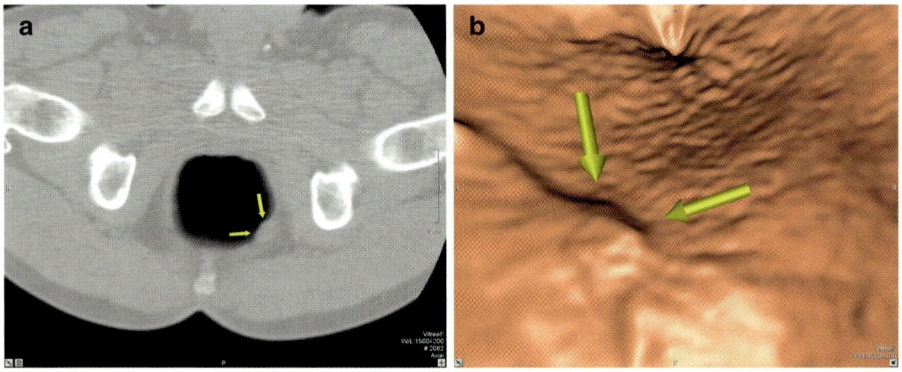

Fig. 10.39. False-positive diagnosis: spasm of the internal sphincter. (**a**) Axial image shows a smoothly delineated (sub)mucosal irregularity, located at the region of the internal sphincter (*arrows*). (**b**) Corresponding endoluminal 3D image shows a wall thickening of the rectal mucosa at the anorectal region (*arrows*). Conventional colonoscopy was normal. Diagnosis: Spasm of the internal sphincter. *Lesson: Submucosal contracted muscle layers may mimic pathology*

CTC. Knowledge of the patient's history could avoid this false-positive diagnosis (Fig. 10.38).

10.3.3.7
Spasm of the Internal Sphincter

Spasm of the internal sphincter causes a smoothly delineated contour irregularity at the anorectal junction and should not be mistaken for a flat lesion (Fig. 10.39).

10.3.3.8
Intermittently Prolapsing Rectal Mucosa

Intermittently prolapsing rectal mucosa appears as a low rectal mass, causing a smooth soft-tissue defect. Sigmoidoscopy shows edematous mucosa due to rectal prolapse (Taylor et al. 2003a–d) (Fig. 10.40).

10.3.3.9
Diverticular Disease

10.3.3.9.1
The Diverticular Fecalith

A pseudo-polypoid lesion occurs when a diverticulum becomes inspissated with fecal matter. As the diverticulum lacks the muscularis propria, the fecal material easily remains in the diverticulum and hardens into fecalith. Imaging findings are unequivocal when they present as hyperdense ring with a hypodense centre on the axial images. The corresponding endoluminal

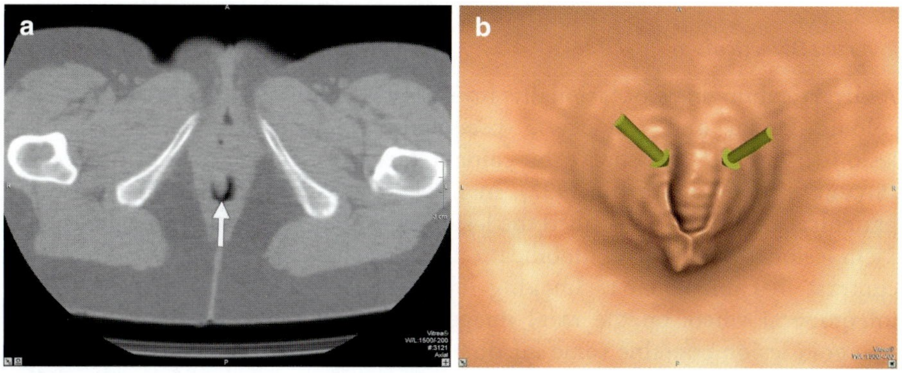

Fig. 10.40. False-positive diagnosis: intermittently prolapsing rectal mucosa. (**a**) Axial image shows a smooth soft-tissue filling defect at the anorectal region (*arrow*). (**b**) Endoluminal 3D image shows an apparent low rectal "mass" (*arrows*). Conventional colonoscopy showed edematous mucosa due to rectal prolapse. *Lesson: Rectal mucosa can appear very prominent, particularly in case of mucosal prolapse, simulating low rectal masses*

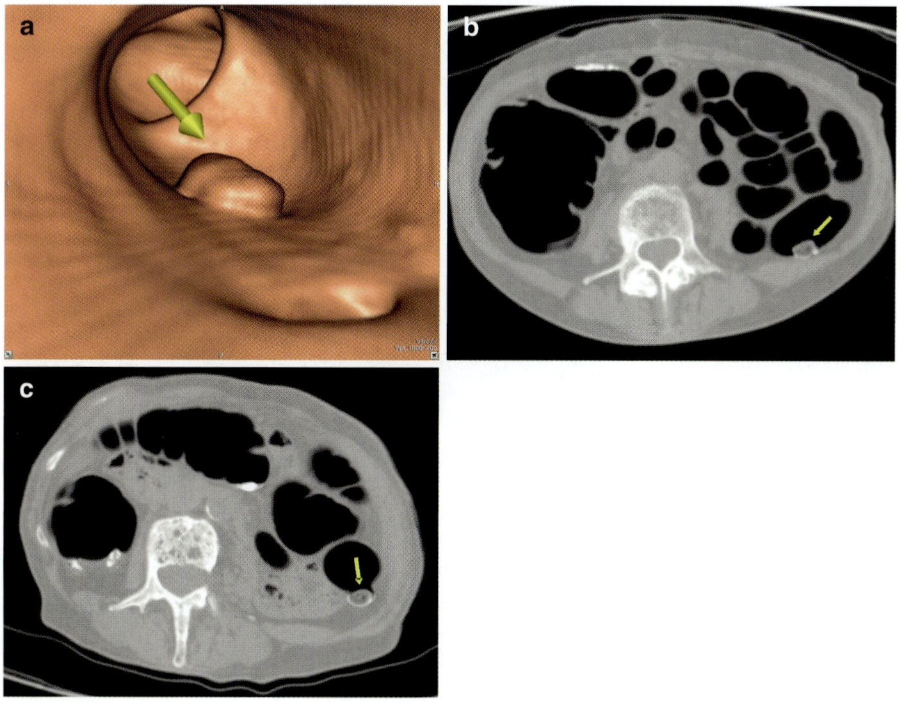

Fig. 10.41. False-positive diagnosis: diverticular fecalith. (**a**) Endoluminal 3D image in prone position shows a polyp-like lesion in the descending colon (*arrow*). (**b**) Corresponding axial image shows that the lesion has a hyperdense ring and a hypodense centre (*arrow*). (**c**) Corresponding axial image in supine position shows that the lesion is incorporated in a diverticulum (*arrow*). Diagnosis: Diverticular fecalith. *Lesson: A polypoid lesion with a hyperdense ring and hypodense centre corresponds to a diverticular fecalith*

3D images show a polypoid lesion. Using conventional colonoscopy, they are recognized as fecal balls falling into the lumen. Furthermore, confusion with polyps has also been described. Some controversy exists over the origin of these image findings. Fletcher et al. (1999) described the hyperdensity as being caused by barium remnants in the diverticulum mixed with a fecalith, rather than by the fecalith itself. However, Lefere et al. (2003) reported that anatomopathological examination of a surgical specimen of a diverishould culum with a fecalith showed that the contents of the diverticulum corresponded to the fecal material. No barium was detected in the diverticulum.

A thrombus filling the diverticulum after an intra-diverticular bleeding has been described as a possible pseudolesion by Keller et al. (1984) (Fig. 10.41).

10.3.3.9.2
Inverted Diverticulum

A diverticulum may occasionally invert into the colonic lumen and produce a pseudopolypoid lesion. It can be the source of colonic bleeding (Silverstein and Tytgat 1997). In a series of 6 patients, Glick (1991) described the lesion as a 1.5–2-cm lesion with a central umbilication on double-contrast barium enema. Imaging findings are unequivocal when, on the axial images, a sessile polypoid lesion contains some air due to a central umbilication in the inverted part of the diverticulum (Posner and Solomon 1995) (Fig. 10.42) or when it presents with a fat attenuation due to an inclusion of perisigmoidal fat (Fenlon 2002). The corresponding endoluminal 3D image invariably has a polypoid aspect and does not help in making the correct diagnosis. Sometimes, imaging findings are equivocal when the inverted diverticulum presents without air or fat. In conventional colonoscopy, inverted diverticula have been described to cause inadvertent diverticulectomy because of their pseudopolypoid appearance (Fenlon 2002; Yusuf and Grant 2000); thus, it is important in case of an additional conventional colonoscopy to inform the endoscopist of this finding.

10.3.3.9.3
C Polyp-Simulating Mucosal Prolapse Syndrome

When diverticular disease progresses, further shortening, thickening, and contraction of the muscular layer and taeniae cause an excess of mucosa to prolapse into the colonic lumen as a redundant fold. This gives rise to a pseudopolypoid or non-neoplastic lesion (Yoshida et al. 1996). These polypoid lesions usually present with a broad base (Kelly 1991).

Edema and erythema are possible due to repetitive trapping of the mucosa in a contraction of the colonic wall. These lesions can be the cause of recurrent bleeding. Imaging findings are equivocal. As they present as a polypoid lesion on the axial and endoluminal 3D images, the polyp-simulating mucosal prolapse syndrome is undistinguishable from the actual polyps. In conventional colonoscopy, these lesions, appearing as a hyperemic mass, are also difficult to distinguish from adenomatous polyps. Sometimes, these ambiguous lesions are only diagnosed after biopsy with histology showing hemosiderin-laden macrophages, capillary thrombi, and congestion with telangiectasia (Mathus-Vliegen and Tytgat 1986).

Kelly (1991) suggested that these lesions were quite common in the population, as they were detected in 8

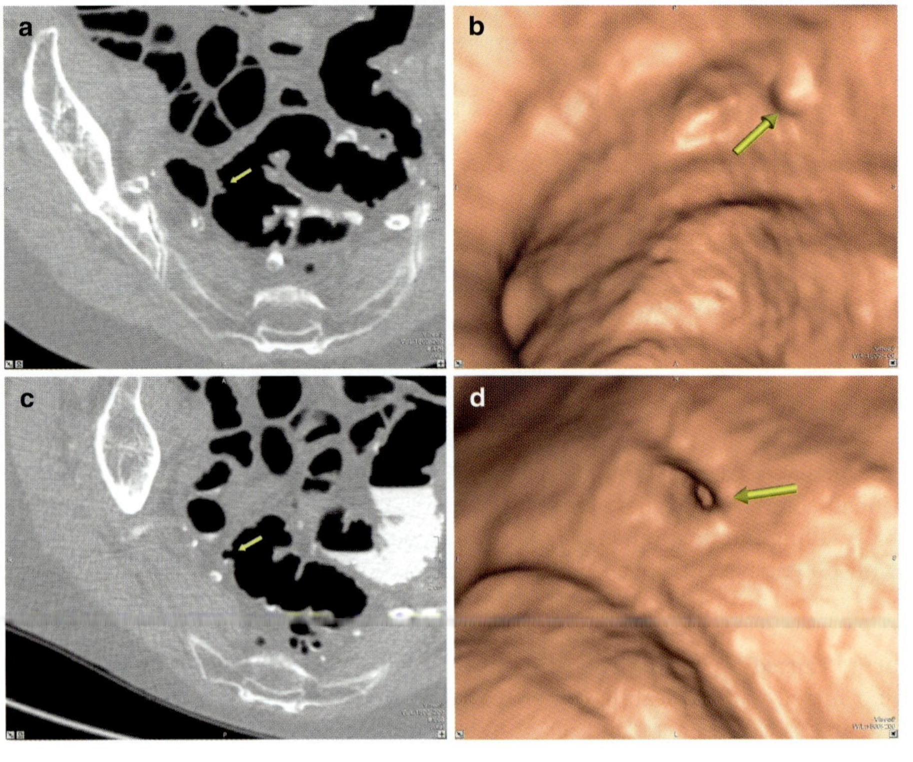

Fig. 10.42. False-positive diagnosis: inverted diverticulum. (**a**, **b**) prone image in a patient with severe diverticular disease shows an endoluminal protruding structure with air inclusion (*arrow* in (**a**)), resulting in a polyp-like structure on axial (*arrow* in (**a**)) and endoluminal 3D view (*arrow* in (**b**)), (**c**, **d**) supine image in the same patient shows the presence of a diverticulum at the same level, seen on axial (*arrow* in (**c**)) and endoluminal 3D image (*arrow* in (**d**)). Diagnosis: Inverted diverticulum. *Lesson: Diverticulae may invert, resulting in pseudopolypoid lesions. The clue to the diagnosis is the presence of air, as in this patient, or fat, included in the lesion*

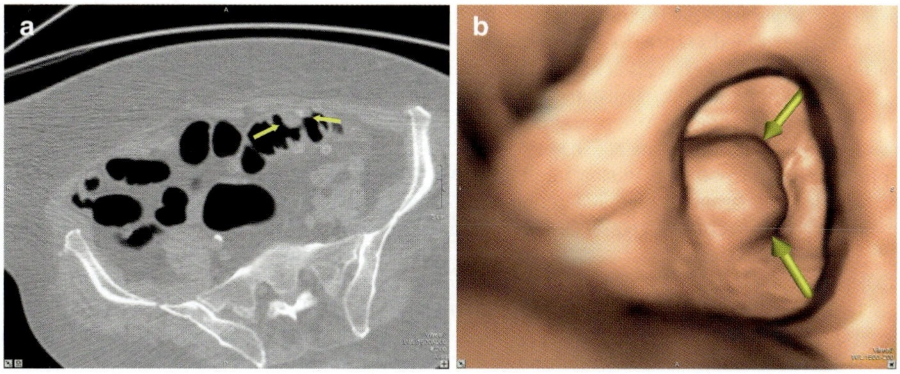

Fig. 10.43. False-positive diagnosis: mucosal prolapse syndrome. Prone image in a patient with severe diverticular disease shows a focal nodular wall thickening on (**a**) axial image (*arrows*) and (**b**) endoluminal 3D images (*arrows*). Biopsy showed hemosiderin-laden macrophages, capillary trombi, and congestion with telangiectasia. Diagnosis of mucosal prolapse syndrome was made. *Lesson: When diverticular disease progresses, shortening, thickening, and contraction of the muscle layer cause an excess of mucosa, prolapsing into the colonic lumen as a redundant fold. Imaging features are equivocal, because on 2D and 3D images, the mucosal prolapse presents as a polypoid lesion*

of a series of 118 resected colonic specimens. The polyp-simulating mucosal prolapse syndrome is histologically similar to the prolapse described in the solitary rectal ulcer syndrome, inflammatory cloacogenic polyps, and gastric antral vascular ectasia (Tendler et al. 2002) (Fig. 10.43).

References

Bielen D, Thomeer M, Vanbeckevoort D et al (2003) Dry preparation for virtual CT colonography with fecal tagging using water-soluble contrast medium: initial results. Eur Radiol 13(3):453–458

Bova JG, Bhattacharjee N, Jurdi R et al (1999) Comparison of no medication, placebo, and hyoscyamine for reducing pain during a barium enema. AJR Am J Roentgenol 172(5): 1285–1287

Bruzzi JF, Moss AC, Brennan DD et al (2003) Efficacy of IV Buscopan as a muscle relaxant in CT colonography. Eur Radiol 13(10):2264–2270

Callstrom MR, Johnson CD, Fletcher JG et al (2001) CT colonography without cathartic preparation: feasibility study. Radiology 219(3):693–698

Dachman AH, Lefere P, Gryspeerdt S et al (2007) CT colonography: visualization methods, interpretation, and pitfalls. Radiol Clin North Am 45(2):347–359

Dachman AH, Schumm P, Heckel B et al (2004) The effect of reconstruction algorithm on conspicuity of polyps in CT colonography. AJR Am J Roentgenol 183(5):1349–1353

Dachman AH, Zalis ME (2004) Quality and consistency in CT colonography and research reporting. Radiology 230(2): 319–323

Embleton KV, Nicholson DA, Hufton AP et al (2003) Optimization of scanning parameters for multi-slice CT colonography: experiments with synthetic and animal phantoms. Clin Radiol 58(12):955–963

Fenlon M (2002) CT colonography: pitfalls and interpretation. Abdom Imaging 27:284–291

Fidler JL, Fletcher JG, Johnson CD et al (2004) Understanding interpretive errors in radiologists learning computed tomography colonography. Acad Radiol 11(7):750–756

Fidler JL, Johnson CD, MacCarty RL et al (2002) Detection of flat lesions in the colon with CT colonography. Abdom Imaging 27(3):292–300

Fletcher JG, Johnson CD, MacCarty RL et al (1999) CT colonography: potential pitfalls and problem solving techniques. AJR Am J Roentgenol 172:1271–1278

Fletcher JG, Booya F, Johnson CD et al (2005) CT colonography: unraveling the twists and turns. Curr Opin Gastroenterol 21(1):90–98

Galdino GM, Yee J (2003) Carpet lesion on CT colonography: a potential pitfall. AJR Am J Roentgenol 180(5):1332–1334

Glick SN (1991) Inverted colonic diverticulum: air contrast barium enema findings in six cases. Am J Roentgenol 156: 961–964

Gluecker TM, Fletcher JG, Welch TJ et al (2004) Characterization of lesions missed on interpretation of CT colonography using a 2D search method. AJR Am J Roentgenol 182(4): 881–889

Gluecker T, Meuwly JY, Pescatore P et al (2002) Effect of investigator experience in CT colonography. Eur Radiol 12(6): 1405–1409

Gryspeerdt SS, Herman MJ, Baekelandt MA et al (2004) Supine/left decubitus scanning: a valuable alternative to supine/prone scanning in CT colonography. Eur Radiol 14(5): 768–777

Gryspeerdt S, Lefere P, Dewyspelaere J et al (2002) Optimisation of colon cleansing prior to computed tomographic colonography. JBR-BTR 85(6):289–296

Goei R, Nix M, Kessels AH et al (1995) Use of antispasmodic drugs in double contrast barium enema examination: glucagon or buscopan? Clin Radiol 50(8):553–557

Hoppe H, Quattropani C, Spreng A et al (2004) Virtual colon dissection with CT colonography compared with axial interpretation and conventional colonoscopy: preliminary results. AJR Am J Roentgenol 182(5):1151–1158

Hwang I, Wong RK (2005) Limitations of virtual colonoscopy. Ann Intern Med 142(2):154–155; author reply 155

Iafrate F, Rengo M, Ferrari R et al (2007) Spectrum of normal findings, anatomic variants and pathology of ileocecal valve: CT colonography appearances and endoscopic correlation. Abdom Imaging 32(5):589–595

Johnson CD, Harmsen WS, Wilson LA et al (2003) Prospective blinded evaluation of computed tomographic colonography for screen detection of colorectal polyps. Gastroenterology 125(2):311–319

Keller CE, Halpert RD, Fecsko PJ et al (1984) Radiologic recognition of colonic diverticula simulating polyps. Am J Roentgenol 143:93–97

Kelly JK (1991) Polypoid prolapsing mucosal folds in diverticular disease. Am J Surg Pathol 15:871–878

Laks S, Macari M, Bini EJ (2004) Positional change in colon polyps at CT colonography. Radiology 231(3):761–766

Lefere P, Gryspeerdt S, Baekelandt M et al (2004) Laxative-free CT colonography. AJR Am J Roentgenol 183(4):945–948

Lefere P, Gryspeerdt S, Baekelandt M et al (2003) Diverticular disease in CT colonography. Eur Radiol 13(Suppl 4): L62–L74

Lefere PA, Gryspeerdt SS, Dewyspelaere J et al (2002) Dietary fecal tagging as a cleansing method before CT colonography: initial results polyp detection and patient acceptance. Radiology 224(2):393–403

Luo MY, Shan H, Yao LQ et al (2004) Postprocessing techniques of CT colonography in detection of colorectal carcinoma. World J Gastroenterol 10(11):1574–1577

Macari M, Bini EJ, Jacobs SL, Lange N et al (2003) Filling defects at CT colonography: pseudo- and diminutive lesions (the good), polyps (the bad), flat lesions, masses, and carcinomas (the ugly). Radiographics 23(5):1073–1091

Macari M, Bini EJ, Jacobs SL et al (2004) Significance of missed polyps at CT colonography. AJR Am J Roentgenol 183(1): 127–134

Macari M, Lavelle M, Pedrosa I et al (2001) Effect of different bowel preparations on residual fluid at CT colonography. Radiology 218(1):274–277

Macari M, Megibow AJ (2001) Pitfalls of using three-dimensional CT colonography with two-dimensional imaging correlation. AJR Am J Roentgenol 176(1):137–143

Mang T, Maier A, Plank C et al (2007) Pitfalls in multi-detector row CT colonography: a systematic approach. Radiographics 27(2):431–454

Mathus-Vliegen EMH, Tytgat GNJ (1986) Polyp-simulating mucosal prolapse syndrome in (pre-) diverticular disease. Endoscopy 18:84–86

McFarland EG (2002) Reader strategies for CT colonography. Abdom Imaging 27(3):275–283

McFarland EG, Zalis ME (2004) CT colonography: progress toward colorectal evaluation without catharsis. Gastroenterology 127(5):1623–1626

Morrin MM, Farrell RJ, Keogan MT et al (2002) CT colonography: colonic distention improved by dual positioning but not intravenous glucagon. Eur Radiol 12(3):525–530

Nio CY, de Vries AH, Stoker J (2007) Perceptive errors in CT colonography. Abdom Imaging 32(5):556–570

Park SH, Ha HK, Kim MJ et al (2005) False-negative results at multi-detector row CT colonography: multivariate analysis of causes for missed lesions. Radiology 235(2):495–502

Park SH, Lee SS, Choi EK et al (2007) Flat colorectal neoplasms: definition, importance, and visualization on CT colonography. AJR Am J Roentgenol 188(4):953–959

Pickhardt PJ (2005) CT colonography (virtual colonoscopy) for primary colorectal screening: challenges facing clinical implementation. Abdom Imaging 30(1):1–4

Pickhardt PJ (2004) Differential diagnosis of polypoid lesions seen at CT colonography (virtual colonoscopy). Radiographics 24(6):1535–1556; discussion 1557–1559

Pickhardt PJ, Choi JR (2005) Adenomatous polyp obscured by small-caliber rectal catheter at low-dose CT colonography: a rare diagnostic pitfall. AJR Am J Roentgenol 184(5): 1581–1583

Pickhardt PJ, Choi JR, Hwang I et al (2003) Computed tomographic virtual colonoscopy to screen for colorectal neoplasia in asymptomatic adults. N Engl J Med 349(23): 2191–2200

Pickhardt PJ, Choi JR, Hwang I et al (2004a) Nonadenomatous polyps at CT colonography: prevalence, size distribution, and detection rates. Radiology 232(3):784–790

Pickhardt PJ, Kim DH, Taylor AJ (2008) Asymptomatic pneumatosis at CT Colonogaphy: a benign self-limited imaging finding distinct from perforation. AJR Am J Roentenol 190:W112–W117

Pickhardt PJ, Nugent PA, Choi JR et al (2004b) Flat colorectal lesions in asymptomatic adults: implications for screening with CT virtual colonoscopy. AJR Am J Roentgenol 183(5): 1343–1347

Pickhardt PJ, Taylor AJ, Johnson GL et al (2005) Building a CT colonography program: necessary ingredients for reimbursement and clinical success. Radiology 235(1):17–20

Pineau BC, Paskett ED, Chen GJ et al (2003) Virtual colonoscopy using oral contrast compared with colonoscopy for the detection of patients with colorectal polyps. Gastroenterology 125 (2):304–310

Posner R, Solomon A (1995) Dilemma of an inverted cecal diverticulum simulating a pedunculated polyp: CT appearance. Abdom Imaging 20:440–441

Reeders J, Rosenbush G (1994) Clinical radiology and endoscopy of the colon. Georg Thieme, Stuttgart

Regge D, Gallo TM, Nieddu G et al (2005) Ileocecal valve imaging on computed tomographic colonography. Abdom Imaging 30(1):20–25

Sala S, Baraldi R, Bighi S et al (2005) Cystic pneumatosis of the colon: imaging findings including virtual Colonoscopy. Eur J Radiol Extra 53:111–114

Silverstein FE, Tytgat GNJ (1997) Gastrointestinal endoscopy, 3rd edn. Mosby, London

Spinzi G, Belloni G, Martegani A, Sangiovanni A et al (2001) Computed tomographic colonography and conventional colonoscopy for colon diseases: a prospective, blinded study. Am J Gastroenterol 96(2):394–400

Taylor SA, Halligan S, Bartram CI (2003a) CT colonography: methods, pathology and pitfalls. Clin Radiol 58(3): 179–190

Taylor SA, Halligan S, Bartram CI et al (2003b) Multi-detector row CT colonography: effect of collimation, pitch, and orientation on polyp detection in a human colectomy specimen. Radiology 229(1):109–118

Taylor SA, Halligan S, Burling D et al (2004) CT colonography: effect of experience and training on reader performance. Eur Radiol 14(6):1025–1033

Taylor SA, Halligan S, Goh V et al (2003c) Optimizing bowel preparation for multidetector row CT colonography: effect of Citramag and Picolax. Clin Radiol 58(9):723–732

Taylor SA, Halligan S, Goh V et al (2003d) Optimizing colonic distention for multi-detector row CT colonography: effect of hyoscine butylbromide and rectal balloon catheter. Radiology. 229(1):99–108

Tendler DA, Aboudola S, Zacks JF et al (2002) Prolapsing mucosal polyps: an underrecognized form of colonic polyp – a clinopathological study of 15 cases. Am J Gastroenterol 97:370–376

Thomeer M, Carbone I, Bosmans H et al (2003) Stool tagging applied in thin-slice multidetector computed tomography colonography. J Comput Assist Tomogr 27(2):132–139

Vos FM, van Gelder RE, Serlie IW et al (2003) Three-dimensional display modes for CT colonography: conventional 3D virtual colonoscopy versus unfolded cube projection. Radiology 228(3):878–885

Yee J (2002) CT colonography: examination prerequisites. Abdom Imaging 27(3):244–252

Yee J, Hung RK, Akerkar GA et al (1999) The usefulness of glucagon hydrochloride for colonic distention in CT colonography. AJR Am J Roentgenol 173(1):169–172

Yoshida M, Kawabata K, Kutsumi H et al (1996) Polypoid prolapsing mucosal folds associated with diverticular disease in the sigmoid colon: usefulness of colonoscopy and endoscopic ultrasonography for the diagnosis. Gastrointest Endosc 44:489–491

Yusuf SI, Grant C (2000) Inverted colonic diverticulum: a rare finding in a common condition? Gastrointest Endosc 52: 111–115

Zalis ME, Perumpillichira J, Del Frate C et al (2003) CT colonography: digital subtraction bowel cleansing with mucosal reconstruction initial observations. Radiology 226(3): 911–917

3D Imaging: Invaluable for the Correct Diagnosis?

Ayso H. de Vries and Jaap Stoker

CONTENTS

Ayso H. de Vries, MD
Jaap Stoker, MD, PhD
Department of Radiology, Academic Medical Centre, University of Amsterdam, Meibergdreef 9, 1105 AZ, Amsterdam, The Netherlands

11.1 Introduction

In the evaluation of computed tomography colonography (virtual colonoscopy) (CTC) examinations, there are basically two principles of reviewing: it can be done two-dimensionally (2D) or three-dimensionally (3D) (Fig. 11.1).

The simplest 2D approach is to view the axial helical or multiplanar reformatting (MPR) CT images without any additional processing. However, in practice this approach will be combined with 3D-rendered images. The method is named *primary* 2D if 3D is only used for problem-solving. Alternatively, evaluation of CTC examinations can be done with a *primary* 3D approach, in which an (endo)luminal 3D view of the colon is combined with a requisite 2D method.

In this chapter, the pros and cons of primary 3D reviewing of CTC examinations are discussed. This discussion will be based on data of CTC only, as no comparative studies on 2D vs. 3D viewing have been published for MR-colonography till date.

11.2 2D and 3D Reading Are Complementary

2D and 3D display methods must be considered as complementary instruments to properly evaluate CTC. If a suspicious area is detected when using a primary 2D review method, a 3D-rendered image can be used to obtain more information about the nature of the abnormality (Figs. 11.2 and 11.3). As 3D information of complex structures (e.g., folds and ileocecal valves) can be difficult to mentally visualize, 3D-rendered images will help reducing the number of false-positive findings.

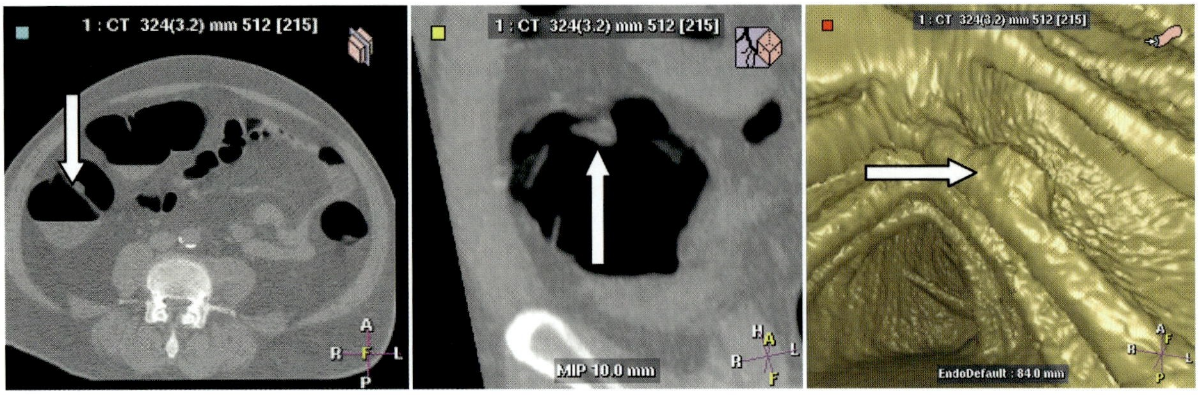

Fig. 11.1. Image of a 14-mm polyp in the cecum displayed at axial 2D (*left*), MPR (*middle*), and 3D (*right*)

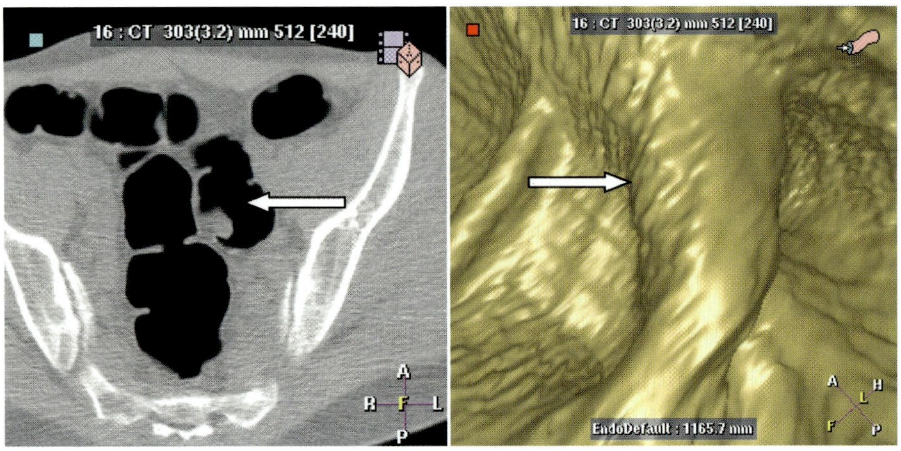

Fig. 11.2. Complex fold that resembles a polyp in the sigmoid colon in axial 2D (*left*), but is not in a conventional 3D view (*right*)

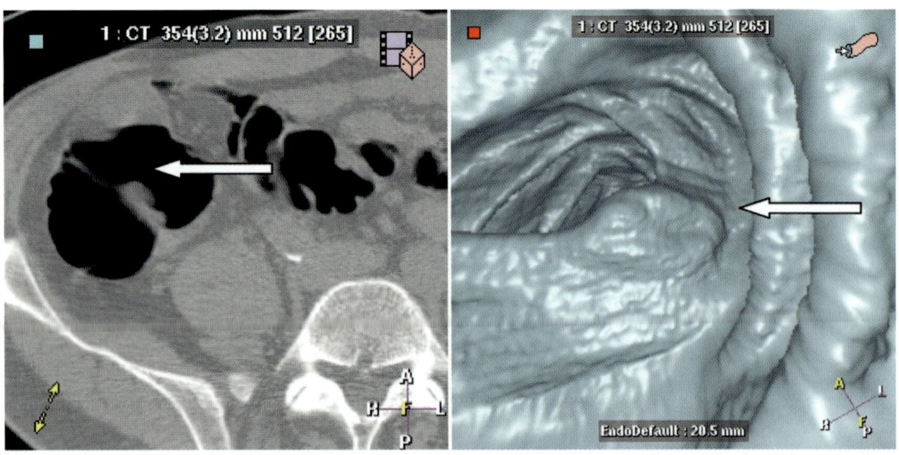

Fig. 11.3. Protruding ileocecal valve seen on axial 2D (*left*) and well recognizable on 3D (*right*)

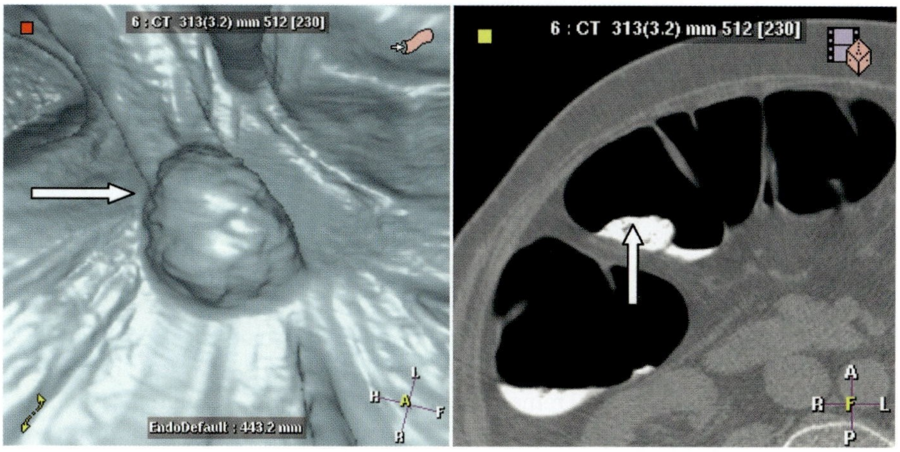

Fig. 11.4. Polyp in the transverse colon, seen on 3D (*left*), proves to be tagged fecal material in a 2D axial view (*right*)

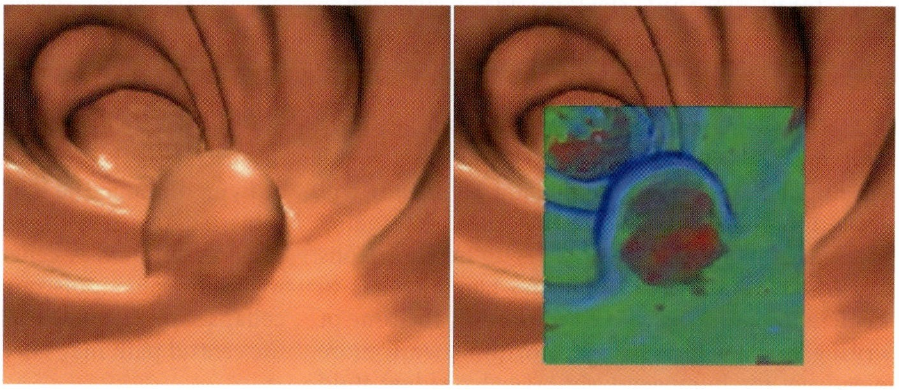

Fig. 11.5. Translucency rendering applied to a 3D image (*right*). The polyp shows a red interior, which is indicative of soft-tissue attenuation

On the other hand, a primary 3D method needs to be complemented by a method that can assess the heterogeneity and level of the attenuation values within an area of interest. Information about the attenuation values of a suspected lesion is mandatory for an accurate differentiation between a polyp and fecal material (Fig. 11.4). Although 3D visualization methods where color display represents attenuation values within the wall have been published (Pickhardt 2004) (Fig. 11.5), most workstations use an axial or MPR 2D method to reduce the number of false-positive findings. Moreover, complementary 2D reading is absolutely mandatory to assess submerged segments of the colon, unless electronic cleansing is used. In this way, the number of false-negative findings is reduced.

Thus, combining these methods will increase both the sensitivity and the specificity of CTC examination.

11.3 Cathartic and Electronic Cleansing

The bowel preparation regime used for CTC will have an effect on the reading method used and the (time) efficiency of that particular method. Some bowel preparations result in a considerable amount of residual fluid, while other preparations lead to a limited fecal residue in the colon. A primary 3D evaluation will be less time-consuming and labor-intensive if the colon is empty, as the fecal material can resemble polyps and fluid levels can hamper polyp detection. Presently, there is widespread use of labeling of fecal remains or fluid with oral iodine or barium-contrast material (i.e., fecal tagging). This will have an impact on the reading method as well. With the use of fecal tagging, submerged lesions can be identified with 2D, but not with a standard 3D approach.

An important disadvantage of extensive *cathartic* cleansing is that many patients experience bowel preparation as burdensome (Lefere et al. 2002; van Gelder et al. 2004a). Therefore, efforts have been made to prepare for CTC with a less-extensive bowel preparation (Iannaccone et al. 2004; Jensch et al. 2008; Lefere et al. 2005). Minimizing bowel preparation may increase patient compliance (Gluecker et al. 2003; Rex 2002; Weitzman et al. 2001), but will result in larger amounts of residual fecal material and therefore hinder proper 3D evaluation of the colon.

Electronic cleansing may overcome this problem by virtually removing the fecal remains that have been labeled with oral contrast. In this way, a 3D evaluation of a virtually cleansed colon is possible. However, specific artifacts of electronic cleansing potentially reducing the accuracy of CTC have been described (Pickhardt and Choi 2003). A specifically noticeable problem is posed by the distracting "ridges" or "pseudo polyps" emanating from locations where air, soft tissue, and tagged material meet. Improved cleansing algorithms may overcome these artifacts (Serlie et al. 2008).

The effectiveness of a cleansing algorithm will depend on the tagging scheme used. A tagging scheme with iodine is associated with homogeneous dense residual fluid, while barium tagging leads to solid, inhomogeneous tagged residue. At the time of writing, electronic cleansing algorithms work more effectively for homogenously tagged residual fluid than for solid, more inhomogenously tagged stool remains (Zalis et al. 2006).

11.4 3D Image Rendering

In general, there are two rendering techniques used to construct 3D images; surface rendering and volume rendering.

Surface rendering uses a threshold value to define the air-lumen interface. Effectively, an opacity value of 0 (complete transparency) is assigned to voxels that have an attenuation coefficient under this threshold, and an opacity value of 1 (no transparency at all) is assigned to voxels above the threshold. Consequently, surface rendering classifies structures either into luminal air or colonic wall, depending on the threshold selected. By raising the threshold, more voxels of the colonic mucosa will be assigned to the lumen, as the attenuation values in the lumen (mucosa) typically remain on the lower side of the transition. Unfortunately, especially after administration of intravenous contrast, the attenuation values of soft tissue vary within the patients, because of which the location of the transition may shift. A second drawback is the method's sensitivity to noise and artifacts (Hopper et al. 2000).

Volume rendering involves a less strict weighting of voxels based on their attenuation coefficient. Unlike surface rendering, volume rendering allows a smoother transition between air and colonic mucosa. Using this technique, colonic mucosa can be reconstructed as a separate, specific structure. Although this technique requires more computer power, it provides a higher visualization quality of the 3D images and the possibility to two-dimensionally assess the structures around the lumen (Hopper et al. 2000). Most of the commercially available software is based on this method.

Until recently, most implementations of both rendering methods did not allow for interactive visualization. However, the increasing gain in computer power over the past decade has allowed the introduction of interactive visualization. Endoluminal 3D images are reconstructed "real time," which generates the illusion of flying through the lumen of the colon. The virtual camera moves along a central path through the colon. This central path is generated in a (semi) automatic way. If the colon is discontinuous because a segment is collapsed or entirely filled with fecal material or fluid, the central path may need to be manually adjusted.

11.5 3D Display Methods

11.5.1 Conventional 3D Display

The first 3D visualization technique for CTC was adopted from conventional endoscopy. The advantage of 3D over 2D (see later) is most likely based on the more intuitive presentation of the colon (Fig. 11.6) and the longer exposure time of the abnormalities (Lee and Pickhardt 2004).

However, the conventional 3D display has similar disadvantages: areas behind the haustral folds are not properly visualized. With a fly-through in one direction, substantial parts of the colonic wall will be obscured by haustral folds, as in optical colonoscopy (Fig. 11.7). Single-pass 3D endoluminal fly-through will leave a quarter of the colorectal mucosa non-visualized (Vos et al. 2003; Pickhardt et al. 2006), which may reduce the accuracy of polyp detection in CTC.

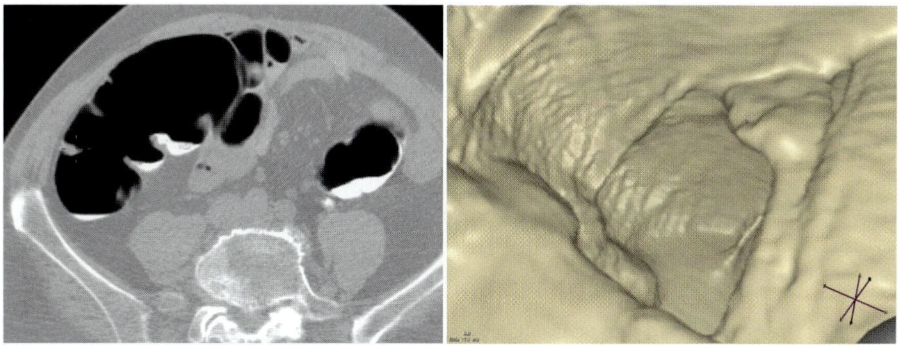

Fig. 11.6. Polyp in cecum, initially missed with an axial 2D method (*right*), but well detectable with 3D (*left*)

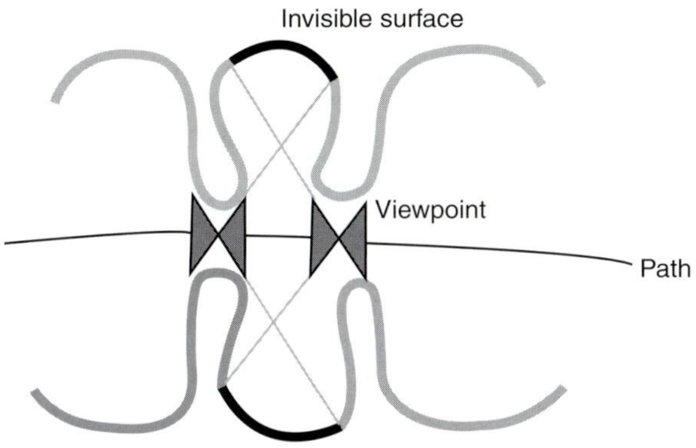

Fig. 11.7. Schematic shows areas in *black* that are missed in conventional 3D view. Reprinted with permission from Vos et al. 2003

Two-directional fly-through evaluation considerably reduces these unseen colonic areas. However, even with a two-directional fly-through, substantial parts of the colonic wall that potentially harbor polyps remain non-visualized (Vos et al. 2003; Pickhardt et al. 2006). Interactive evaluation can overcome this problem at the expense of additional increase in reading time.

A solution to the problem of unseen areas is to use an algorithm that identifies areas that are not visualized during two-directional evaluation. These areas, indicated by color, are presented to the observer after completing the two-directional evaluation (Fig. 11.8). For practical purposes, the areas can be presented in descending order of size.

An alternative approach to reduce unseen areas is to increase the viewing angle of the virtual camera. Consequently, more colonic surface is displayed (East et al. 2007). A major drawback is the resulting distortion, especially at the edges, that prevents the use of these large viewing angles (Fig. 11.9).

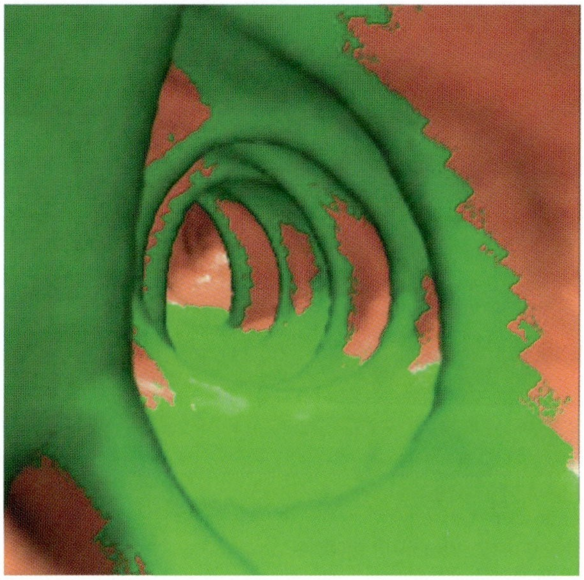

Fig. 11.8. Endoluminal view with "Missed Region Tool". This feature allows the reader to investigate areas (*indicated in pink*) that were not previously viewed during conventional fly-through (Figure courtesy: Viatronix, Stony Brook, NY)

11.5.2 Alternative Enhanced 3D Display Methods

To overcome the problems of unseen colonic areas and inefficiency, alternative enhanced 3D techniques have been introduced. The ideal 3D display mode shows the complete colonic surface (hence, in theory no polyps can be missed) in a time efficient way and without image distortion (thus, polyps can be recognized as such).

Several groups have studied alternative 3D methods, all of which have in common a less "colonoscopy"-like representation of the colonic surface than the conventional 3D endoluminal fly-through.

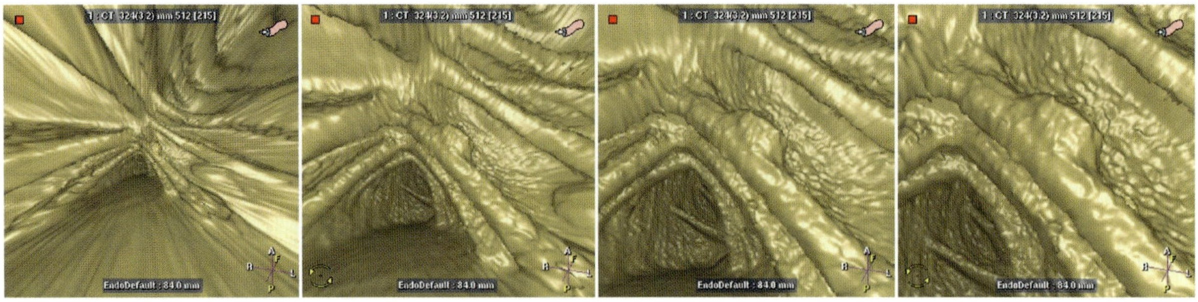

Fig. 11.9. Distortion illustrated of a polyp at four different endoluminal views of 160°, 120°, 90°, and 60°

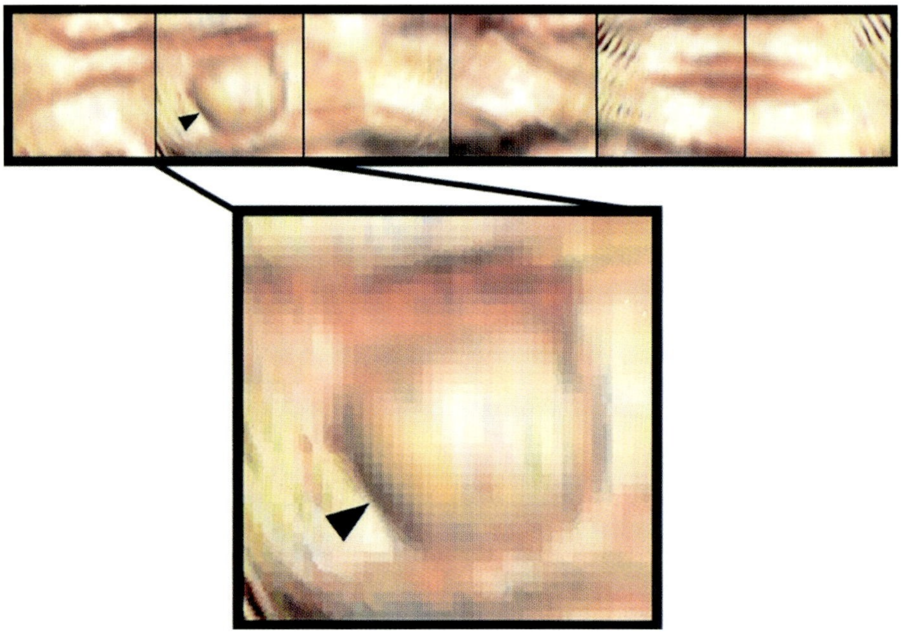

Fig. 11.10. "Panoramic endoscopy" display. Reprinted with permission from Beaulieu et al. 1999

Beaulieu et al. (1999) evaluated the "Panoramic endoscopy" method (Fig. 11.10). The technique depicts the inner colonic surface as a flattened structure. The camera is rotated around the path in 60° increments, which generates six image panels along the central path. The images are reconstructed with an interval along the central path of 3 mm. When these image panels are displayed side by side, they depict a panoramic view of the colonic wall.

"Virtual colon dissection" (also named "filet view") is an improvement of this method, and was evaluated by Hoppe et al. (2004). The virtual camera captures 90° of the circumference of the complete colon length at 45° increments. Thus, eight overlapping contiguous panels displaying the colonic circumference were generated.

In a later stage, the number of panels evolved to one (Fig. 11.11). In this approach, the entire colon is opened and straightened along the longitudinal axis with a 45° overlap on each side. The potential advantage of these "flattening methods" is the easy overview over a substantial part of the colonic surface. This leads to a reduction in interpretation time (see Sect. 11.7).

A drawback of the method is that straightening of a curved structure like the colon, results in distortion of the colonic surface. Moreover, it does not display the forward and backward viewing directions. Consequently, the frontal and back sites of the structures may not be visible and a lesion or polyp on a fold could be easily missed.

The latter problem can be reduced by pushing the panel across a virtual tube, rounding the centre of the viewing area, as shown in Fig. 11.12. This approach allows the user to see both the retrograde and the antegrade sides of the fold.

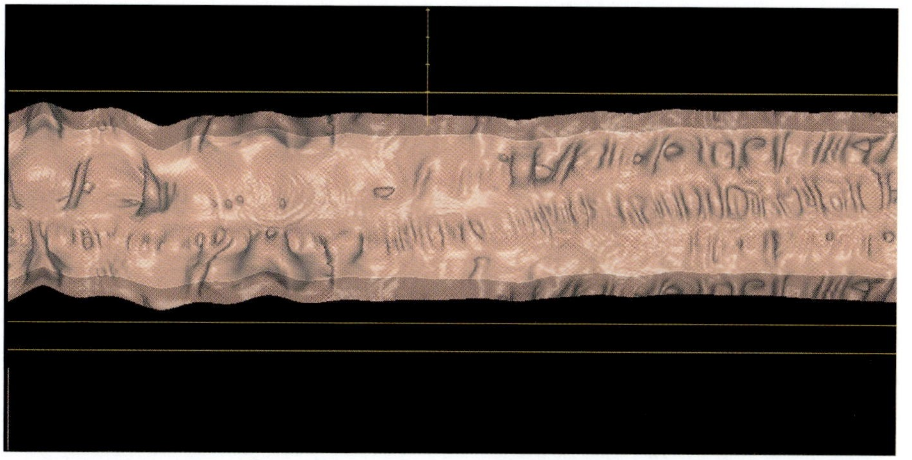

Fig. 11.11. Virtual dissected colon (Courtesy of GE Medical Systems, Milwaukee, USA)

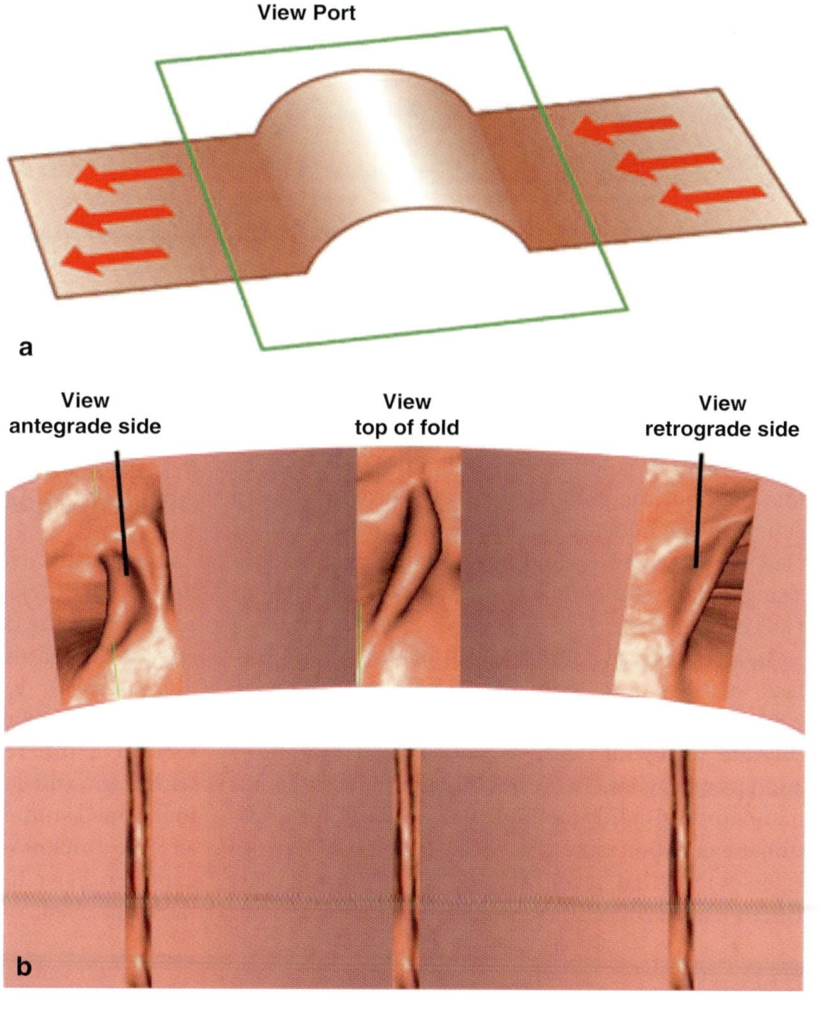

Fig. 11.12. Principles of 3D virtual colon-dissection viewing. (**a**) The dissected colon is viewed as if the viewing area is pushed across a tube, rounding the centre of the viewing area. (**b**) *Top*: As a result of this viewing algorithm, the colon dissection software allows the user to see both the retrograde and the antegrade sides of the fold. *Bottom*: In contrast, with other dissection methods, the view of the colon is flat and shows only the top of the folds. Consequently, these methods do not allow the user to see around and between the colon folds; thus, a lesion or polyp on a fold could be easily missed

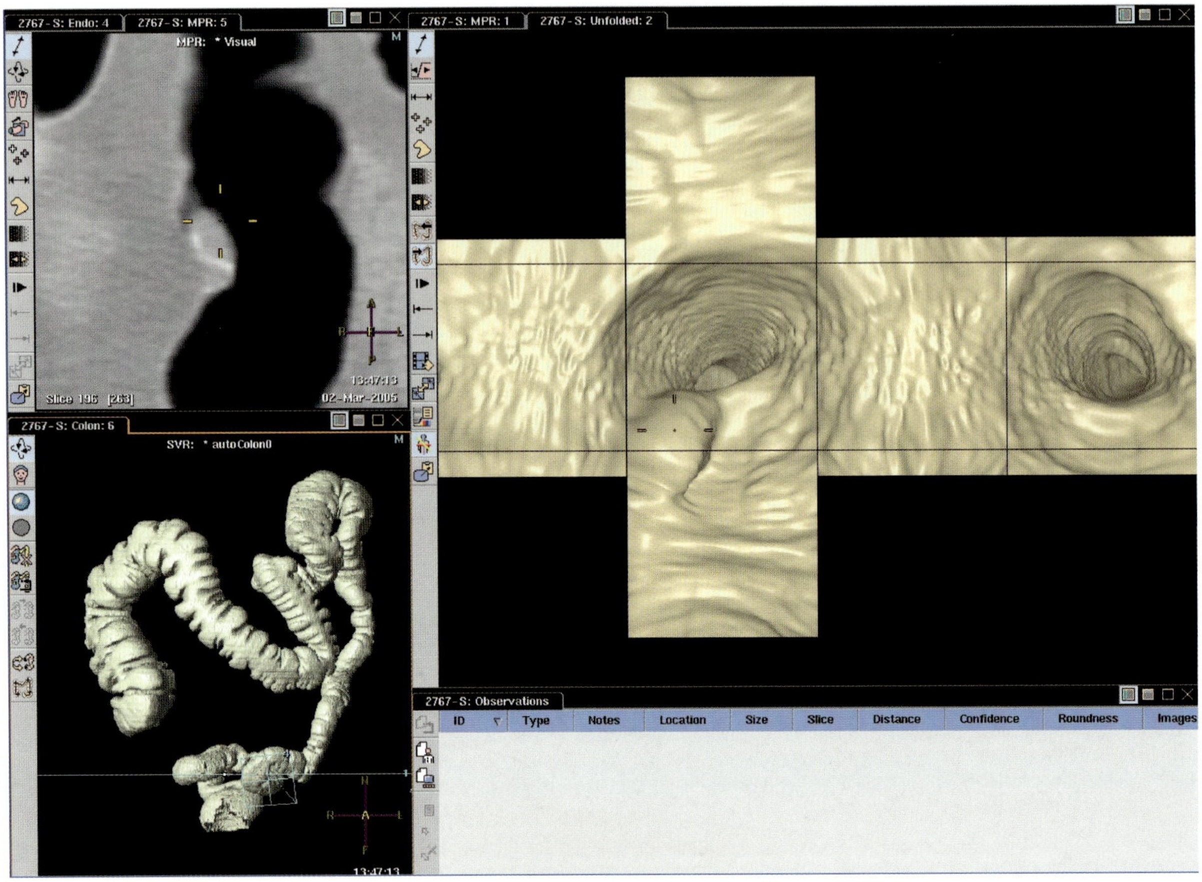

Fig. 11.13. Screen panel that combines an unfolded cube display (*right*), an axial 2D display (*top left*), and an overview of the colon (*bottom left*)

The "unfolded cube" method (Fig. 11.13), developed by Serlie et al. (2001), is a solution that tackles the problem of colon coverage in a different way. In this method, the colonic surface is projected on a cube. On the cube faces, images with a 90° field of view are projected. By folding out the six images onto a single plane (unfolded cube display), a 360° field of view is rendered.

In a comparative series, 99.5% of the colonic surface was displayed with this technique (Vos et al. 2003) compared with 93.8% with antegrade and retrograde reviewing with a conventional 3D (120°) endoluminal view. Two-directional reviewing is not mandatory with this method and, therefore, the additional evaluation time compared with 2D reviewing is lesser than that of *conventional* 3D reviewing (van Gelder et al. 2004c).

11.6 Primary 2D and Primary 3D Methods: Difference in Accuracy?

As the sensitivity per polyp is a derivative of the visibility of a polyp, it can be used as a criterion for the accuracy of the different review methods. The accuracy of a diagnostic tool can vary with the prevalence of a disease or disorder. This may apply for both primary 2D and primary 3D methods. Therefore, in this section, a differentiation is made between studies with high and low polyp prevalence. Although the mentioned studies differ in a number of aspects, such as slice thickness, use of oral contrast, or reader's experience, we have focused on the different review methods used.

11.6.1 High-Prevalence Population

A population was considered a high (polyp)-prevalence population if the a priori chance of abnormalities was relatively high. Thus, a population that (merely) consisted of symptomatic patients with positive fecal occult blood screening test, a personal or familial history of polyps or colorectal cancer, or known lesions was considered a high-prevalence group.

11.6.1.1 3D Methods

van Gelder et al. (2004b) evaluated CTC with an enhanced primary 3D approach, using the unfolded cube display method (Fig. 11.13). The study included 249 increased risk patients, 20 patients having a history of mild symptoms. CTC reported a sensitivity and specificity of 76 and 92% for large polyps, respectively, and 70% each for medium polyps. Van Gelder et al. concluded that CTC and colonoscopy have a *similar* ability to identify individuals with large polyps in patients at increased risk for colorectal cancer.

11.6.1.2 2D Methods

Pineau et al. (2003) conducted a comparative study with optic colonoscopy to assess the diagnostic accuracy of virtual colonoscopy. The colonography examination was carried out using a primary 2D method with 3D problem solving. In a population of 205 patients, the sensitivity for large colorectal polyps (≥10 mm) was 78%. The reported specificity was 95%. For medium-sized polyps (6–9 mm), these figures were 75 and 83%, respectively.

Johnson et al. (2003b) conducted a multi-centre accuracy study (18 radiologists) using a primary axial 2D method with MPR and 3D for problem solving. The average sensitivity for large polyps was 75% with a corresponding specificity of 73%; for polyps ≥6 mm, these figures were 54 and 72%, respectively. Experienced readers, however, performed better.

Iannaccone et al. (2004) used a primary axial 2D method for the detection of colorectal polyps in a population of 203 patients who had not been cathartically prepared; however, oral contrast was added to a low-fiber diet 2 days prior to the colonography examination. The average sensitivity per polyp for three observers was 100% for large polyps and 86% for polyps ≥6 mm, while the specificity per patient was 100% for large polyps and 94% for polyps ≥6 mm.

These studies show that in a high-prevalence population, primary 2D studies report relatively good results for large polyps.

11.6.1.3 2D vs. 3D Method

Kim et al. (2007a) compared a 3D virtual dissection technique (with an antegrade and retrograde viewing direction) with primary 2D method in 96 patients. The datasets were examined with at least a 2-month interval, by two observers. The per-reader sensitivity for primary 3D virtual dissection ranged from 69 to 77% for polyps larger than 6 mm. The sensitivity for primary 2D method varied from 63 and 69%, respectively. However, this difference was not statistically significant. All the large lesions were detected by all observers using both the techniques. The specificity did not statistically differ between both the techniques.

van Gelder et al. (2007) compared the primary 2D evaluation with a primary 3D evaluation method (unfolded cube projection) in a series of 77 patients. The mean sensitivity for large polyps for the primary 3D and 2D review methods were 83 and 72%, respectively, and the specificity was 92 and 94%, respectively. Fewer perceptive errors were made with the primary 3D method than with the primary 2D method, although they were not statistically significant ($p = 0.06$).

Iannaccone et al. (2004) compared the diagnostic performance of primary 2D and primary 3D display techniques in a selected population of 50 patients. The mean per-polyp sensitivity for lesions ≥6 mm and false-positive rate were 73.3 and 21.4% for primary 2D, and 76.6 and 23.3% for primary 3D, respectively. Similar to Kim et al. and van Gelder et al., Iannaccone et al. concluded that for polyps measuring ≥6 mm in size, there was no significant difference in the sensitivity between a primary 2D or 3D technique.

In summary, these studies in high-prevalence populations reported a good sensitivity for both primary 2D and 3D review methods, and in none of the comparative studies of 2D and 3D, a significant difference was detected.

11.6.2
Low-Prevalence Population

A population was considered as a low (polyp)-prevalence population if the a priori chance of abnormalities was low, as can be seen in an asymptomatic (screening) population.

11.6.2.1
3D Methods

Pickhardt et al. (2003) studied the accuracy of CTC in an asymptomatic screening population of 1,233 patients with an average risk for colorectal cancer. A primary 3D endoluminal two-directional fly-through was used for detection of polyps, after electronic cleansing. Non-visualized areas were presented to the observers after the fly-through (Fig. 11.9). Pickhardt reported a sensitivity and specificity for large adenomatous polyps of 92 and 96%, respectively. For adenomatous polyps larger than 6 mm, the results were 86 and 80%, respectively. The authors concluded that CTC with the use of a 3D approach is an accurate screening method for the detection of colorectal neoplasia. It could even be compared *favorably* with optical colonoscopy.

Kim et al. (2007b) compared the diagnostic yield of CTC and colonoscopy in two parallel studies of 3,120 and 3,163 asymptomatic screening patients, respectively. A primary 3D endoluminal two-directional fly-through was used for the detection of polyps. One of the main outcome measures included the detection of advanced neoplasia. Advanced neoplasia can be defined as large lesions or lesions with a (pre)malignant histology.

Patients with one or two medium polyps (6–9 mm) were offered the option of CTC surveillance or referral for polypectomy during colonoscopy. Advanced neoplasia was confirmed in 100 of the 3,120 patients in the CTC group (3.2%) and in 107 of the 3,163 patients in the colonoscopy group (3.4%). Primary CTC and colonoscopy screening strategies resulted in similar detection rates for advanced neoplasia.

These studies have consistently shown that using a 3D review method results in a very good polyp detection rate.

11.6.2.2
2D Methods

Less favorable results were reported in studies performed by Johnson et al. and Cotton et al. Johnson et al. (2003a) studied the accuracy of CTC in a population of 703 asymptomatic patients. In contrast to the latter two primary 3D studies, CTC was reviewed with a primary axial 2D method combined with 2D MPR and 3D for problem solving. This was done by three reviewers. The sensitivity reported for the detection of large polyps was between 32 and 73%, depending on the reader. The specificity ranged from 97 to 98%. For medium-sized polyps, the sensitivity ranged from 29 to 57%, and the specificity ranged from 88 to 95%. Thus, the author concluded that in this low-prevalence population, the detection rates of CTC were *inferior* to colonoscopy.

Cotton et al. (2004) reported a sensitivity of 52% for large polyps and 32% for medium-sized polyps in a population of 615 patients, while the specificity was 96 and 93%, respectively. As in the study performed by Johnson, the detection rates of CTC were *inferior* to colonoscopy.

Although both studies differed in a number of aspects from the above-mentioned low-prevalence 3D studies (see later), a clear difference in polyp detection can be observed.

11.6.2.3
2D vs. 3D Technique

Johnson et al. (2007) compared the performance of a primary 3D technique using 360° virtual dissection (without an antegrade and retrograde viewing direction) and a primary 2D technique in 492 asymptomatic patients. They concluded that no advantage exists for either CTC technique in the detection of large or medium-sized lesions.

In a large comparative screening study of CTC and colonoscopy in 2,531 patients (Johnson et al. 2008), data were randomly assigned to be read independently with the use of either a primary 2D review method or a primary 3D review method. The pooled sensitivities for detecting large lesions with the use of primary 2D conventional software and primary 3D endoluminal fly-through software were similar: 0.87 (95% CI 0.75–0.95) and 0.88 (95% CI, 0.76–0.95), respectively. The results showed similar performance with the two image-display methods.

In a comparative study of primary 2D and conventional two-directional 3D by Pickhardt et al. (2007), 10 radiologists blinded to polyp findings retrospectively interpreted 730 consecutive colonoscopy-proven CTC cases using a primary 2D technique. Primary 2D performance was compared with the primary 3D results from the original trial of 1,233 asymptomatic adults (Pickhardt et al. 2003). The ten 2D reviewers were significantly more experienced in CTC interpretation than the six reviewers from the initial 3D trial. Primary 2D sensitivity for adenomas ≥6 and ≥10 mm was significantly higher using 3D (44.1 vs. 85.7% and 75.0 vs. 92.2%). Based on these results, Pickhardt et al. concluded that primary 2D is less sensitive than primary 3D for polyp detection in low-prevalence screening cohorts.

In contrast to Johnson et al., Pickhardt et al. concluded that 3D review of CTC seems to improve polyp detection as fewer perceptive errors are made.

11.6.3 Discussion on Accuracy

In this section on accuracy, a distinction between high and low prevalence has been made. The difference that is made in this spectrum is of course arbitrary, and is not absolute. However, by drawing this line, a difference in the performance of both methods is apparent. Though, one must keep in mind that the studies mentioned differ in various aspects like reader's experience, type of 3D technique, the scan parameters used, the use of oral contrast material, or primary outcome measures.

In studies with a high prevalence for colorectal polyps or cancer, primary 2D and 3D reviewing performed equally well (Pineau et al. 2003; Johnson et al. 2003b; Iannaccone et al. 2004), and in comparative studies of primary 2D vs. primary 3D (Kim et al. 2007; van Gelder et al. 2007; Iannaccone et al. 2004), no difference in sensitivity was detected between both review methods. It is noteworthy that in the study by van Gelder et al., more polyps were detected using an optimized 3D visualization technique (unfolded 3D), although this difference did not reach statistical significance ($p=0.06$).

In the low-prevalence group, a discrepancy can be seen between studies with good results (Pickhardt et al. 2003; Kim et al. 2007) and moderate outcomes (Johnson et al. 2003a; Cotton et al. 2004). These controversial results have resulted in speculations about its cause; the review method (primary 2D or primary 3D), the bowel preparation (with or without oral contrast), scanning parameters (5 mm vs. thinner), and the role of the reviewer's experience.

Although we cannot determine the definite cause for the differences in the above-mentioned papers, it is striking that the two low-prevalence studies that reported the highest sensitivity used primary 3D review methods to detect polyps, whereas the two studies with the lower sensitivity used a primary 2D review method.

However, the studies that have addressed this issue in a comparative study report conflicting data; Pickhardt et al. (2007) reported a superiority of 3D in detecting lesions, while Johnson et al. (2008) reported good results for both 2D and 3D methods in detecting the lesions. Experience of the reading radiologists may be a reason for this difference. The 2D data in the study by Pickhardt were read by reviewers who had observed at least 100 CTC studies verified by colonoscopy. The 3D images in this study were read by less-experienced observers. In the study by Johnson et al., the reviewers of both techniques had at least seen 500 CTC studies or had participated in a specialized 1.5-day training session. In addition, all participating radiologists were required to complete a qualifying examination in which they achieved a detection rate of 90% or more for polyps measuring 10 mm or more in diameter in a reference image set. This may indicate that a learning curve of 2D may be less steep than a learning curve of 3D.

The superior performance of 3D in some aspects is most likely based on the more intuitive presentation (Fig. 11.7) and the longer exposure time to polyps (Lee and Pickhardt 2004). Lee and Pickhardt compared the exposure time of 20 polyps in an axial 2D method with a conventional endoluminal 3D method. Lee concluded that the opportunity of polyp detection, including both exposure time and distance of polyp visualization, is significantly greater for the 3D endoluminal display. A consequence may be that less perceptive errors are made by the reviewer.

11.7 Review Time

A 3D image gives a more intuitive presentation of the colonic wall than a 2D image, resulting in an easier characterization of complex structures (e.g., folds, ileocecal valve; Fig. 11.3). Moreover, the exposure time of polyps is longer, which may facilitate detection. However, there were historic barriers to use 3D evaluation as the primary strategy for review, as it was initially time-consuming and labor-intensive (Macari et al. 2000; McFarland et al. 2001).

The first factor for its time-consuming nature is the additional processing time that is needed to create a 3D-rendered view. In 1999, Fenlon et al. (1999) reported an average time of 30 min for endoluminal reconstruction. However, large improvements in the processing speed reduced this processing time to a matter of seconds. Second, processing may not be fully automated due to interrupting fecal material or collapsed parts of the colon that may lead to a discontinuous colon. Attaching colon parts may require manual interaction. On the other hand, an insufficient ileocecal valve may lead to insufflation and segmentation of small bowel segments. These segments need to be manually removed. Recent data on manual intervention time are sparse.

The third cause of its time-consuming nature is the extra time needed to examine a colon when compared with the 2D method. The cause of this problem lies within the fact that to cover as much colonic surface as possible with conventional 3D methods, evaluation in both antegrade and retrograde direction is mandatory. Johnson et al. (2008) compared the interpretation times of primary 2D and conventional 3D on several different working stations. The study revealed a 23% increase in the interpretation time when using a conventional 3D method (111.4 vs. 25.3 min).

Studies that used display modes that do not require two-directional fly-through demanded less extra time or were even faster compared with the 2D evaluation. van Gelder et al. (2007) who used an unfolded cube display, only used an additional 16% evaluation time compared with the 2D evaluation (approximately 14 vs. approximately 12 min).

In two comparative studies of 2D and 3D virtual dissection (Kim et al. 2007; Johnson et al. 2007), the latter technique revealed a significant shorter interpretation time: 9.5–10.4 vs. 14.1–14.5 min. Both studies reported similar polyp detection rates compared with the primary 2D method.

11.8 Conclusion and Future Development

In populations with high polyp prevalence, the use of primary 3D method does not seem to be advantageous compared with the primary 2D method. However, CTC studies in a low-prevalence population using a primary 3D method reported a better polyp detection rate than studies using a primary 2D method. Though the comparative studies of both the methods reported conflicting results, a superiority of primary 3D was reported in a retrospective comparison by Pickhardt et al. (2007), while Johnson et al. (2008), on the other hand, did not report any differences in the polyp detection. Based on the studies described earlier, we can conclude that a primary 3D technique is at least equally good in detecting polyps when compared with the primary 2D technique, and possibly superior. For less-experienced readers, a primary 3D read may be advantageous over a primary 2D read, probably because of the longer exposure time to polyps and the more intuitive representation of the colonic wall. When employing a primary 3D reading method, the use of an enhanced 3D method is recommended from a time efficiency point of view.

An important topic in CTC is the reduction of ionizing radiation. This topic is of particular interest when CTC is used as a potential screening tool in the prevention of colorectal cancer. Although the imaging of structures with a high-contrast difference (e.g., colon wall, air, or tagged stool) allows a higher noise level and therefore, a lower radiation exposure, noise-related artifacts may still arise. This noise in the data can be counteracted by smoothing the images with a smooth reconstruction filter. However, this is at the expense of image resolution.

2D images seem less affected by this noise than 3D images. Noise on a 3D endoluminal image appears as floating endoluminal debris or results in a coarsened mucosal texture. This may obscure more subtle wall abnormalities and make the detection of small or flat polyps difficult (Johnson and Dachman 2000). However, in an experimental setting, the radiation dose in a 3D setting could be reduced to ultra-low levels without negative effect on sensitivity for large polyps (van Gelder et al. 2004c).

An important factor that may influence the discussion of 2D and 3D methods is the use of computer-aided diagnosis (CAD), which will be discussed in the following chapter. Currently, CAD is a standard accessory in many working stations, and CAD hits can be presented in 2D and 3D. CAD has the potential to increase the diagnostic performance of especially inexperienced observers and to reduce inter-reader variability. Although data of prospective studies in low-prevalence studies are sparse, it may have the potential to level out differences in polyp detection of both methods.

Acknowledgments Frans M. Vos is acknowledged for his comments.

References

Beaulieu CF, Jeffrey RB, Karadi C et al (1999) Display modes for CT-colonography – part II. Blinded comparison of axial CT and virtual endoscopic and panoramic endoscopic volume-rendered studies. Radiology 212:203–212

Cotton PB, Durkalski VL, Benoit PC et al (2004) Computed tomographic colonography (virtual colonoscopy)–a multicenter comparison with standard colonoscopy for detection of colorectal neoplasia. J Am Med Assoc 291:1713–1719

East JE, Saunders BP, Burling D et al (2007) Surface visualization at CT colonography simulated colonoscopy: effect of varying field of view and retrograde view. Am J Gastroenterol 102:2529–2535

Fenlon HM, Nunes DP, Schroy PC et al (1999) A comparison of virtual and conventional colonoscopy for the detection of colorectal polyps. N Engl J Med 341:1496–1503

Gluecker TM, Johnson CD, Harmsen WS et al (2003) Colorectal cancer screening with CT-colonography, colonoscopy, and double-contrast barium enema examination: prospective assessment of patient perceptions and preferences. Radiology 227:378–384

Hoppe H, Quattropani C, Spreng A et al (2004) Virtual colon dissection with CT-colonography compared with axial interpretation and conventional colonoscopy: preliminary results. Am J Roentgenol 182:1151–1158

Hopper KD, Iyriboz AT, Wise SW et al (2000) Mucosal detail at CT virtual reality: surface versus volume rendering. Radiology 214:517–522

Iannaccone R, Laghi A, Catalano C et al (2004) Computed tomographic colonography without cathartic preparation for the detection of colorectal polyps. Gastroenterology 127:1300–1311

Jensch S, de Vries AH, Peringa J et al (2008) CT-colonography with limited bowel preparation: performance characteristics in an increased-risk population. Radiology 247:122–132

Johnson CD, Harmsen WS, Wilson LA et al (2003a) Prospective blinded evaluation of computed tomographic colonography for screen detection of colorectal polyps. Gastroenterology 125:311–319

Johnson CD, Toledano AY, Herman BA et al (2003b) Computerized tomographic colonography: performance evaluation in a retrospective multicenter setting. Gastroenterology 125:688–695

Johnson CD, Fletcher JG, MacCarty RL et al (2007) Effect of slice thickness and primary 2D versus 3D virtual dissection on colorectal lesion detection at CT-colonography in 452 asymptomatic adults. AJR Am J Roentgenol 189: 672–680

Johnson CD, Chen MH, Toledano AY et al (2008) Accuracy of CT-colonography for detection of large adenomas and cancers. N Engl J Med 359:1207–1217

Kim SH, Lee JM, Eun HW et al (2007a) Two- versus three-dimensional colon evaluation with recently developed virtual dissection software for CT-colonography. Radiology 244:852–864

Kim DH, Pickhardt PJ, Taylor AJ et al (2007b) CT-colonography versus colonoscopy for the detection of advanced neoplasia. N Engl J Med 357:1403–1412

Lee A, Pickhardt P (2004) Polyp visualization at CT-colonography: comparison of 2D axial and 3D endoluminal displays. In: Proceedings of the 90th Scientific Assembly and Annual Meeting of the Radiological Society of North America, Chicago

Lefere PA, Gryspeerdt SS, Dewyspelaere J et al (2002) Dietary fecal tagging as a cleansing method before CT-colonography: initial results–polyp detection and patient acceptance. Radiology 224:393–403

Lefere P, Gryspeerdt S, Marrannes J et al (2005) CT-colonography after fecal tagging with a reduced cathartic cleansing and a reduced volume of barium. AJR Am J Roentgenol 184: 1836–1842

Macari M, Milano A, Lavelle M et al (2000) Comparison of time-efficient CT-colonography with two- and three-dimensional colonic evaluation for detecting colorectal polyps. Am J Roentgenol 174:1543–1549

Macari M, Lee J, Garcia Figueiras R et al (2004) Primary 2D versus 3D interpretation techniques using thin section multi-detector row CT-colonography (CT-colonography). In: Proceedings of the 90th Scientific Assembly and Annual Meeting of the Radiological Society of North America, Chicago

McFarland EG, Brink JA, Pilgram TK et al (2001) Spiral CT-colonography: reader agreement and diagnostic performance with two- and three-dimensional image-display techniques. Radiology 218:375–383

Pickhardt PJ, Choi JH (2003) Electronic cleansing and stool tagging in CT-colonography: advantages and pitfalls with primary three-dimensional evaluation. AJR Am J Roentgenol 181:799–805

Pickhardt PJ, Choi JR, Hwang I et al (2003) Computed tomographic virtual colonoscopy to screen for colorectal neoplasia in asymptomatic adults. N Engl J Med 349:2191–2200

Pickhardt PJ (2004) Translucency rendering in 3D endoluminal CT colonography: a useful tool for increasing polyp specificity and decreasing interpretation time. Am J Roentgenol 183:429–436

Pickhardt PJ, Taylor AJ, Gopal DV (2006) Surface visualization at 3D endoluminal CT-colonography: degree of coverage and implications for polyp detection. Gastroenterology 130:1582–1587

Pickhardt PJ, Lee AD, Taylor AJ et al (2007) Primary 2D versus primary 3D polyp detection at screening CT-colonography. AJR Am J Roentgenol 189:1451–1456

Pineau BC, Paskett ED, Chen GJ et al (2003) Virtual colonoscopy using oral contrast compared with colonoscopy for the detection of patients with colorectal polyps. Gastroenterology 125:304–310

Rex DK (2002) Current colorectal cancer screening strategies: overview and obstacles to implementation. Rev Gastroenterol Disord 2(Suppl 1):S2–S11

Serlie I, Vos FM, van Gelder RE et al (2001) Improved visualization in virtual colonoscopy using image-based rendering. In: Proceedings of the Joint Eurographics and IEEE TCVG Symposium on Visualization, Switzerland

Serlie IWO, de Vries AH, van Vliet LJ et al (2008) Lesion conspicuity and efficiency of CT colonography with electronic cleansing based on a three-material transition model. AJR Am J Roentgenol 191:1493–1502

Taylor SA, Laghi A, Lefere P et al (2007) European Society of Gastrointestinal and Abdominal Radiology (ESGAR): consensus statement on CT-colonography. Eur Radiol 17: 575–579

van Gelder RE, Birnie E, Florie J et al (2004a) CT-colonography and colonoscopy: assessment of patient preference in a 5-week follow-up study. Radiology 233:328–337 van Gelder RE, Nio CY, Florie J et al (2004b) Computed tomographic colonography compared with colonoscopy in patients at increased risk for colorectal cancer. Gastroenterology 127: 41–48

van Gelder RE, Venema HW, Florie J et al (2004c) CT-colonography: feasibility of substantial dose reduction–comparison of medium to very low doses in identical patients. Radiology 232:611–620

van Gelder RE, Florie J, Nio CY et al (2007) A comparison of primary two- and three-dimensional methods to review CT-colonography. Eur Radiol 17:1181–1192

Vos FM, van Gelder RE, Serlie IWO et al (2003) Three dimensional display modes for CT-colonography: conventional 3D virtual colonoscopy versus unfolded cube projection. Radiology 228:878–885

Weitzman ER, Zapka J, Estabrook B et al (2001) Risk and reluctance: understanding impediments to colorectal cancer screening. Prev Med 32:502–513

Zalis ME, Perumpillichira JJ, Magee C et al (2006) Tagging-based, electronically cleansed CT colonography: evaluation of patient comfort and image readability. Radiology 239: 149–159

The Challenge: Detection of Early-Stage Superficial Colorectal Lesions

Gen Iinuma, Mototaka Miyake, Kaori Uchida, Yasuaki Arai, Yukio Muramatsu, and Noriyuki Moriyama

CONTENTS

12.1 Introduction

Early-stage colorectal carcinoma has been conventionally diagnosed mainly on the basis of colonoscopy and barium enema study. Particularly in Japan, where colonoscopic technique is remarkably advanced, colonoscopy is the principal modality for early detection of colorectal carcinomas. A detailed investigation on superficial type of lesions, so called "flat lesion," has been conducted with the development of electronic video colonoscopy(Kudo 1996). More recently, detecting colorectal lesions by electronic video colonoscopy also became possible with narrow band imaging (NBI) of mucosal capillary blood flow(Sano et al. 2006). Moreover, with the advancements of therapeutic techniques, including endoscopic submucosal dissection (ESD), simultaneous diagnosis and treatment of superficial type of lesions has been made possible(Saito et al. 2005).

The recent proliferation of multi-detector row computed tomography (MDCT) has revolutionized the efficiency of CT scanning and image enhancement (Nakajima et al. 2008). In addition, digital imaging technology has enabled three-dimensional (3D) imaging of various organs that can also be used for diagnosing gastrointestinal tract. Especially, 3D imaging of the large intestine is globally referred to as computed tomography colonography CTC. This modality has been thoroughly investigated with regard to its application in colorectal screening in Western countries and is now accepted worldwide for diagnosing colorectal lesions(Johnson et al. 2008). Also in Japan, CTC has been gradually admitted as an option for evaluation of colorectum in preoperative staging. For future proliferation of CTC in colorectal screening, the diagnosis of superficial type of lesions should be scrutinized and established based on Japanese experiences in the advanced colonoscopic diagnosis.

Gen Iinuma
Mototaka Miyake
Kaori Uchida
Yasuaki Arai
Diagnostic Radiology, Division National Cancer Center Hospital, 1-1 Tsukiji 5-chome, Tokyo, Chuo-ku, 104-0045, Japan
Yukio Muramatsu
Noriyuki Moriyama
Cancer Screening Division, Research Center for Cancer Prevention and Screening, 1-1 Tsukiji 5-chome, Tokyo, Chuo-ku, 104-0045, Japan

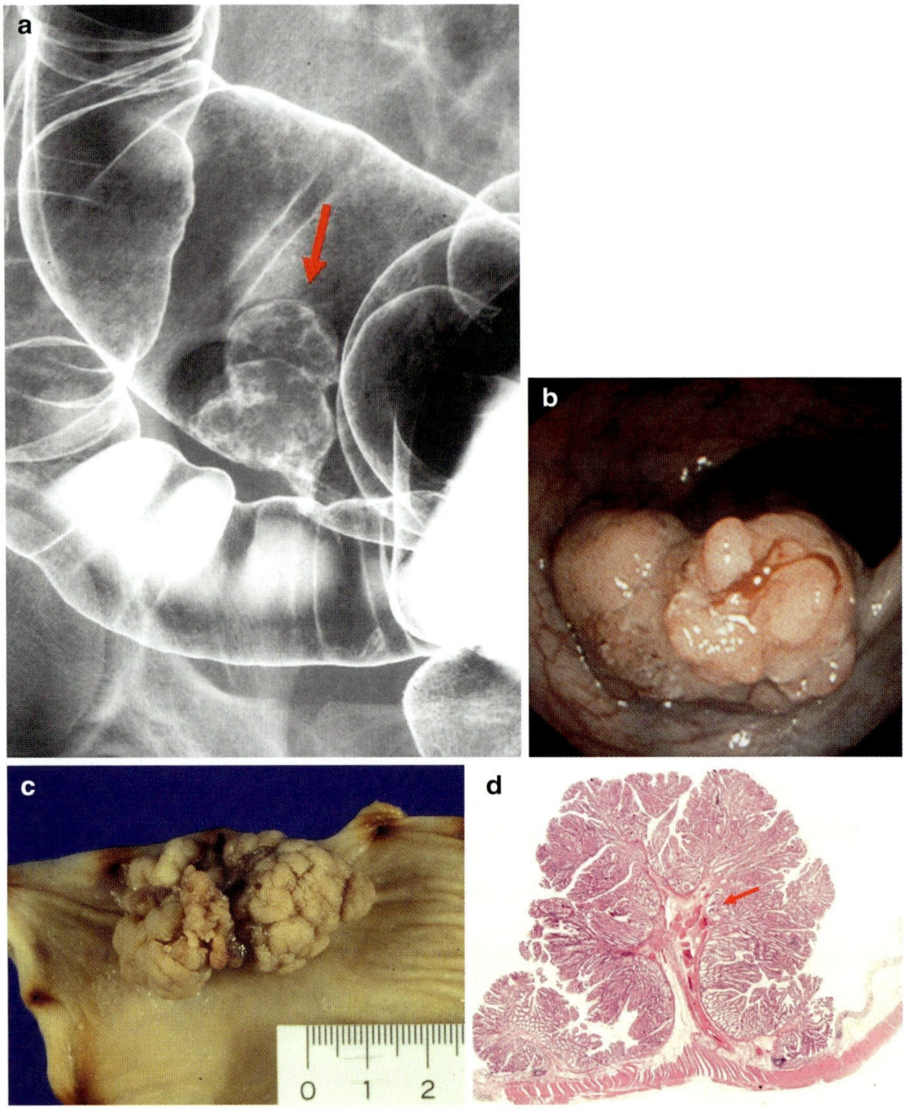

Fig. 12.1. A 66 year-old male. A polypoidal cancer, 30 mm in size, with submucosal invasion in the sigmoid colon. (**a**) Barium enema image. A subpedunclated polypoid mass with lobular surface was found in the sigmoid colon (*arrow*). (**b**) Colonoscopic view. (**c**) Surgically removed specimen. (**d**) Histopathological findings. The muscular mucosa layer is lost in a part of the mucosal lesion to allow a minute invasion to the submucosal layer (*arrow*)

The present chapter describes the characteristics of superficial type of colorectal lesions observed in CTC cases at the National Cancer Center in Japan, and compares these observations with colonoscopic and pathologic findings to evaluate the contribution of CTC to the diagnosis and screening of superficial type of colorectal carcinomas.

12.2 Current Diagnosis of Early-Stage Colorectal Carcinomas

The advent of electronic endoscope and improvement in bowel preparation methodology using GoLYTELY® oral solution have allowed revolutionary advancements of colonoscopy in 1990s, enabling the diagnosis of many superficial type of colorectal lesions such as flat and/or depressed lesions in Japan(Kudo et al. 1995). Protruding type of early-stage colorectal cancers is easy to diagnose with barium enema examination if attention is paid to barium-repelled and radiolucent component in colorectum (Fig. 12.1) (Levine et al. 2000). Most of these lesions are accompanied by adenoma and the degree of depth of invasion into colorectal wall is always minute or small, so protruding lesions are considered detectable with barium enema screening. On the other hand, colonoscopy permits direct observation of abnormalities on the mucosal surface and comprehensive evaluation of the lesions,

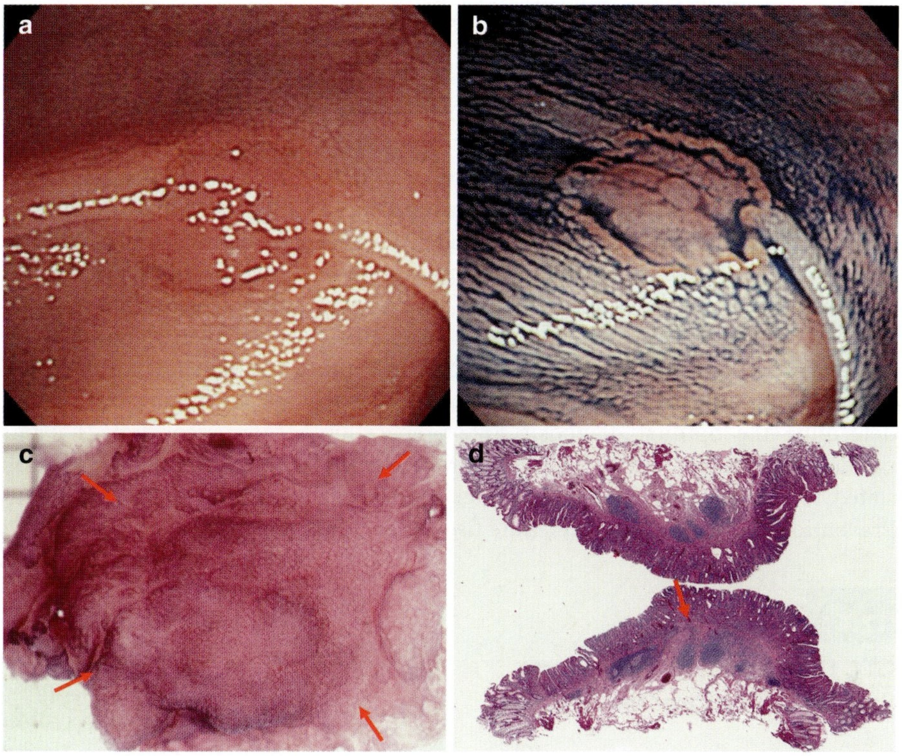

Fig. 12.2. A 60 year-old male. A depressed cancer, 7 mm in size, with submucosal invasion in the ascending colon. (**a**) Colonoscopic view. A small reddish area is observed in the transverse colon. (**b**) Colonoscopic view (dye sprayed). Dye spraying distinguishes the area from surrounding normal mucosa which can be diagnosed as a depressed cancer. (**c**) Endoscopically resected sample (cresyl violet stained). Irregular pit patterns can be observed in the depressed area. (**d**) Histopathological findings. Intramucosal lesion matching the depressed surface is confirmed. A part of the lesion has broken the muscular layer to allow minute invasion (*arrow*)

including the surface colors. These features facilitate the easy identification of superficial lesions. Furthermore, dye spraying method (indigo carmine method) enables more detailed observation of slight asperities on mucosa, making the accurate diagnosis of small flat and/or depressed lesions possible (Fig. 12.2). Additionally, recent progress in imaging engineering has promoted the proliferation of colonoscopy using a specific light source, such as NBI. Thus, colonoscopy is an excellent modality for detecting the presence of early colorectal neoplasms, but the possibility of overlooking lesions may still be a problem. A recent study reported miss rates of 27% for colorectal polyps ≤5 mm, 13% for colorectal polyps 6–9 mm, and 6% for colorectal polyps ≥10 mm and found that missed lesions were mostly located within the tract curves and ascending colon where the lumen forms many haustral folds (Rex et al. 1997). Under colonoscopic examination, even when sufficient attention is paid to blind spots, observing the entire colorectal mucosal surface with complete discovery is impossible. Therefore, methods to compensate for this shortcoming of colonoscopy should be investigated in the colorectal examination protocol.

12.3 Introduction of CT Colonography in National Cancer Center, Japan

The history of CTC in National Cancer Center dates back to the era of single-slice CT. The first report on CTC originated in the United States during the same period of time as when the East Hospital of the Center located in Kashiwa, Chiba, began its investigation and evaluated usefulness in colorectal diagnosis. Single-slice CT of that era had a minimal slice width of approximately 5 mm and a long scanning time and produced a CTC image with insufficient quality for clinical application of detecting colorectal flat lesions. However, the advent of MDCT completely changed the expectation towards CTC in colorectal diagnosis. The Central Hospital of the Center in Tokyo introduced a four-row MDCT in 2000 and has since investigated the effectiveness of CTC in colorectal preoperative diagnosis and its fundamental ability to visualize early invasive lesions(Iinuma et al. 2005). In 2003, the Hospital introduced 16-row MDCTs in clinical CT examinations and began investigating 3D visualization of colorectum with the goal of not only providing preoperative diagnosis but also screening. In 2005, the Center introduced a 64-row MDCT (Aquilion 64, Toshiba, Otawara) with high-speed scanning capability with a slice width of 0.5 mm, which produced high-resolution CTC images. The Center further added automatic CO_2 insufflation system (Protocol, Bracco, Italy) and implemented a high-speed CT three-dimensional imaging network (ZIO1000, Ziosoft, Tokyo) to complete a colorectal preoperative diagnosis system for the clinical setting. This preoperative CTC protocol was highly regarded among colorectal surgeons and completely eliminated the preoperative enema study in the Hospital. Studies to determine the optimal diagnosis and preparation methods for CTC screening of colorectal cancer are slated to begin in the Research Center for Cancer Prevention and Screening in 2009 the fiscal year.

12.4 CTC Diagnosis of Early-Stage Superficial Colorectal Lesions

Studies in Western countries involving numerous imaging interpretation results have validated the effectiveness of CTC for diagnosing colorectal polyps (McFarland et al. 1997; Hara et al. 1997). However, these results used the adenoma-carcinoma sequence (Muto et al. 1975) as the predominant transformation pattern, thereby always identifying the lesions by early detection as polypoid tumors. Flat and/or depressed lesions, possibly originating denovo, have not been recognized as important in the West (Fujii et al. 1998; Shimoda et al. 1989). In Japan, colonoscopic research has established diagnostic criteria for superficial tumors (Fig. 12.3) (Anon 2003), including

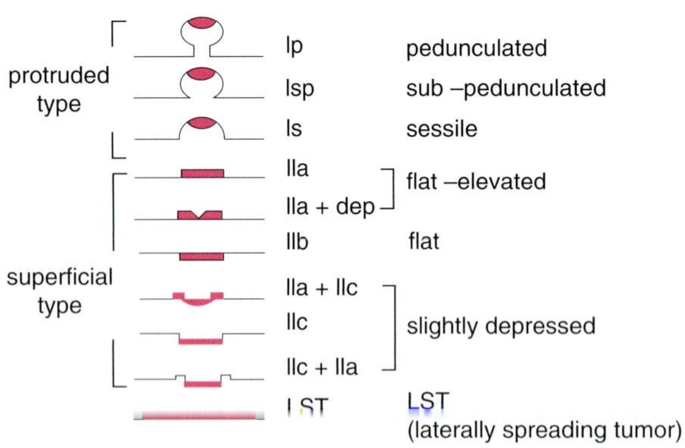

Fig. 12.3. Schematic representation of the various morphologies of superficial colorectal neoplasia

laterally spreading type (LST), and some recent studies with CTC in the West include findings on superficial lesions(Pickhardt et al. 2004). Those lesions classified by the colonoscopist as superficial types, depth of penetration no greater than the submucosa-type 0, are sub-classified as either polypoidal, protruding above the surrounding mucosa (type 0–I) or flat (nonpolypoidal), slightly elevated (height less than twice width; type 0–II). Type 0–II tumors are then further subclassified as type 0–IIa (minimally elevated), type 0–IIb (completely flat), or type 0–IIc (depressed). Lesions showing a mix of these features were classified as such(Anon 2003), depending on the predominant component. Type II–a and type II–b lesions were classified as "laterally spreading" if their estimated maximal dimension was greater than 20 mm.

Park et al. reported CTC findings of "flat lesions" characterized by (i) nodular mucosal surfaces, (ii) plaque-shaped mucosal elevations, and (iii) thickened haustral folds(Park et al. 2007). But in CTC diagnosis, superficial lesions are naturally hard to detect because they sometimes don't look like lesions. They have no obviously avulsed tissue, no bulges, and not even any cracks in the surface. They don't look bad like polypoidal cancers, just out of place. So first we need to know the "geography": to know what bumps, dimples, and folds are supposed to be there; and when they are absent, we need to look again for a reason, because any of them might be a flat or depressed lesion. Furthermore, correct diagnosis of superficial lesions is especially important, because they look flat on the surface because they are growing not "up" into the bowel cavity but "down" into bowel tissue and sources of nutrition and routes for early metastasis, despite a smaller size(Iinuma et al. 2003).

In our experience with the staging use of CTC for early colorectal cancers, even flat LST lesions are relatively easy to detect if they have slight elevation. LSTs including ones with large diameters, in more than 2 cm, are mostly adenomas or in situ cancers that can be eradicated by ESD(Matsuda et al. 2004). Lesions with prominent nodules of varied sizes may present with submucosal (SM) invasion, which can be treated with additional surgical dissection after diagnosis. Imaging an entire large LST lesion existing in the tract curve is challenging for colonoscopy, but CTC can easily depict the entire lesion using various imaging controls (Fig. 12.4). CTC is also useful in determining the feasibility of colonoscopic treatment. A small-size, low-elevation, superficial tumor is often difficult to identify even if its presence is known. As Park et al. indicated most of these lesions are located

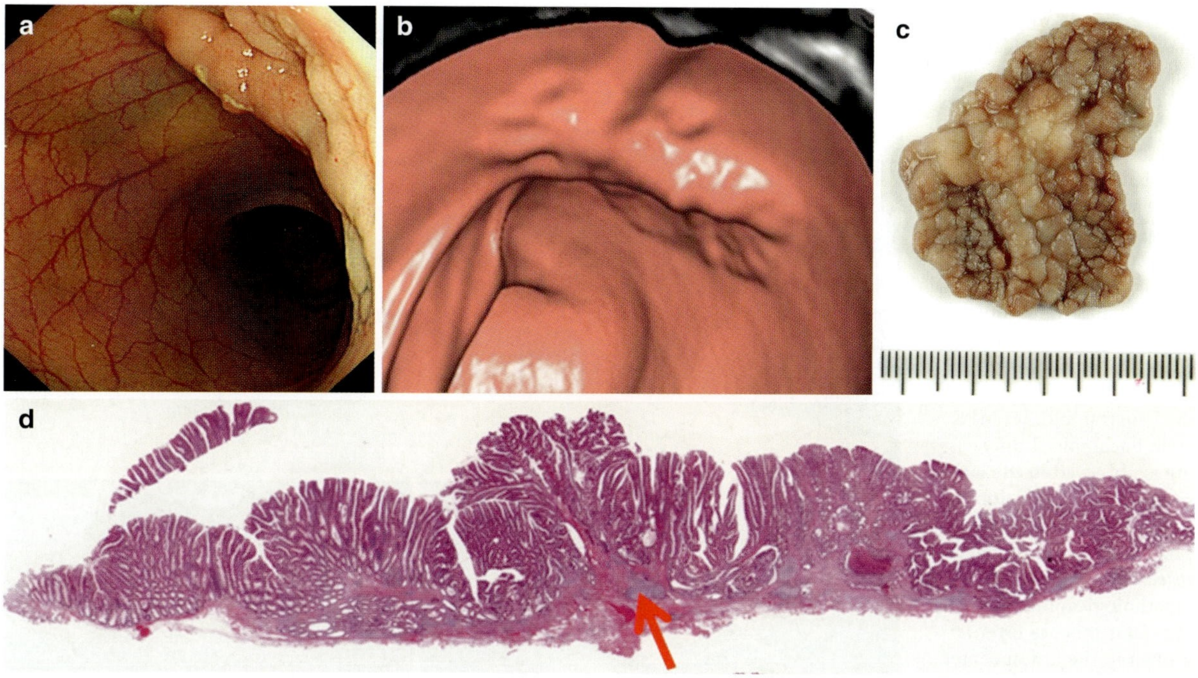

Fig. 12.4. A 67 year-old female. A type IIa (LST) lesion, 45 mm in size, with submucosal invasion in the sigmoid colon. (**a**) Colonoscopic view. The lesion shows an aggregation of small nodules. (**b**) Virtual colonoscopic view shows findings similar to those with colonoscopy. The lesion can be observed more clearly in its entirety, which is useful for evaluation preceding colonoscopic dissection. (**c**) Endoscopically resected specimen. The lesion was completely resected with endoscopic dissection (ESD). (**d**) Histopathological findings. Moderate submucosal invasion was confirmed within the central large nodules (*arrow*)

in haustral folds; therefore, the fold images should be carefully examined(Park et al. 2006). Superficial tumors with moderate SM invasion are usually accompanied by slight elevations independent of tumor diameter and thus can be recognized on CTC as focal, irregular thickening of the haustral folds (Fig. 12.5). These lesions may be difficult to definitively diagnose. When an irregularly thickened fold is identified, the presence or absence of the central depression should be confirmed, and the mural thickening should be viewed in multi-planar reconstruction (MPR) mode to correctly diagnose superficial tumors with CTC. Superficial tumors with advanced SM invasion are relatively easy to diagnose. Such tumors are observed as a flat elevation with focal mural thickening and a distinct border on virtual endoscopic and MPR views (Fig. 12.6).

As shown in the aforementioned studies, the superficial tumors that are challenging for CTC diagnosis are also difficult for colonoscopy to correctly diagnose with no failure. However, CTC may have greater potential for diagnosing superficial lesions with moderate to advanced SM invasion (Fig. 12.7). CTC diagnosis of superficial lesions may experience higher demand in the future, and the precise characteristics of superficial lesions should be further elucidated to improve more and more the diagnostic accuracy.

12.5 Potential of Computer-Assisted Detection for Superficial Lesions in CTC

Computer-assisted detection (CAD) in CTC provides the automatic detection of lesions protruding into the lumen by digitally perceiving the lumen surface in the colorectal tracts(Summers et al. 2001). The potential of CAD has been actively investigated in the West since the era of single-slice CT, and the utility of CAD systems for detecting colorectal polyps has achieved a clinically applicable level. However, here again, the problem is that the target of CAD for CTC in the West is colorectal polyps because of the respect for the adenoma-carcinoma sequence. Recent recognition of the importance of a superficial tumor identified as a flat lesion on CTC will demand the development of CAD that can detect flat/depressed lesions on CTC.

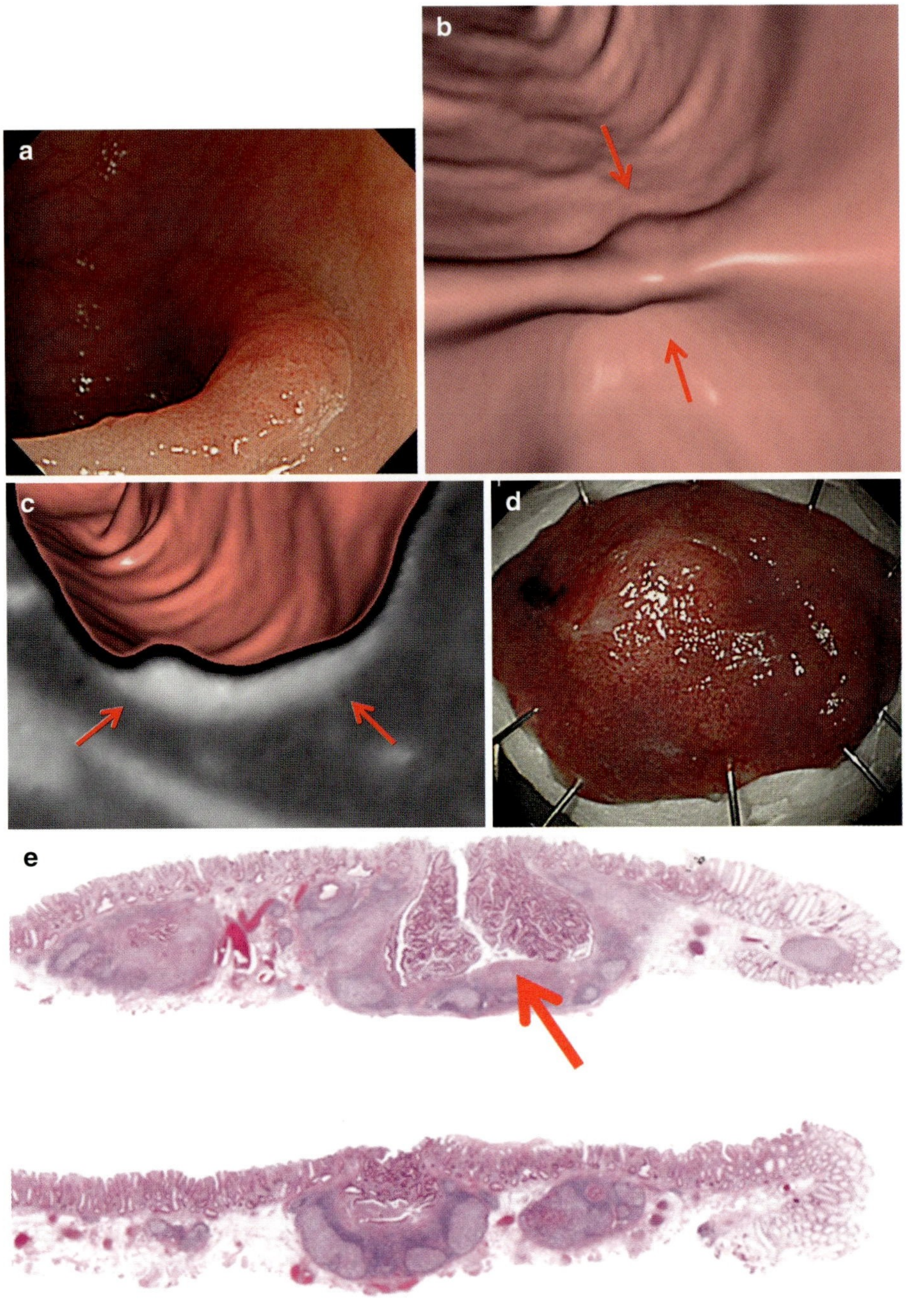

Fig. 12.5. A 44 year-old male. A type IIa + IIc lesion, 18 mm in size, with submucosal invasion in the transverse colon. (**a**) Colonoscopic view. A small, slightly elevated flare is observed in the transverse colon. The entire lesion, situated on a haustral fold, cannot be observed with colonoscopy. (**b**) Virtual colonoscopic view. Irregular focal thickening and a slight central depression are observed on the haustral fold. (**c**) MPR view. Focal mural thickening is observed in the lesion site (arrows). (**d**) Colonoscopic resection sample. The lesion was completely resected with ESD. (**e**) Histopathological findings. The muscular mucosa layer is broken in the lesion center, and moderate submucosal invasion is distinctly shown (arrows)

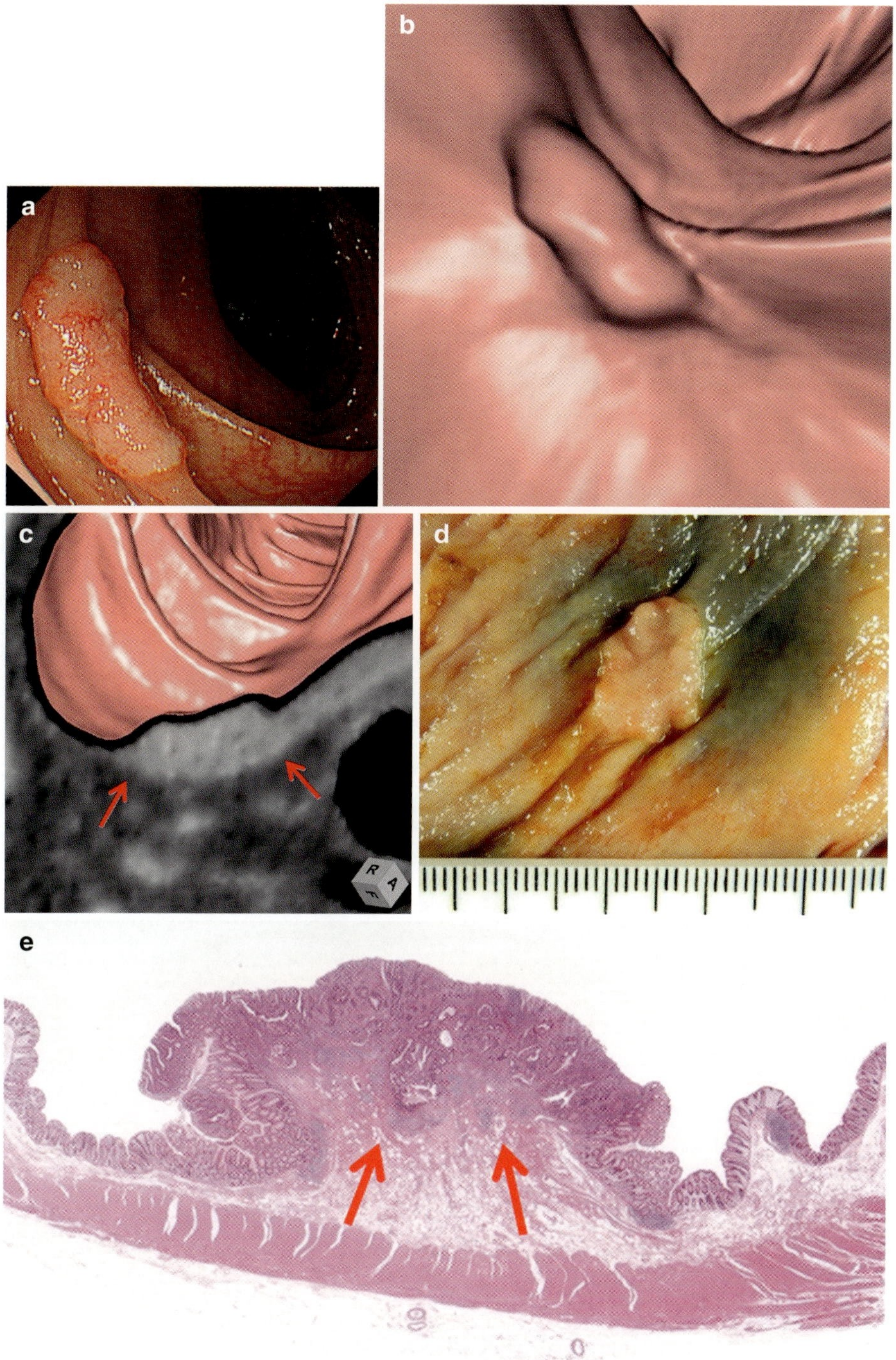

Fig. 12.6. A 65 year-old female. A type IIa + IIc lesion, 12 mm in size, with submucosal invasion in the ascending colon. (**a**) Colonoscopic view. A flat elevation with a shallow central depression is observed on a haustral fold. (**b**) Virtual colonoscopic view. The lesion is shown as a relatively distinct plaque-like elevation. A slight central depression is depicted, similar to colonoscopic observation. (**c**) MPR view. Distinct mural thickening corresponding to the lesion is observed on the colon wall. (**d**) Surgically removed specimen. Typical type IIa + IIc lesion showing a plaque-like elevation with a depressed center. (**e**) Histopathological findings. The mucosal lesion virtually disappeared with the submucosal layer exposed due to cancer invasion

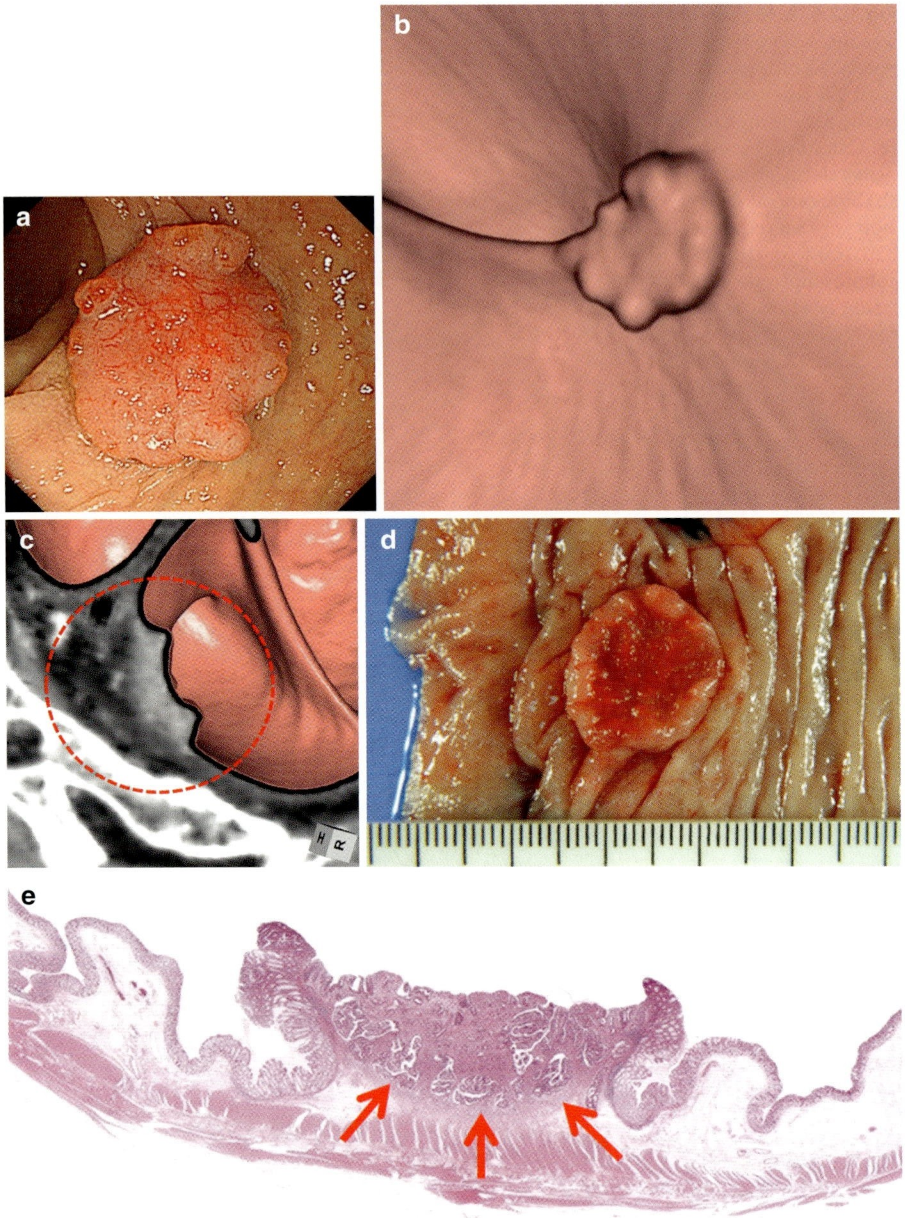

Fig. 12.7. A 62 year-old-male. A type IIa+IIc lesion, 20 mm in size, with submucosal invasion in the upper rectum. (**a**) Colonoscopic view. A nodular elevation with a irregularly shaped central depression is observed. (**b**) Virtual colonoscopic view. The lesion is shown as a distinct plaque-like elevation. A central depression is clearly depicted, similar to colonoscopic observation. (**c**) MPR view. Distinct mural thickening corresponding to the lesion is observed on the colon wall. (**d**) Surgically removed specimen. Typical IIa+IIc lesion showing a nodular elevation with irregularly shaped central depression. (**e**) Histopathological findings. The massive invasion in the submucosa nearly reached proper muscle layer

Our Center is presently engaged in formal joint research with London University through a British corporation, Medicsight PLC, to develop CAD for CTC(Taylor et al. 2008). This research focuses specifically on clarifying the characteristics of superficial tumors on CTC and developing detection algorithms. We evaluated the current CAD performance regarding 92 early-stage cancers with SM invasion. Colorectal lesions destroying muscularis mucosae and invading the SM layer are more dangerous than intramucosal adenoma or cancer, because these invasive lesions are considered likely to develop into advanced carcinomas. Therefore, we believe that SM cancers are clearly more important than colonic adenomas as a target for early diagnosis. It is essential to clarify the characteristics of the CTC images and reliably detect them in CTC examinations. Eighty of 92 lesions (86.9%) were detected as well as 100% of elevated lesions and nearly 80% of superficial lesions, which was a favorable result beyond our expectation

Table 12.1. CAD detection rates in 93 cases with submucosal cancers. Eighty of 92 lesions (86.9%) were detected. Hundred percent of elevated lesions and nearly 80% of superficial lesions were detected, yielding favorable results beyond expectation. Development of a new algorithm to detect lesions, including superficial types, will contribute to the improved analytic performance of CAD.

	Type	Number	Detection (%)
Protruded type (42 lesions)	Ip+IIc	2/2	100
	Isp	12/12	100
	Is	7/7	100
	Is+IIa	13/13	100
	Is+IIc	8/8	100
Flat/depressed type type (50 lesions)	IIa	7/9	77.8
	IIa+IIc	31/40	77.5
	IIc	0/1	0
	Total	80/92	86.9

2005~2007, NCCH

(Table 12.1). CAD succeeded in detecting type IIa and IIa+IIc flat lesions that are challenging for colonoscopy, which suggests the great potential for CTC diagnosis with CAD. To detect a lesion, CAD captures an extremely small focal elevation (Fig. 12.8) or a small nodule in a shallow central depression (Fig. 12.9). We are further planning to develop a high-precision CAD algorithm that is also applicable to superficial tumors to be used clinically for colorectal screening in Japan.

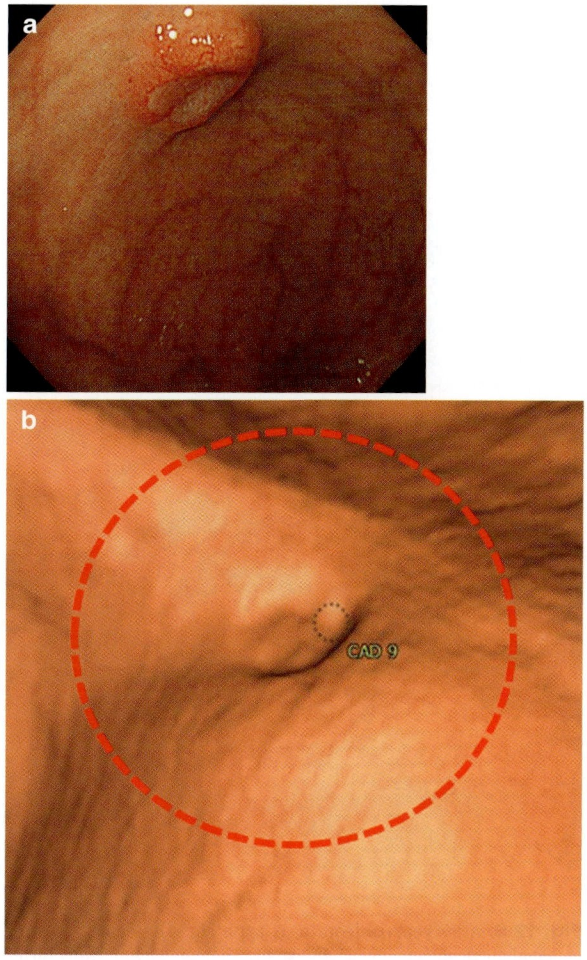

Fig. 12.8. A 39 year-old-male. A type IIa+IIc lesion, 5 mm in size, with submucosal invasion in the upper rectum. (**a**) Colonoscopic view. A small elevated lesion with a distinct central depression is observed in the upper rectum. The lesion was confirmed histopathologically to have deep submucosal invasion. (**b**) CAD analysis results. CAD detected marginal protruded component

12.6 Future Prospects of CTC Diagnosis for Early-Stage Colorectal Cancer

Using CTC for diagnosing colorectal lesions has become a universally accepted practice in the West and has now advanced from the research setting to the clinical setting. Academic and research meetings are organizing numerous events for hands-on training using an imaging work station applicable for clinical diagnosis. Presently in Japan, the standard modality for colorectal diagnosis is colonoscopy. The CTC approach is not widespread because of some resistance toward applying CT in colorectal diagnosis. However, the proliferation of MDCT systems and remarkable advances in imaging technology have elevated preoperative CTC performance to a clinically applicable level and eliminated the necessity of preoperative enema studies. CTC is a user-friendly and minimally invasive method for evaluating both local lesions and the entire organ. Our Center has experienced a significant contribution of CTC performed following colonoscopy to the improved efficiency in preoperative diagnosis. CTC takes full advantage of CT images to allow optimized 3D views and CAD. The research investigating digital preprocessing of bowel preparation by tagging feces with oral contrast agent is also advancing(Lefere et al. 2002). Such advances will contribute to the increased potential of CTC for screening colorectal lesions. Certainly some superficial lesions are difficult to diagnose with CTC and they should be targeted in investigation for future screening. When both CTC and colonoscopy have difficulty in identifying these superficial lesions, CTC, which has no blind spots, will likely become superior to colonoscopy in diagnostic

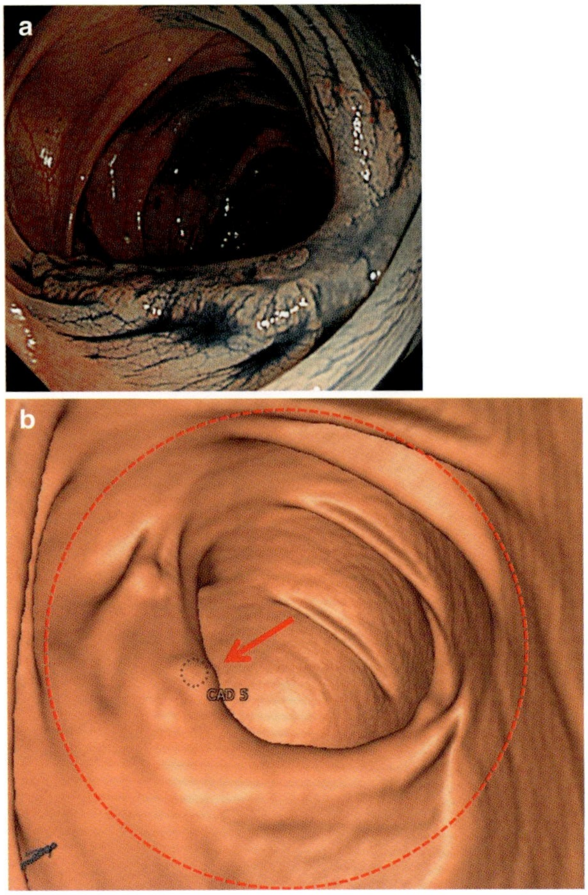

Fig. 12.9. A 59 year-old-male. A type IIa+IIc lesion, 55 mm in size, with submucosal invasion in the ascending colon. (**a**) Colonoscopic view (dye sprayed). The lesion was situated on a haustral fold in the ascending colon and could not be visualized in its entirety with colonoscopy. It is an extremely flat, mostly depressed lesion. Histopathology of the colonoscopically resected sample showed moderate submucosal invasion. (**b**) CAD analysis. CAD detected a nodule component within the depression

accuracy. Our experience with the excellent diagnostic performance of colonoscopy will support CTC performance to increase the diagnostic accuracy and early detection of early-stage colorectal cancer.

The present modality used in Japan for colorectal screening is the fecal occult blood test (FOBT), which has low sensitivity for detecting early-stage cancer(Lefere et al. 2002). Therefore, a more effective method with higher sensitivity is desired. Colonoscopy has limitations as a screening modality because of its potential risks, complex preparation, and low throughput. Developing an effective colorectal diagnosis system that incorporates the advantages of digital image diagnosis with CTC for early detection of colorectal cancer is essential. However, some superficial lesions are still impossible to find with CTC, some are difficult but some of these high probability killers can be found and stopped, if we have the right techniques. Early detection of colorectal cancer will surely advance with more reliable screening system that utilizes full advantage of digital CT data(Pickhardt 2007).

12.7 Conclusion

CTC has great potential for diagnosing early-stage colorectal cancer. The inexorable progress in CT image quality and digital imaging processing will make it the primary modality for colorectal examination and screening. Diagnostic expertise derived from our experience with colonoscopy will contribute to achieving a higher level of performance in the diagnosis of early-stage colorectal lesions using CTC. The key is to clarify the remaining limitations and also the most effective settings for finding small protrusions or other irregularities by standard methods on the colorectal cancer screening with CTC.

12.8 Topics

12.8.1 Superficial Tumor

In the *General Rules for Clinical Pathological Studies on Cancer of the Colon, Rectum, and Anus*, early cancers are grossly categorized into two large types: protruded type (type I) and superficial type (type II). The protruded lesion is divided into three subtypes: (i) Ip or pedunculated type, (ii) Isp or subpedunculated type, and (iii) Is or sessile type. Superficial lesions are further divided into three subtypes: (i) IIa or elevated type, (ii) IIb or flat type, and (iii) IIc or depressed type. For a lesion with multiple morphologic types, applicable types should be connected with "+" in the order of the prominence of findings, such as IIa+IIc or IIa+Is. The LST is divided into a granular type (LST-G) and a nongranular type (LST-NG). LST-G is further subdivided into a uniform type that comprises homogenous nodules and the nodule mixed type that comprises large nodule(s) within the lesion. A significant number of studies reported characteristic histopathological findings of these types, which are effectively utilized for clinical colonoscopic diagnosis.

12.8.2 Endoscopic Submucosal Dissection (ESD)

The conventional endoscopic treatment technique for early colorectal cancer has been endoscopic mucosal resection (EMR), but ESD has recently begun to be used for colorectal sites. ESD has already been widely used in practice as a standard treatment method for early-stage gastric cancer. It is also a practical treatment option for colorectal lesions because en bloc dissection is possible regardless of lesion size or location, which is a useful feature for LST lesion treatment. Compared with gastric lesions, ESD of colorectal sites requires a higher degree technical skill and has a higher accident rate. Further improvement of the ESD device and establishing procedural standards will allow it to become an efficient treatment option for superficial colorectal tumors.

Acknowledgements The works were supported by Grants for Scientific Research Expens es for Health and Welfare Programs and the Foundation for the Promotion of Cancer Research, and by the 3rd-term Comprehensive 10-year Strategy for Cancer Control from the Ministry of Health, Labor and Welfare.

References

Anon (2003) The Paris endoscopic classification of superficial neoplastic lesions: esophagus, stomach, and colon. Gastrointest Endosc 58:S3–S43

Fujii T, Rembacken BJ, Dixon MF et al (1998) Flat adenomas in the United Kingdom: Are treatable cancers being missed? Endoscopy 30:437–443

Hara AK, Johnson CD, Reed JE et al (1997) Detection of colorectal polyps with CT colography: initial assessment of sensitivity and specificity. Radiology 205:59–65

Iinuma G, Moriyama N, Miyakawa K et al (2003) Early invasive colorectal carcinomas with submucosal invasion: ?Radiographic characteristics with barium double contrast. Abdom Imaging 28:492–504

Iinuma G, Moriyama N, Satake M et al (2005) Vascular virtual endoluminal visualization of invasive colorectal cancer on MDCT colonography. AJR 184:1194–1198

Johnson CD, Chen MH, Toledano AY, et al (2008) Accuracy of CT colonography for detection of large adenomas and cancers. N Engl J Med 359:1207–1217

Kudo S (1996) Early colorectal cancer, detection of depressed type of colorectal carcinomas. Igaku-Shoin, Tokyo, Japan, pp166

Kudo S, Tamura S, Nakajima T et al (1995) Depressed type of colorectal cancer. Endoscopy 27:54–57

Lefere PA, Gryspeerdt SS, Dewyspelaere J et al (2002) Dietary fecal tagging as a cleansing method before CT colonography: Initial results – polyp detection and patient acceptance. Radiology 224:393–403

Levine MS, Rubesin SE, Laufer I et al (2000) Diagnosis of colorectal neoplasms at double-contrast barium enema examination. Radiology 216:11–18

Matsuda T, Fujii T, Emura F et al (2004) Complete closure of a large defect after EMR of a lateral spreading colorectal tumor when using a two-channel colonoscope. Gastrointest Endosc 60:836–838

McFarland EG, Brink JA, Loh J et al (1997) Visualization of colorectal polyps with spiral CT colography: evaluation of processing parameters with perspective volume rendering. Radiology 205:701–707

Muto T, Bussey HJR, Morson BC (1975) The evolution of cancer of the colon and rectum. Cancer 36:2251–2270

Nakajima Y, Yamada K, Imamura K et al (2008) Radiologists supply and workload: international comparison – Working Group of Japanese College of Radiology. Radiat Med 26: 455–465

Park S, Ha H, Kim A et al (2006) Flat polyps of the colon: detection with 16-MDCT colonography – preliminary results. AJR 186:1611–1617

Park S, Lee SS, Choi EK et al (2007) Flat colorectal neoplasms: definition, importance, and visualization on CT colonography. AJR 188:953–959

Pickhardt PJ (2007) Screening CT colonography: How i do it. AJR 189:290–298

Pickhardt PJ, Choi JR, Hwang I et al (2004) Nonadenomatous polyps at CT colonography: prevalence, size distribution, and detection rates. Radiology 232:784–790

Rex DK, Cutler CS, Lemmel GT et al (1997) Colonoscopic miss rates of adenomas determined by back-to-back colonoscopy. Gastroenterology 112:24–28

Saito H, Soma Y, Koeda J et al (1995) Reduction in risk of mortality from colorectal cancer by fecal occult blood screening with immunochemical hemagglutination test; a case-control study. Int J Cancer 61:465–469

Saito Y, Emura F, Matsuda T et al (2005) A new sinker-assisted endoscopic submucosal dissection method for colorectal tumors. Gastrointest Endosc 62:297–301

Sano Y, Horimatsu T, Fu KI et al (2006) Magnifying observation of microvascular architecture of colorectal lesions using a narrow band imaging system. Dig Endosc 18: S44–S51

Shimoda T, Ikegami M, Fujisaki J, Matsui M, Aizawa S, Ishikawa. E (1989) Early colorectal carcinoma with special reference to its development de novo. Cancer 64:1138–1146

Summers RM, Johnson CD, Pusanik LM et al (2001) Automated polyp detection at CT colonography: Feasibility assessment in the human population. Radiology 219:51–59

Taylor SA, Iinuma G, Saito Y et al (2008) CT colonography: computer-aided detection of morphologically flat T1 colonic carcinoma. Eur Radiol 18:1666–1673

Extracolonic Findings

Francesca Turini, Francesca Cerri, and Emanuele Neri

CONTENTS

13.1 Introduction

Computed tomography colonography (CTC), also referred to as virtual colonoscopy, is a noninvasive CT examination of the colon that has shown promise as a tool for colorectal cancer screening.

In most cases, CTC is performed without i.v. contrast at a reduced radiation dose. Therefore, in addition to intraluminal images of the colon, a noncontrast CT of the entire abdomen and pelvis, and often the lower thorax, is obtained. This allows CTC to image many organs other than the colon during a routine study, unlike other colon screening examinations such as endoscopy or barium enema. This ability can be seen as a double-edged sword (Hara 2005). In fact, the ability to evaluate extracolonic structures can present a clinical dilemma. On the one hand, CTC may incidentally demonstrate asymptomatic malignant diseases or other clinically important conditions, thus possibly decreasing morbidity or mortality. On the other hand, CTC may reveal numerous findings of no clinical relevance. This could result in costly additional diagnostic examinations with an increase in morbidity and an overall negative effect on a patient's health (Sosna et al. 2005). Only a minority of the extracolonic findings observed by means of CTC are clinically important (Zalis et al. 2005; Pickhardt et al. 2003; Hara et al. 2000). Excessive caution and ambiguity in the description of findings, which are almost certainly benign, can lead to considerable follow-up examination costs and unnecessary anxiety for the patient (Zalis et al. 2005). But there are also technical considerations to put forth. In fact, it is also important for the interpreting radiologist to remain cognizant of the diagnostic limitations imposed by the reduced X-ray dose and infrequent use of intravenous contrast material that are typical when screening colorectal cancer via CTC.

Francesca Turini, MD
Francesca Cerri, MD
Emanuele Neri, MD
Department of Oncology, Diagnostic and Interventional Radiology, Transplants and Advanced Technologies in Medicine, University of Pisa, Via Roma 67, 56100, Pisa, Italy

13.2 Definitions of Extracolonic Findings

Incidental extracolonic findings (ECFs) may be defined as findings on CTC that have potential deleterious health effects and are asymptomatic, unsuspected, and unrelated to the colon. This excludes findings such as anatomic anomalies or variations and post-surgical or post-traumatic abnormalities (Berland 2009).

ECFs at CT are often classified by their clinical relevance into major, moderate, or minor significance (Sosna et al. 2005; Hara et al. 2000; Gluecker et al. 2003; Rajapaksa et al. 2004; Hellstrom et al. 2004; Ginnerup Pedersen et al. 2003; Edwards et al. 2001).

A major important finding is typically defined as a finding requiring immediate medical or surgical attention, including indeterminate solid organ lesions, previously undiagnosed abdominal aortic aneurysms greater than 3.5 cm, and uncalcified pulmonary nodules, lymphadenopathy, and suspected osseous metastasis (Fig. 13.1).

A finding of moderate importance is defined as a condition that does not require immediate evaluation, but could cause medical problems in the future. Examples include gallstones, renal stones, uterine or ovarian enlargements, fatty liver, and coronary artery calcifications (Fig. 13.2).

Findings of minor importance are considered benign and unlikely to require any additional medical treatment. Examples of these include abdominal vascular calcifications, granulomas (in the lung or the abdomen), diverticulosis, simple cysts of solid organs, and small to medium hiatal hernias (Fig. 13.3).

Another classification of the ECF is the one proposed by Zalis et al. (2005) to have a standardized reporting system that can better assist patients and referring physicians in making decisions. This categorization system is provided in Table 13.1.

13.3 Prevalence of the Extracolonic Findings

Studies aimed at assessing primarily ECFs at CTC present a wide variation in the prevalence of ECF.

The variation is because different studies have considered different populations and used different study protocols. Regarding the choice of populations, there are studies on young or elder people, average risk or high risk of developing colorectal cancer patients, symptomatic or asymptomatic patients (Gluecker et al. 2003; Rajapaksa et al. 2004; Hellstrom et al. 2004; Edwards et al. 2001; Pickhardt et al. 2003; Yee et al. 2005; Ng et al. 2004; Chin et al. 2005; Khan et al. 2007).

Low radiation dose protocols do not greatly affect the evaluation of the colon, owing to the high contrast between the air in the lumen and the density of the colonic wall (Bechtold et al. 1997). However, a decrease in tube current will result in an increase in image noise that limits the ability to evaluate extracolonic soft tissue. Thus, detection and characterization of abnormalities in the solid abdominal organs is compromised (Fig. 13.4). At very low tube current, the opportunity to evaluate the extracolonic solid organs will decrease or get lost, possibly resulting in an examination of only the colon (Iannaccone et al. 2004; van Gelder et al. 2002).

Identification and characterization of findings also depend on the use of intravenous contrast medium that allows a consistent increase in the number of identified findings and better characterization within a single exam. However, the use of intravenous contrast medium increases the examination cost and the patient's risks, which is not effective especially in the case of using CTC in the screening of colorectal cancers (Morrin et al. 2000; Spreng et al. 2005; Kim et al. 2008).

In considering the results of assessing the prevalence, attention must be paid to the possible bias in publications, as for example the fact that some findings could be already known at least to the patient before the CTC, and hence generating neither additional cost nor additional anxiety to the patients. Another bias can be caused by false-positive findings.

Finally, different authors have used different thresholds for their classification and they have tended to classify "major" in terms of the need for a clinical response (i.e., before further investigations had been carried out), rather than whether detection was likely to have been beneficial in retrospect (i.e., in the light of knowledge gleaned from further investigations) (Xiong et al. 2005).

Table 13.2 reports the results of the most relevant studies, published in the last years and reporting data about the prevalence of ECFs and their follow-up.

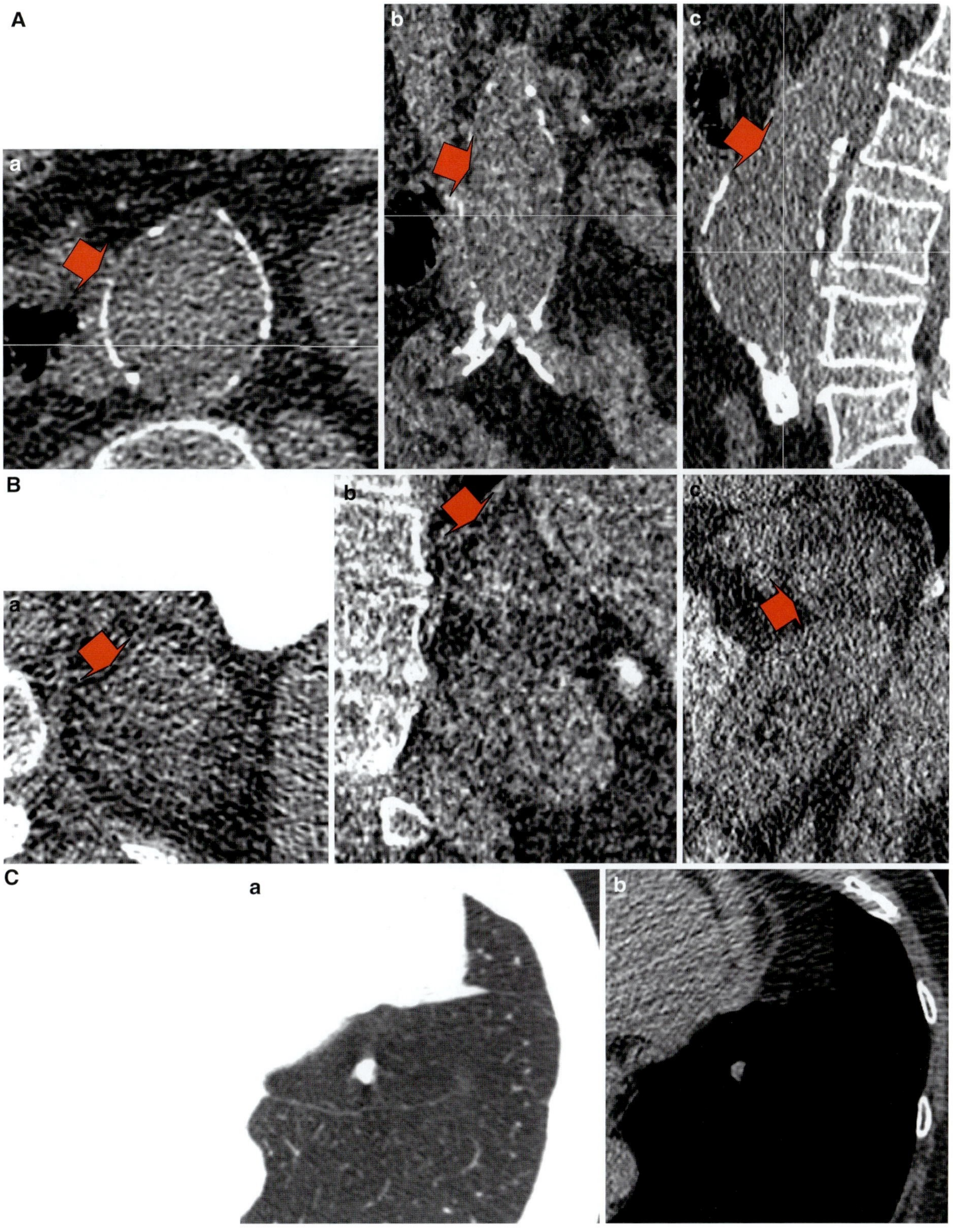

Fig. 13.1. (**A**) Nonenhanced transverse (**a**), coronal (**b**), and sagittal (**c**) CT scan obtained at 50 mA for CT colonography demonstrate a 35 mm diameter subrenal abdominal aortic aneurysm (*arrow*), which was previously unknown. (**B**) Nonenhanced transverse (**a**), coronal (**b**), and sagittal (**c**) CT scan obtained at 50 mA for CT colonography demonstrate a left adrenal mass (*arrow*). (**C**) Nonenhanced transverse CT scan obtained through the lower chest visualized on lung (**a**) and abdominal (**b**) window show a lung nodule

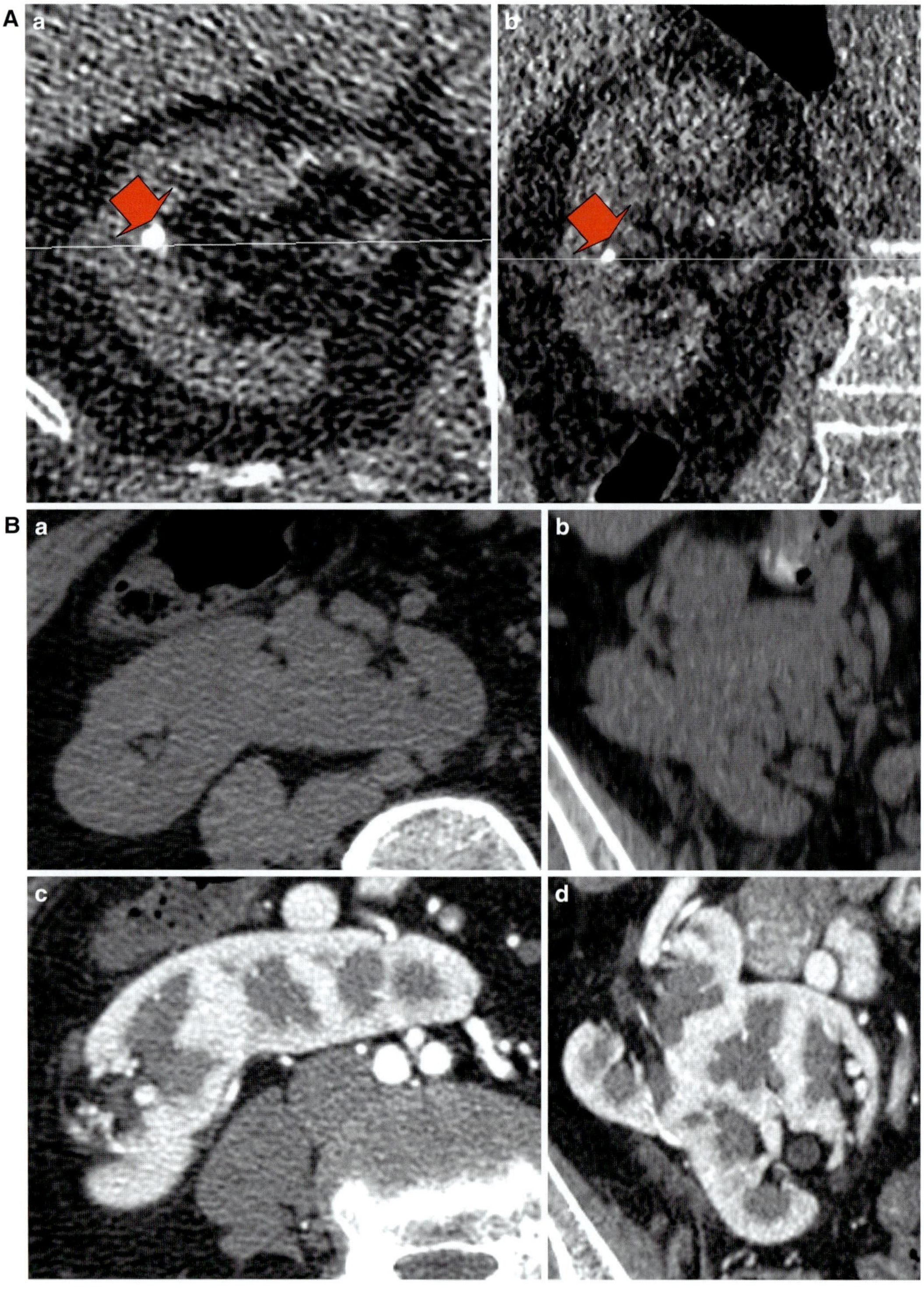

Fig. 13.2. (**A**) Nonenhanced axial and coronal CT scan obtained at 50 mA show a small radiopaque calculus (*arrow*) in the right renal pelvis. (**B**) Nonenhanced transverse (**a**) and coronal (**b**) CT scan demonstrate kidney fusion anomaly, better demonstrated in the transverse (**c**) and coronal (**d**) scan after contrast medium administration

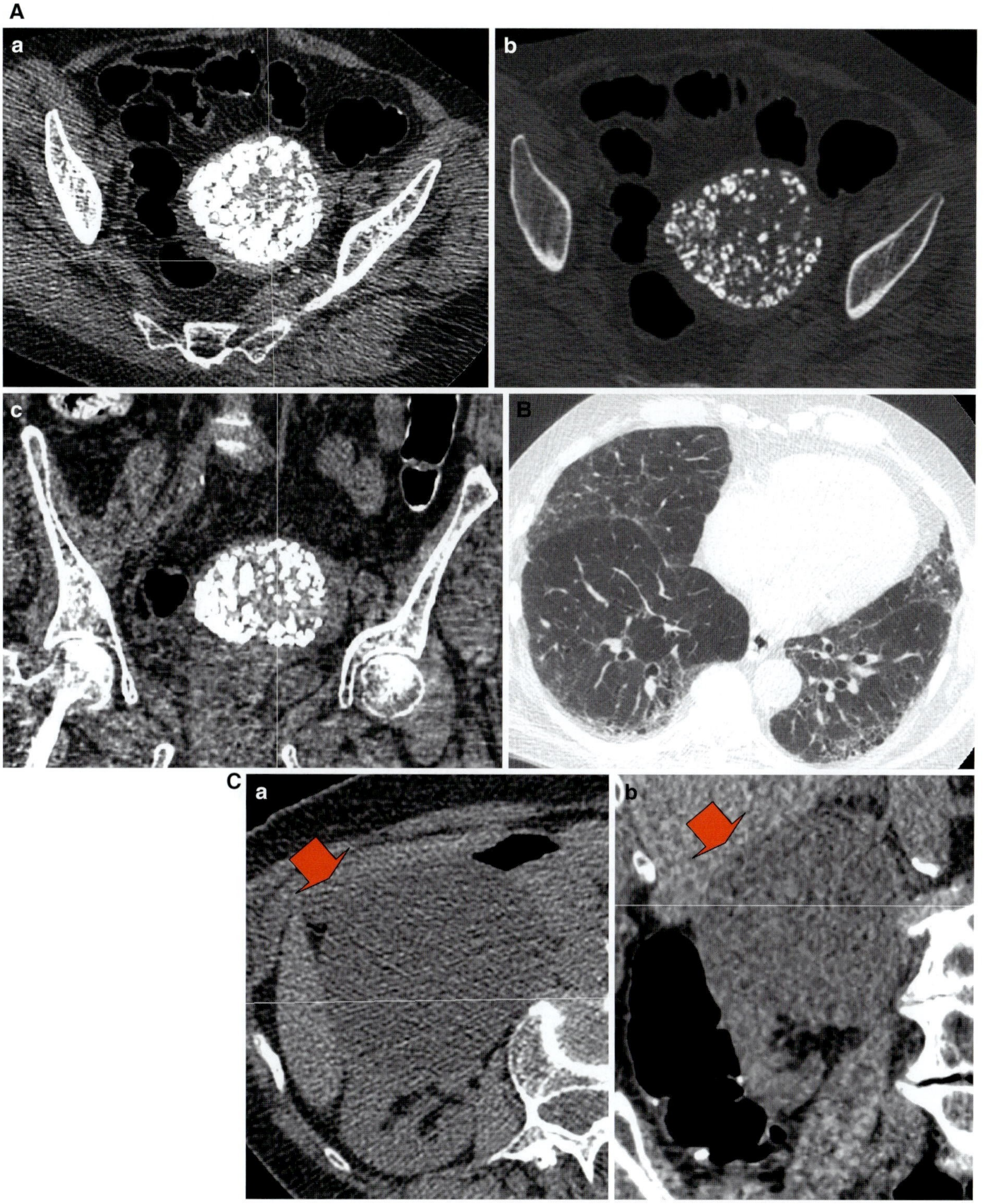

Fig. 13.3. (A) Nonenhanced axial (**a**, **b**) and coronal (**c**) CT scans show a large calcified uterine fibroma. (**B**) Nonenhanced transverse CT scan obtained through the lower chest shows ground-glass opacification with little evidence of honeycombing. (**C**) Nonenhanced transverse (**a**) and coronal (**b**) CT scan obtained at 50 mA demonstrate a voluminous right renal cyst (*arrow*)

Table 13.1. Categorization system for ECFs proposed by Zalis et al. 2005

E0	Limited exam. Compromised by artifacts; evaluation of extracolonic soft tissues is severely limited
E1	Normal exam or anatomic variant. No extracolonic abnormalities visible Anatomic variant: e.g., retroaortic left renal vein
E2	Clinically unimportant finding. No work-up indicated. Examples: Liver, kidney: simple cysts Gallbladder: cholelithiasis without cholecystitis Vertebra: hemangioma
E3	Likely unimportant finding, incompletely characterized. Subject to local practice and patient preference, work-up may be indicated. Examples: Kidney: minimally complex or homogeneously hyperattenuating cyst
E4	Potentially important finding. Communicate to referring physician as per accepted practice guidelines Kidney: solid renal mass Lymphadenopathy Vasculature: aortic aneurysm Lung: nonuniformly calcified parenchymal nodule ≥1 cm

In general, the prevalence of ECF is quite high, with an average of 40% up to 87–89% when considering all different types of ECF, from minor to major clinical relevance.

Focusing only on the major findings, notwithstanding the high variability of the results among different studies, the average prevalence is around 10–12%. However, the patients who need an immediate treatment present a percentage much lower, around 1%.

Among the major findings, a 2–3% of cancers and 0.9–1% of abdominal aortic aneurisms were found (Xiong et al. 2005).

The average prevalence when considering very inhomogeneous populations changes if patients are stratified into several groups. In particular, when considering a screening population (Gluecker et al. 2003; Edwards et al. 2001; Pickhardt et al. 2003; Chin et al. 2005), it comes out that both extracolonic findings of major relevance and extracolonic findings requiring further diagnostic inquiries and neoplastic pathologies show a lower prevalence.

Further analysis allows us to see that, as expected, the population studied by Pickardt et al. (2003) is also the youngest among the ones considered for the evaluation of extracolonic findings.

This shows that the number of extracolonic findings increases with the age of the population.

In fact, the prevalence increases up to 24% in old patients and when the general conditions are poor not only with respect to the total percentage of ECF, but also with respect to the number of major findings that require surgery (12%) (Ng et al. 2004).

An important feature affecting the percentage of ECF prevalence is the usage of the intravenous contrast media. In fact, it is usually administered to symptomatic patients, who are supposed to have a

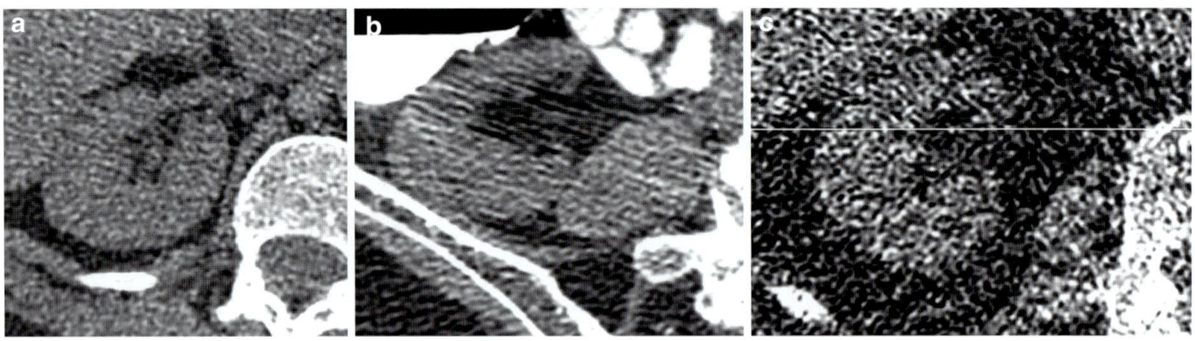

Fig. 13.4. Effect of dose reduction on axial CT images; image noise increases with decreasing quality of imaging: (**a**) 100 mA, (**b**) 80 mA, (**c**) 50 mA

colorectal cancer. In these patients, the contrast media administration is necessary for staging the probable cancer. As a consequence, the likelihood of discovering an ECF (e.g., liver metastases) is much higher (Morrin et al. 2000; Spreng et al. 2005). There is also a technical reason that explains the increase in the number of ECF when using intravenous contrast media: in this case, it is necessary to use a standard radiation dose, thus excluding all the limitations enforced by the low-dose protocols, and facilitating the identification and characterization of parenchymal lesions.

Kim et al. (2008) showed in a recent study that a virtual colonoscopy performed using the intravenous contrast medium can be useful for asymptomatic patients too. In fact, it reduces the number of noncharacterized ECF, and it increases the number of diagnosed neoplastic lesions, which would be impossible to characterize in the only basal condition. It increases the number of neoplastic pathologies discovered in an early stage, thus reducing the morbidity and mortality of the population under examination.

The routine use of intravenous contrast medium in CTC would likely decrease the number of false-positive major findings; however, there would be an added risk of contrast medium-induced renal failure and hypersensitivity reactions. Thus, routinely adding intravenous contrast to CTC does not seem to be indicated (Sosna et al. 2005). Furthermore, the use of contrast medium in a screening population would increase the cost of the single examination. For all the above reasons, the guidelines of the European Society of Gastrointestinal and Abdominal Radiology (ESGAR) do not recommend its use (Taylor et al. 2007).

13.4 Monetary Cost

One of the most critical issues of ECF concerns its monetary cost. Only a small number of studies have examined the added cost of additional examinations performed as a consequence of ECF at CTC (Sosna et al. 2005).

In general, such a cost was considered rather low compared with the cost of CTC and quantifiable in the range of 24–34$ (Hara 2005; Gluecker et al. 2003; Yee et al. 2005; Chin et al. 2005) depending on the percentage of findings requiring further work-up. The datum furthermore is proved independent from risk factors of the population. The percentage of total ECF and also of the clinically relevant ones is the same in asymptomatic patients that is in a screening population, both with respect to average risk and high risk for developing a colorectal cancer (Hara 2005; Yee et al. 2005).

Another interesting result (Yee et al. 2005) is the lack of morbidity and mortality increase due to the diagnostic–therapeutic follow-up of patients with ECF.

However, this methodological approach has been contrasted by new considerations (Hassan et al. 2008) based on the potential impact of ECF on the efficacy and cost-effectiveness of the colorectal cancer by means of CTC, when compared with alternative strategy including optical colonoscopy and abdominal ecography performed only once in 50 years old patients for the screening of abdominal aortic aneurysm.

In other words, the study determines whether the ECF, and in particular the identification of the abdominal aortic aneurysm and other extracolonic cancers, can be considered an advantage for the usage of CTC for screening rather than a cost. More specifically, the additional identification of these pathologies can give the use of CTC for screening a better cost-effectiveness ratio with respect to a situation in which the ECF are not considered at all. This study shows that the simultaneous analysis of the colon and of the abdominal aorta is the best strategy for cost-effectiveness ratio, compared with the alternative strategy that uses optical colonoscopy and abdominal ecography after the age of 50.

In conclusion, besides considering the pure monetary cost, it is also important to consider the value of patients and informal care-giving time and resources devoted to treatment and long-term follow-up examinations that may result. In fact, other benefits and harms associated with follow-up and management of ECF also need to be taken into account, such as patient anxiety and concern, long-term morbidity, mortality, and quality of life outcomes. Even findings of moderate or minor importance can create distress for the patients (Sosna et al. 2005).

Table 13.2. Description of papers regarding ECFs on CTC

Study	Number of patients	Population	Age	Radiation dose	Contrast media	ECF (%)	Clinical relevance			Percentage of ECF patients with workup	Percentage of treatment	Percentage of tumors
							Minor	Moderate	Major			
Hara et al. 2000	264	Symptomatic /high risk	64	Low dose	No	41	21	17	11	7	2	0.7
Edwards et al. 2001	100	Symptomatic /high risk	65	Low dose	No	15	1	11	3	11	2	1
Gpedersen et al. 2003	75	Asymptomatic /surveillance	61	Low dose	No	65	–	–	–	12	3	1.3
Gluecker et al. 2003	681	Asymptomatic /screening	64	Low dose	No	87	50	27	10	–	1.3	1
Hellstrom et al. 2004	111	Symptomatic /high risk	66	Standard	No	85	41	52	23	13	–	3.6
Ng et al. 2004	1,077	Symptomatic/elderly	80	Standard	No	24	–	24				–
Rajapaksa et al. 2004	250	Symptomatic	64	Low dose	No	33	48	39	12	24	–	–
Chin et al. 2005	432	Asymptomatic/screening	58	Low dose	No	27	–	–	7	7	–	–
Spreng et al. 2005	102	Symptomatic	66	Standard	Yes	89	–	–	10	30	18	6.9
Yee et al. 2005	500	Asymptomatic /screening	62	Low dose	No	63	85		14	8	1.3	–
Kim et al., 2008	2,230	Asymptomatic	57	Standard	Yes	66	–	–	5	4.5	2	0.5

References

Bechtold RE, Chen MY, Ott DJ et al (1997) Interpretation of abdominal CT: analysis of errors and their causes. J Comut Assist Tomogr 21:681–685

Berland LL (2009) Incidental extracolonic findings on CT colonography: the impending deluge and its implications. J Am Coll Radiol 6:14–20

Chin M, Mendelson R, Edwards J et al (2005) Computed tomographic colonography: prevalence, nature, and clinical significance of extracolonic findings in a community screening program. Am J Gastroenterol 100(12):2771–2776

Edwards JT, Wood CJ, Mendelson RM et al (2001) Extracolonic findings at virtual colonoscopy: implications for screening programs. Am J Gastroenterol 96:3009–3012

van Gelder RE, Venema HW, Selie IW et al (2002) CT colonography at different radiation dose levels: feasibility of dose reduction. Radiology 224:25–33

Ginnerup Pedersen B, Rosenkilde M, Christiansen TE et al (2003) Extracolonic findings at computed tomography colonography are a challenge. Gut 52:1744–1747

Gluecker TM, Johnson CD, Wilson LA et al (2003) Extracolonic findings at CT colonography: evaluation of prevalence and cost in a screening population. Gastroenterology 124: 911–916

Hara AK, Johnson CD, MacCarty RL et al (2000) Incidental extracolonic findings at CT colonography. Radiology 215:353–357

Hara AK (2005) Extracolonic findings at CT colonography. Semin Ultrasound CT MRI 26:24–27

Hassan C, Pickhardt PJ, Laghi A et al (2008) Computed tomographic colonography to screen for colorectal cancer, extra-

colonic cancer, and aortic aneurysm: model simulation with cost-effectiveness analysis. Arch Intern Med 168(7):696–705
Hellstrom M, Svensson MH, Lasson A (2004) Extracolonic and incidental findings on CT colonography (virtual colonoscopy). AJR 182:631–638
Iannaccone R, Laghi A, Catalano C et al (2004) Computed tomography colonography: colon examination or Pandora's box. Gut 53:915
Khan KY, Xiong T, McCafferty I et al (2007) Frequency and impact of extracolonic findings detected at computed tomographic colonography in a symptomatic population. Br J of Surg 94:355–361
Kim YS, Kim N, Kim SY et al (2008) Extracolonic findings in asymptomatic screening population undergoing intravenous contrast-enhanced computed tomography colonography. J Gastroenterol Hepatol 23(7 Pt 2):e49–e57
Morrin MM, Farrell RJ, Kruskal BJ et al (2000) Utility of intravenously administered contrast material on CT colonography. Radiology 217:765–771
Ng CS, Doyle TC, Courtney HM et al (2004) Extracolonic findings in patients undergoing abdomino-pelvic CT for suspected colorectal carcinoma in the frail and disabled patient. Clin Radiol 59(5):421–430
Pickhardt PJ, Choi JR, Hwang I et al (2003) Computed tomographic virtual colonoscopy to screen for colorectal neoplasia in asymptomatic adults. N Engl J Med 349: 2191–2200
Rajapaksa RC, Macari M, Bini EJ (2004) Prevalence and impact of extracolonic findings in patients undergoing CT colonography. Clin Gastroenterol 38:767–771
Sosna J, Kruskal JB, Bar-Ziv J et al (2005) Extracolonic findings at CT colonography. Abdom Imaging 30(6):709–713
Spreng A, Netzer P, Mattich J et al (2005) Importance of extracolonic findings at IV contrast medium-enhanced CT colonography versus those at non enhanced CT colonography. Eur Radiol 15:2088–2095
Taylor SA, Laghi A, Lefere P et al (2007) European Society of Gastrointestinal and Abdominal Radiology (ESGAR): consensus statement on CT colonography. Eur Radiol 17(2): 575–579
Xiong T, Richardson M, Woodroffe R et al (2005) Incidental lesions found on CT colonography: their nature and frequency. Br J Radiol 78(925):22–29
Yee J, Kumar NN, Godara S et al (2005) Extracolonic abnormalities discovered incidentally at CT colonography in a male population. Radiology 236(2):519–526
Zalis ME, Barish MA, Choi JR, Working Group on Virtual Colonoscopy et al (2005) CT colonography reporting and data system: a consensus proposal. Radiology 236(1): 3–9

The Future: Computer-Aided Detection

H. Yoshida

CONTENTS

H. Yoshida, PhD
Deapartment of Radiology, Massachusetts General Hospital, 75 Blossom Court, Boston, MA 02114,USA

14.1 Introduction

During the past decade, computer-aided diagnosis (CAD) has been shown to be of clinical benefit in fields such as detection of microcalcifications and classification of masses in mammograms (Astley and Gilbert 2004). The concept of CAD is not unique to these fields; indeed, it is more important and beneficial for examinations in which a large quantity of images need to be interpreted rapidly for finding a lesion with low incidence, such as the detection of polyps in CT colonography (CTC) and the detection of lung nodules in thoracic CT scans. In its most general form, CAD can be defined as a diagnosis made by a radiologist who uses the output of a computerized scheme for automated image analysis as a diagnostic aid (Doi 2004). Conventionally, CAD acts as a "second reader," pointing out abnormalities to the radiologist that otherwise might have been missed. The final diagnosis is made by the radiologist. This definition emphasizes the intent of CAD to support rather than substitute the human reader in the detection of polyps.

CAD for CTC typically refers to a computerized scheme for automated detection of polyps and masses in CTC data. It provides the locations of suspicious polyps and masses to radiologists. This offers a second opinion that has the potential to improve radiologists' detection performance and to reduce variability of the diagnostic accuracy among radiologists, without significantly increasing the reading time. Such a CAD scheme should be distinguished from semi-automated computer applications in radiology that automate only one of these components and depend on user interaction for the remaining tasks. A typical example is the 3D visualization of semi-automatically segmented organs (e.g., segmentation of the liver, endoluminal visualization of the colon and bronchus), or image

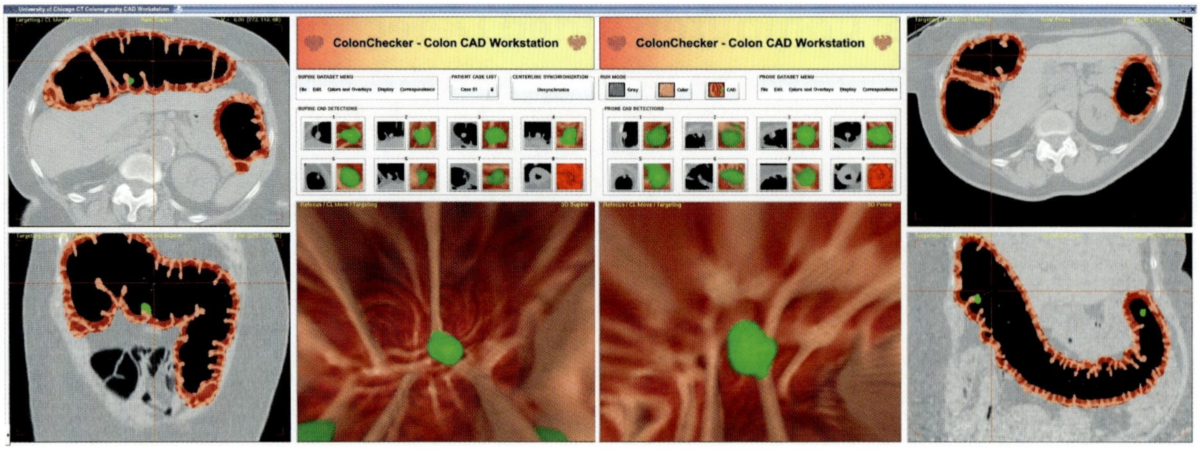

Fig. 14.1. Prototype colon CAD workstation

processing of a part of an organ for generation of an image that is more easily interpreted by human readers (e.g., peripheral equalization of the breast in mammograms, digital subtraction bowel cleansing in virtual colonoscopy).

Despite its relatively short history, CAD is becoming a major area of investigation and developments in CTC. Rapid technical developments have established the fundamental CAD scheme for the detection of polyps during the last several years. Prototype CAD systems have been demonstrated at conferences (Näppi et al. 2005b; Yoshida et al. 2004b) (Fig. 14.1) and commercial systems that implement the full CAD scheme or a part of it are becoming available in the market with names such as the Poly Enhanced View (Siemens Medical Solutions) and Colon Computer-Assisted Rader (MedicSight Inc.).

In the colon CAD workstation shown in Fig. 14.1, for example, the left and right images show the 2D multiplanar reconstruction (MPR) views of the supine and prone scans of a patient, respectively, with the computer-extracted colonic wall superimposed. The bottom middle two images show the corresponding 3D endoluminal views of the colon. Polyps detected by CAD are shown as a list of icons on the middle row of the screen. By clicking on one of the icons, one can jump to the corresponding polyp on a 3D endoluminal view and/or an MPR view. The polyp (green) is displayed in both supine and prone views if it is found in the corresponding regions in these two views (see Sect. 14.5.2). CAD output is integrated into the 2D MPR and 3D endoluminal views by use of the coloring scheme that delineates the detected polyps and the normal structures in the colonic lumen (see Sect. 14.2).

The latest prototype CAD systems yield a clinically acceptable high sensitivity and a low false-positive rate (see Sect. 14.4), and they are becoming integrated into the 3D workstation for CTC examinations and thus into clinical workflow. However, some technical and clinical challenges still remain as open problems for CAD to become a clinical reality.

The remainder of this chapter describes the benefits of CAD, the fundamental CAD scheme, the detection performance of CAD, the pitfalls in CAD, and the current and future challenges in CAD.

14.2 Why CAD?

Although CTC is a promising alternative screening tool for colon cancer (Dachman and Yoshida 2003; Pickhardt 2005; van Gelder et al. 2005), currently three key obstacles have held the clinical practicality of CTC at bay: (1) the variable diagnostic performance of CTC across studies (Dachman 2002; Mulhall et al. 2005), (2) the need for a full colon cleansing preparation, which is one of the major sources of poor patient compliance in colon cancer screening (Gluecker et al. 2003; Ristvedt et al. 2003), and (3) expertise required of the readers for interpreting the examination (Bodily et al. 2005; Fletcher et al. 2005).

The first problem was partly addressed by Pickhardt et al. (2003), who showed that, based on 1,233 asymptomatic patients, CTC could have a high by-polyp sensitivity of 93.9% for polyps >8 mm. This was superior even to that of optical colonoscopy. However, other large trials showed much lower sensitivity: a prospective trial on 703 asymptomatic patients reported by Johnson et al. (2003a), a multicenter trial at 8 hospitals on 314 patients also reported by Johnson et al. (2003b), a prospective multicenter trial at 9 hospitals on 615 patients by Cotton et al. (2004), and the most recent prospective multicenter trial at 15 hospitals on 617 patients by Rockey et al. (2005). Therefore, a larger clinical trial with the state-of-the art CT scanner and interpretation method needs to be conducted to address the first concern.

The second problem was partly addressed by Lefere et al. (2002, 2004a, b), who showed that dietary fecal-tagging CTC could be a viable alternative to full colon cleansing. However, the third obstacle remains problematic. In particular, the detection performance among readers can be quite variable, which may be one of the factors for the large variation in the results of reported large-scale clinical trials (Fletcher et al. 2005).

CAD for CTC is attractive because it has the potential to overcome the third obstacle, i.e., polyps and masses detected by CAD have the potential to increase radiologists' detection performance and to reduce variability of the detection accuracy among readers.

An improvement in the detection performance can be achieved because CAD can reduce radiologists' perceptual errors during the detection of polyps. These perceptual errors may be caused by the presence of normal structures that mimic polyps or by variable conspicuity of polyps, depending on the display method (Beaulieu et al. 1999; Fletcher et al. 1999; Johnson and Dachman 2000; Karadi et al. 1999; McFarland 2002). The absence of visual cues that normally exist with colonoscopy, such as mucosal color changes and a large number of images for each patient, also makes image interpretation tedious and susceptible to perceptual error.

A reduction of variability can be achieved because CAD can provide objective and consistent results. The performance of a radiologist may be influenced by his or her skill and experience. Moreover, a variety of circumstances, including distraction, fatigue, as well as time constraints in a busy clinical practice, influence the diagnostic performance. Although radiologists may detect a type of polyp in the majority of cases, the same persons may miss the same type of polyp under different circumstances. Use of CAD can potentially overcome this lack of consistency of radiologists, and thus it can be useful for reducing variability among readers in identifying polyps in CTC, as demonstrated by CAD for mammography and chest radiography (Jiang et al. 2001; Kobayashi et al. 1996) as well as the studies described in Sect. 14.4.2.

14.3 CAD Techniques for Detection of Polyps

To date, most of the CAD schemes developed in academia and in industry comprise the following four fundamental steps: (1) extraction of the colonic wall from the CTC images, (2) detection of polyp candidates in the extracted colon, (3) characterization of false-positives, and (4) discrimination between false-positives and polyps. A brief description of each of these steps is provided here. More technical details on the fundamental CAD scheme can be found in recent review articles (Yoshida and Dachman 2004, 2005).

In the first step of the extraction of the colonic wall, either fully automated (Masutani et al. 2001; Näppi et al. 2002a, 2004b; Wyatt et al. 2000) or semi-automated (Chen et al. 2000; Iordanescu et al. 2005; Summers et al. 2000) methods are used. Most of these methods use the thresholding of the CTC data based on the CT values characteristic of the colonic wall and the contrast between the colonic wall and the air in the colonic lumen as a means of extracting the colon.

In the second step, polyp candidates are detected by use of morphologic features that characterize the shape differences among polyps, folds, and the colonic wall. Figure 14.2a shows an example colonoscopy image of a 6-mm polyp in the sigmoid colon. As schematically shown in the middle column, polyps tend to appear as bulbous, cap-like structures adhering to the extracted colonic wall, whereas folds appear as elongated, ridge-like structures, and the colonic wall itself appears as a large, nearly flat, cup-like structure. To characterize these morphologic differences, various methods have been developed, including use of a volumetric shape index and curvedness (Yoshida et al. 2002a; Yoshida and Näppi 2001), surface curvature with a rule-based filter (Summers et al. 2000), sphere fitting (Kiss et al. 2002), and overlapping surface normal method (Paik et al. 2004). Figure 14.2b shows pseudo-coloring of the colonic lumen that visualizes the result of the shape analysis based on the volumetric shape index. The shape index determines to which of the following five topologic classes a voxel belongs: cup, rut, saddle, ridge, or cap. Color coding of the anatomic structures in the colonic lumen based on these classes can thus differentiate among polyps (green), folds (pink), and colonic walls (brown) effectively (Näppi et al. 2005b).

Typically, the polyp candidates thus detected include a large number of false-positives, many of which are caused by prominent folds and by feces

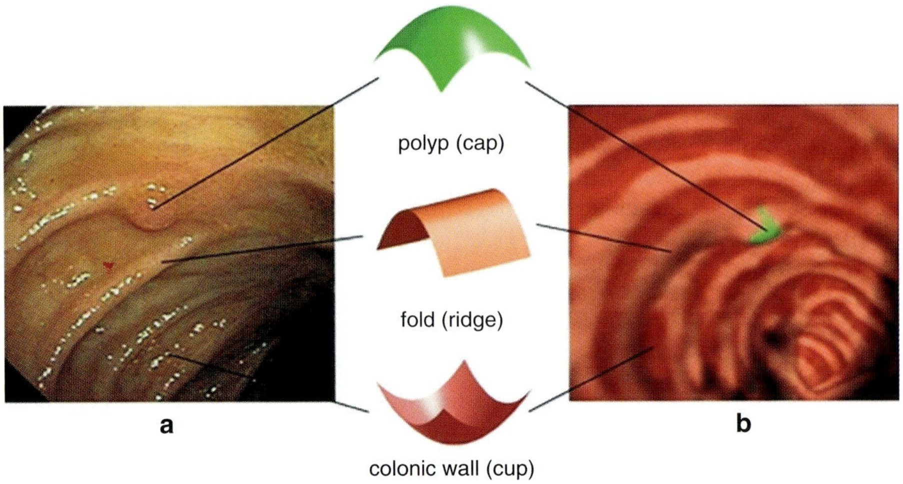

Fig. 14.2. (**a**, **b**) Schematic illustration of the geometric modeling of the structures in the colonic lumen (Reprint, with permission, from Yoshida and Dachman 2004)

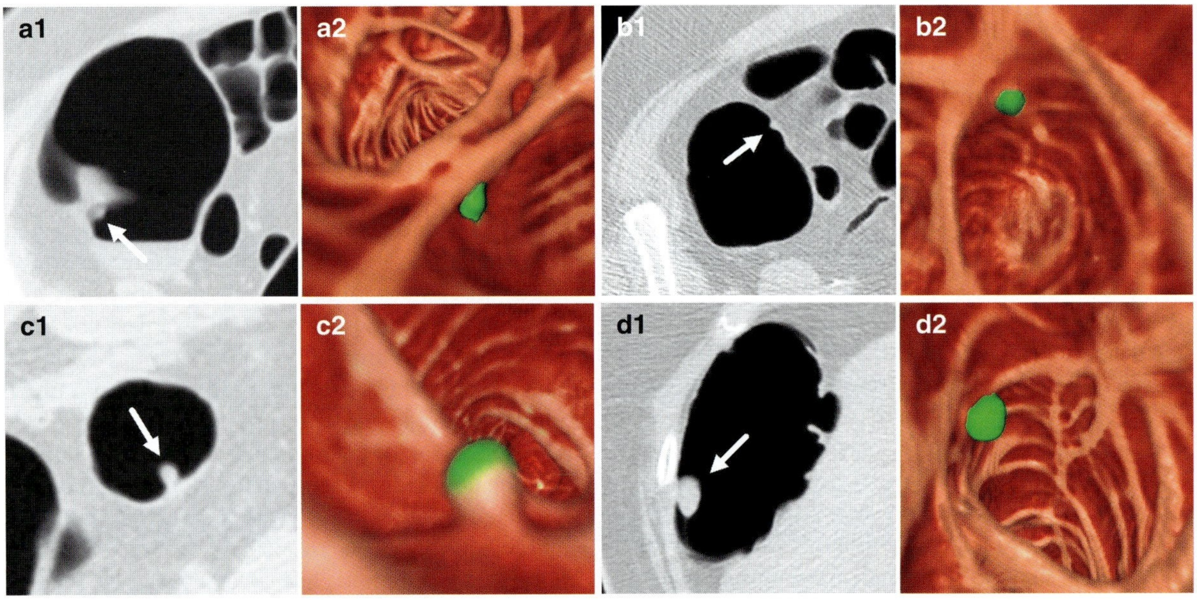

Fig. 14.3. (**a–d**) Example of polyps detected by CAD (Reprint, with permission, from Yoshida and Dachman 2005)

(Yoshida et al. 2002a, b). Various methods characterizing false-positives based on geometric and texture features have been developed for reduction of their number and include volumetric texture analysis (Näppi and Yoshida 2002), CT attenuation (Summers et al. 2001), random orthogonal shape section (Gokturk et al. 2001), and optical flow (Acar et al. 2002).

The final detected polyps are obtained by application of a statistical classifier based on the image features to the differentiation of polyps from false-positives. Investigators use parametric classifiers such as quadratic discriminant analysis (Yoshida and Näppi 2001), nonparametric classifiers such as artificial neural networks (Jerebko et al. 2003b; Kiss et al. 2002; Näppi et al. 2004b), a committee of neural networks (Jerebko et al. 2003a), and a support vector machine (Gokturk et al. 2001). In principle, any combination of features and a classifier that provides a high classification performance should be sufficient for the differentiation task.

The CAD output is displayed, in a 3D workstation, as a list of detected polyps (Yoshida et al. 2004b) (Fig. 14.1) or integrated in 2D MPR and 3D endoluminal views of the colon by use of, for example, the coloring scheme that delineates the detected polyps and the normal structures in the colonic lumen (Näppi et al. 2005b) as shown in Fig. 14.3. For each pair in this figure, the left image shows an axial CT image containing a polyp (arrow), and the right image shows its 3D endoscopic view by perspective volume rendering. The color coding is based on the above shape index analysis (Fig. 14.2). Figure 14.3a shows a 6-mm sessile polyp in cecum and Fig. 14.3b shows a 5.3-mm polyp in cecum, both of which were missed by a radiologist at first reading. Figure 14.3c shows a 7-mm polyp in the transverse colon, and Fig. 14.3d shows an 11-mm sessile polyp in the hepatic flexure. All these polyps are clearly segmented from folds and the colonic wall by use of CAD.

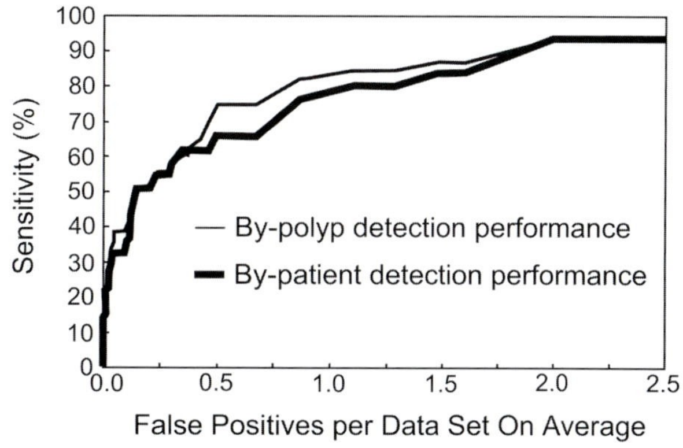

Fig.14.4. Free-response receiver-operating characteristic curve showing the performance of CAD in the detection of polyps

14.4 Performance in the Detection of Polyps

14.4.1 Performance of CAD

Several academic institutions have conducted clinical trials to demonstrate the performance of their CAD systems (Kiss et al. 2002; Näppi et al. 2004b; Näppi and Yoshida 2003; Paik et al. 2004; Summers et al. 2001; Yoshida et al. 2002a, b; Yoshida and Näppi 2001) that implement the full CAD scheme in the previous section or a part of it. In these studies, optical colonoscopy was used as the gold standard, i.e., the locations of the polyps detected by CAD were compared with the "true" locations of polyps that were determined visually in CTC data sets based on colonoscopy reports. In most of these studies, the performance of CAD was evaluated on CTC cases that were collected retrospectively at a single institution, and that were acquired with a protocol that is currently widely used for CTC, i.e., standard precolonoscopy cathartic bowel cleansing, insufflation of the colon with room air or carbon dioxide, and standard-dose CT scanning with CT parameter settings such as the following: a collimation of 2.5–5.0 mm, pitch of 1–2, a tube current of 50–200 mA, and a reconstruction interval of 1.25–3.0 mm.

Among the studies published in peer-reviewed journals that describe a full CAD scheme, the CAD scheme developed at the University of Chicago yielded a 95% by-polyp sensitivity, with an average of 1.5 false-positives per patient (0.7 false-positives per data set), based on 72 patients (144 data sets), including a total of 21 polyps ≥5 mm in 14 *patients.* In a by-patient analysis, the sensitivity was 100%, with 1.3 false-positives per patient (Näppi and Yoshida 2003). The same group reported, in a follow-up study that was published in a conference proceedings paper, a 93% by-polyp sensitivity with 4.0 false-positives per patient (2.0 false-positives per data set) based on 121 patients (242 data sets), including a total of 42 polyps ≥5 mm in 28 patients (Näppi et al. 2004b). Figure 14.4 shows a free-response receiver-operating characteristic (FROC) curve that shows the sensitivity of this CAD scheme as a function of the average number of false-positives per data set. Generally, sensitivity of CAD increases as the number of false-positives increases.

The CAD system at the University Hospital Gasthuisberg achieved an 80% by-polyp sensitivity, with 8.2 false-positives per patient (4.1 false-positives per data set), based on 18 patients, with 15 polyps ≥5 mm in 9 patients (Kiss et al. 2002). In this study, fecal tagging was used for most of the cases. A group at Stanford reported a 100% sensitivity with 7.0 false-positives per data set (only the supine data set of each patient was used) based on 8 patients that included a total of 7 polyps >10 mm in 4 patients (Paik et al. 2004). The sensitivity was less than 50% at the same false-positive rate for 11 polyps between 5 and 9 mm that were found in 3 of the above 8 patients. A group at the NIH reported a 90% sensitivity with 15.7 false-positives per data set, based on 40 patients (80 data sets) that included a total of 39 polyps ≥3 mm in 20 patients (Jerebko et al. 2003b). In a separate study, they reported that multiple artificial neural networks could potentially be employed to increase the sensitivity by an average of 6.9% and to reduce the false-positive rate by 30–36% (Jerebko et al. 2003a, Yao et al. 2004).

These studies indicate that CAD is promising in detecting polyps with high sensitivity and a low false-positive rate. It appears that the detection performance can reach up to 100% by-patient sensitivity with 1.3 false-positives per patient for polyps ≥5 mm (Näppi and Yoshida 2003). Generally, however, the performance of CAD systems appears to range between 70 and 100% by-patient sensitivity for polyps ≥6 mm, with 2–8 false-positives per patient. A meta-analysis of the reported performance of CTC showed that for human readers, the pooled by-patient sensitivity for polyps ≥10 mm and for those 6–9 mm was 85 and 70%, respectively (Mulhall et al. 2005). Comparing this performance with that of CAD, it appears that the performance, especially the sensitivity, of CAD is approaching that of an average human reader.

14.4.2 Improvement of Radiologists' Detection Performance

The ultimate goal of CAD is to improve the performance of radiologists in the detection of polyps and masses. Thus, establishing the sensitivity and specificity of CAD is only the first step in the evaluation of the benefit of CAD; CAD must be shown to improve the performance of radiologists.

It should be noted that CAD does not have to be as accurate as are expert radiologists to improve the detection performance of human readers. Computers make detection errors, as do human beings. However, together they can improve the diagnostic performance. Such a tendency can be found in an early clinical study by Summers et al. (2002), who examined the complementary role of CAD in radiologists' detection performance based on 25 polyps >10 mm in 40 asymptomatic high-risk patients. Two radiologists participated in the study. The sensitivity of both the two radiologists and that of CAD was only 48%; however, CAD showed that 4 of 13 polyps were missed by radiologists, thus increasing the potential sensitivity to 64%.

A recent observer performance study, which evaluated the effect of CAD on radiologists in an environment that closely resembles a clinical interpretation environment of CTC, showed that CAD could substantially improve radiologists' detection performance (Dachman et al. 2004; Okamura et al. 2004). Four observers with different levels of reading skill (two experienced radiologists, a gastroenterologist, and a radiology resident) participated in the study, in which an observer read 20 CTC data sets (including 11 polyps 5–12 mm in size), first without and then with CAD. The observer rated the confidence level regarding the presence of at least one polyp ≥5 mm in the colon. As shown in Fig. 14.5, the

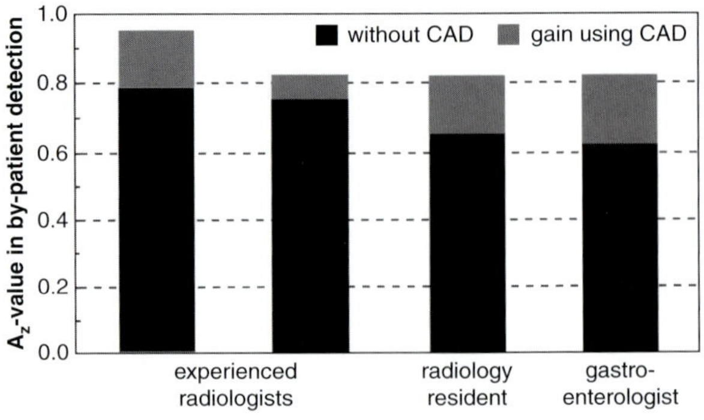

Fig. 14.5. Improvement of detection performance of human reader by use of CAD in the detection of polyps

detection performance, measured by the area under the receiver-operating characteristic curve (*Az*) (Metz 2000), increased for all the observers when they used CAD, regardless of the different levels of their reading skill. The average *Az* values without and with CAD were 0.70 and 0.85, respectively, and the difference was statistically significant ($p = 0.025$). The increase in the *Az* value was the largest for the gastroenterologist (0.21) among the four observers.

Another observer study was conducted by Mani et al. (2004) based on 41 CTC cases, in which the average by-polyp and by-patient detection performance for three observers increased from 63 to 74% and from 73 to 90%, respectively, for 12 polyps ≥10 mm in ten subjects, although the differences were not statistically significant.

These small-scale studies show the potential of CAD in increasing radiologists' detection performance, especially for those with less experience as indicated by the second study. A larger scale study needs to be conducted to show convincingly the benefits of CAD in improving the detection performance, in reducing the variability of the detection accuracy among readers, and in bringing the detection accuracy of inexperienced readers up to that of experienced readers.

14.5 CAD Pitfalls

14.5.1 CAD False-Negatives

Knowing the pattern of the false-negatives in CAD is important for improved sensitivity when the output of CAD is used as a detection aid. The types of false-negatives included in CAD results are similar to those encountered by radiologists (Yoshida et al. 2002a, b). Most of the CAD techniques depend on a shape analysis that assumes that polyps appear to have a cap-like shape, i.e., they appear as polypoid lesions. Therefore, polyps that do not protrude sufficiently into the lumen (e.g., diminutive polyps and flat lesions), whose shape deviates significantly from polypoid (e.g., infiltrating carcinoma), those that lose a portion due to the partial volume effect, those that are located in a collapsed region of the colon, or those that are submerged in fluid, may be missed by CAD. Improvement of the CAD techniques for reliable detection of these types of polyps remains for future investigation.

Representative examples of CAD false-negatives are shown in Fig. 14.6. Figure 14.6a shows a magnified view of a 6-mm polyp at the proximal transverse colon (white arrow), and Fig. 14.6b shows its 3D endoscopic view (white arrow). This polyp was located in a narrow valley where two folds merge, and thus the shape of the polyp was distorted. Moreover, a motion artifact made the polyp appear blurred, and thus it was a false-negative polyp. The neighboring polyp (black arrow), located below the convergence of the two folds, was detected by CAD because it was less distorted than the above polyp. Figure 14.6c shows a 7-mm polyp in the sigmoid colon, and Fig. 14.6d shows an 8-mm polyp in the sigmoid colon. These polyps appear smaller than expected from their size, mainly because they lost a portion due to the partial volume effect, and thus these polyps were false-negative polyps in CAD.

14.5.2 CAD False-Positives

False-positives may lead to unnecessary further workups such as polypectomy by colonoscopy; therefore, knowledge about the pattern of CAD false-positives is important for dismissing them. Studies showed that most of the false-positives detected by CAD tend to exhibit polyp-like shapes, and the major causes

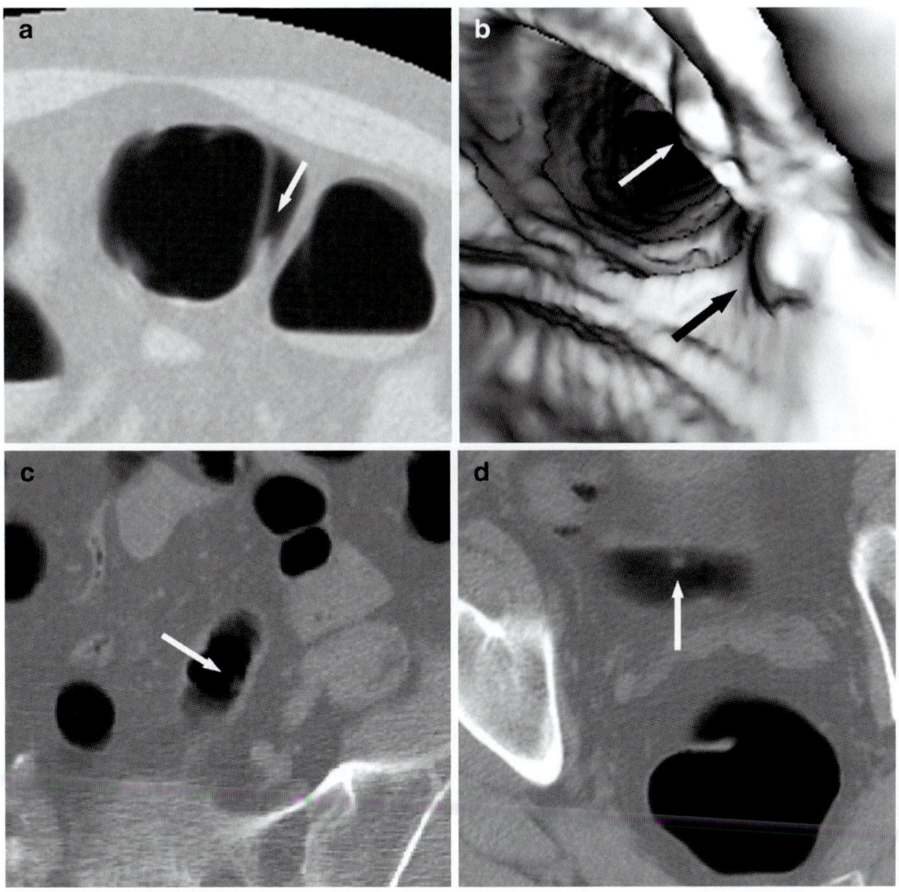

Fig. 14.6. (a–d) Example of CAD false-negatives (Reprint, with permission, from Yoshida and Dachman 2005)

of CAD false-positives are the following (Yoshida et al. 2002a, b). Approximately half (45%) of the false-positives are caused by folds or flexural pseudotumors. They consist of sharp folds at the sigmoid colon, folds prominent on the colonic wall, two converging folds, ends of folds in the tortuous colon, and folds in the not-well-distended colon. One-fifth (20%) are caused by solid stool, which is often a major source of error for radiologists as well. Approximately 15% are caused by residual materials inside the small bowel and stomach, and 10% are caused by the ileocecal valve. Among other causes of false-positives are rectal tubes, elevation of the anorectal junction by the rectal tube, and motion artifacts, each amounting to less than 3%.

Representative examples of CAD false-positives are shown in Fig. 14.7. Figure 14.7a shows a prominent fold (arrow). The tip of the fold appeared to be a cap-like structure, and thus it was incorrectly identified by CAD as a polyp. Figure 14.7b shows a piece of solid stool (*arrow*). This polyp-mimicking stool has a cap-like appearance and a solid internal texture pattern, and thus it was detected incorrectly as a polyp. Figure 14.7c shows an ileocecal valve (*arrow*). The tip of the ileocecal valve often has the cap-like appearance of a polyp and thus can be a cause of false-positives in CAD. Figure 14.7d shows the residual materials (*arrow*) inside the small bowel and stomach. Although a majority of the small bowel and stomach is removed in the colon extraction step, a small piece of them may be extracted along with the colon, and thus residual materials in the small bowel and stomach can cause false-positive detections.

Studies show that radiologists can dismiss the majority of these false-positives relatively easily based on their characteristic locations and appearance (Dachman et al. 2002). For example, false-positives due to ileocecal valves and the rectal tube can easily be dismissed based on their anatomic location and shape; a semi-automated recognition of ileocecal valves may make this already easy task even easier (Summers et al. 2004). Solid stool can be distinguished from polyps by visual correspondence analysis between prone and supine views; this relatively elaborate process can be facilitated by a computer aid (see Sect. 14.5.2).

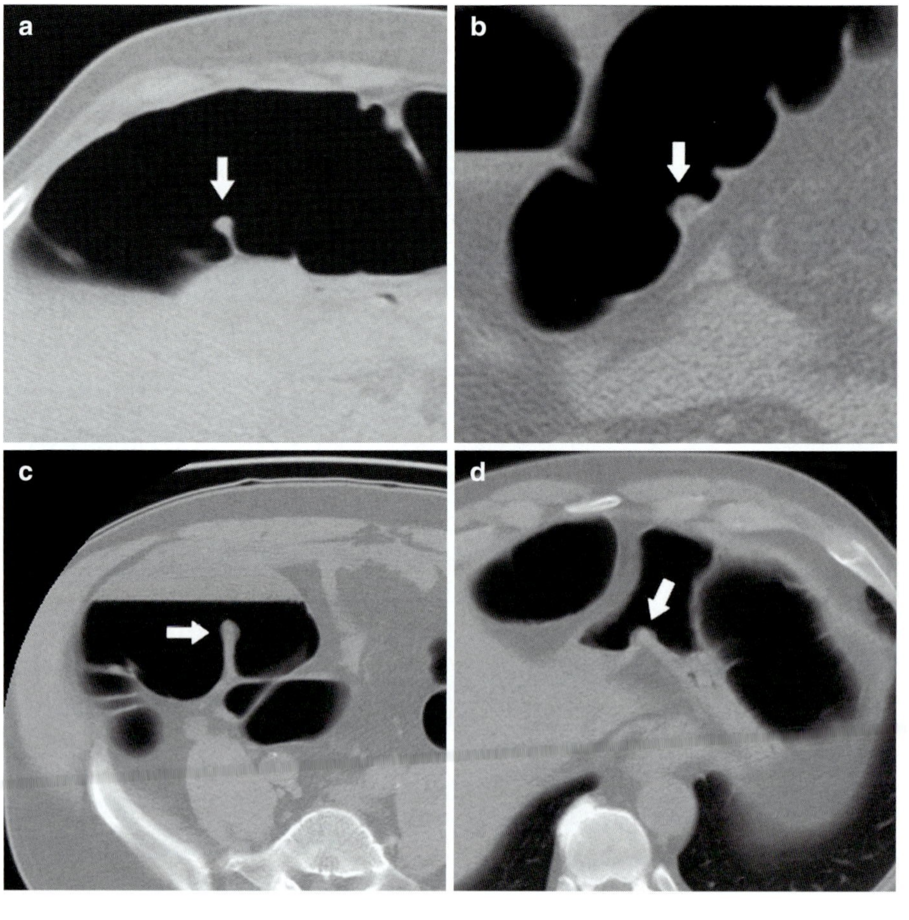

Fig.14.7. (a–d) Example of CAD false-positives (Reprint, with permission, from Yoshida and Dachman 2005)

However, there are types of false-positives, such as solid stool that mimics the shape of polyps and adheres to the colonic wall, which are difficult to differentiate from polyps even for an experienced radiologist. Moreover, the pattern of the false-positives may differ as new CAD techniques are developed. More research is required for establishing how radiologists can remove these false-positives to make a correct final diagnosis reliably.

14.6 Current and Future Challenges

During the past several years, many of the challenges that were facing CAD in its early stage of development (Summers and Yoshida 2003; Summers 2002) have been extensively investigated and partially solved. However, some challenges remain as open problems. Also, new challenges are facing CAD as the methods for acquisition and interpretation of CTC images evolve. Some of the current and future challenges of CAD are described in the following sections.

14.6.1 Detection and Extraction of Colorectal Masses

Despite the importance of the detection of cancers, only a very small number of CAD schemes have been developed for detection of colorectal masses that are likely to be cancers. This is probably because colorectal masses are generally considered to be easily seen by radiologists owing to their size and invasiveness. On the contrary, it is not easy for CAD to detect and accurately delineate entire mass regions; instead, CAD tends erroneously to report local surface bumps of a mass as several polyps.

The detection of both polyps and masses by CAD would be a more efficient computer aid in the interpretation of CTC examinations than is the detection of polyps alone. If masses are not detected by CAD, radiologists need to perform a careful and complete review of all CTC cases for the presence of masses, which may increase the reading time. Moreover, accurate detection of masses may depend on radiologists' experience and on how rapidly they read the cases (Morrin et al. 2003). Therefore, the application of CAD to the detection of masses could improve the diagnostic accuracy of CTC by reducing potential reading errors due to reader fatigue, inexperience, or a too rapid reading. Furthermore, without explicit mass detection, CAD could also confuse radiologists by presenting portions of masses as several polyps.

Automated detection of masses poses challenges for CAD because they may appear as intraluminal types (lobulated, polypoid, or circumferential) or nonintraluminal types (mucosal wall-thickening type of growth pattern or masses that block the colon), both of which have a wide variation in shape characteristics. Only a few CAD schemes for the detection of colorectal cancers have addressed this challenge (Näppi et al. 2002b, 2004a). One of these studies (Näppi et al. 2004a) used a fuzzy merging method and wall-thickening analysis for delineation of intraluminal and nonintraluminal masses, respectively. The CAD scheme detected 93% of masses (13 of the 14 masses) in 82 patients and extracted their regions, with 0.21 false-positives per patient on average. Figure 14.8a shows a 50-mm intraluminal circumferential mass with apple-core morphology, and Fig. 14.8b shows its endoscopic view. The entire mass region was extracted by the mass detection method, as indicated by the white regions in Fig. 14.8c, d.

Preliminary results indicate that CAD has the potential to detect colorectal masses in CTC with high accuracy. However, further research and a large-scale evaluation are needed for development of a CAD scheme that detect and delineate various types of masses reliably.

14.6.2 Use of Correspondence Between Supine and Prone Views

Use of both supine and prone data sets of a patient is important for improving the specificity in the detection of polyps, because the mobility of a suspicious lesion between supine and prone views can differentiate polyps from stool (Chen et al. 1999; Morrin et al. 2002). A real polyp tends to stay at the same location in the supine and prone views of the colon, whereas a piece of stool tends to move around in the colon, and thus, the stool can be found in different locations when supine and prone views are compared.

However, for CAD to find such a movement, it is necessary to establish a location correspondence between the supine and prone views. This is often a challenging task because the colon can be substantially deformed when the patient's position is changed from supine to prone. Moreover, some parts of the colon can be displaced and collapsed at this positional change.

Fig.14.8. (a–d) Detection of masses

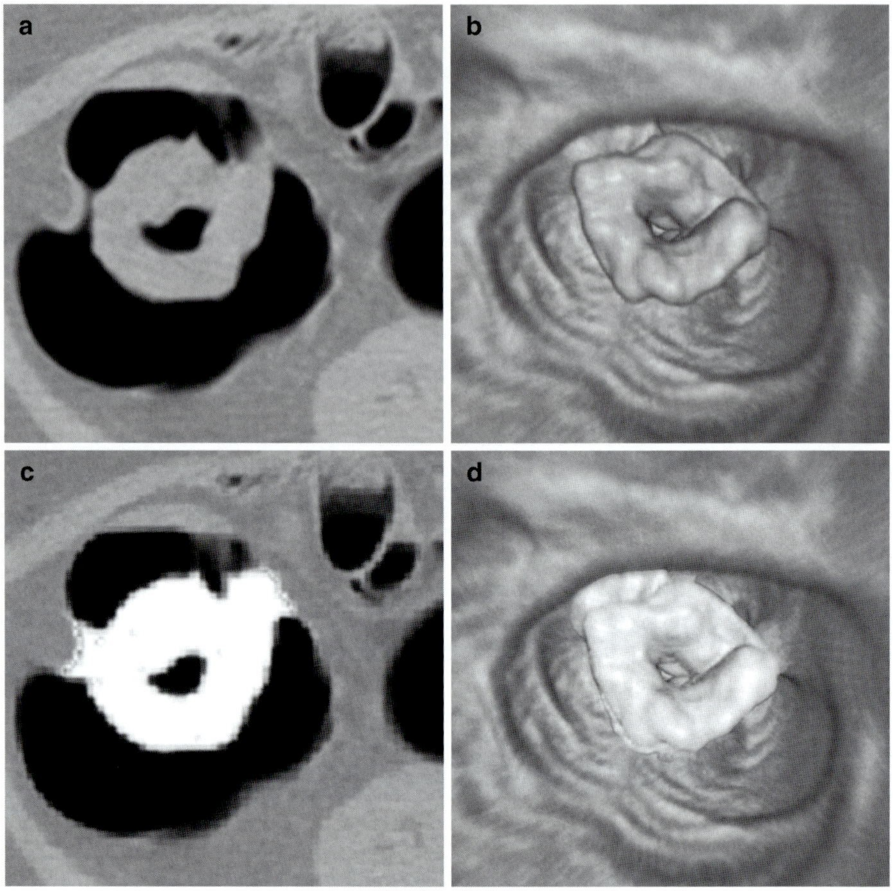

Most of the previous studies on correspondence between the supine and prone views were aimed at matching the polyp pairs after they are detected (Iordanescu and Summers 2003; Li et al. 2004; Nain et al. 2002). Such a method would permit radiologists easily to identify the matched polyps in both views for subsequent detailed examination. For example, the CAD user interface in Fig. 14.1 provides such a polyp matching function as shown in the middle two windows on the screen.

Only a few studies have addressed the challenge of using the supine-prone correspondence for improving the detection performance of CAD. One of these established a regional correspondence between supine and prone data sets of a patient by dividing the colon into overlapped regions (Näppi et al. 2005a). Figure 14.9 shows an example of the overlapped regions, in which a narrow region (light gray) indicates the overlap between the two neighboring regions (dark gray and black). In this study, a polyp candidate was kept as a detected polyp if both of the corresponding regions in the supine and prone views contain the polyp candidate (gray circle). On the other hand, if only one of the corresponding regions contains a polyp candidate, it was removed as a false-positive detection (white circle). Use of this region-based correspondence method in CAD reduced the number of false-positive detections by 20% while maintaining a 90% by-patient detection sensitivity (Näppi et al. 2005a).

The preliminary result is encouraging; however, further investigations need to be conducted for demonstrating that the use of both the prone and supine views is truly useful for CAD to achieve a high specificity.

14.6.3 Effect of Fecal Tagging and Digital Bowel Cleansing

Tagging of feces, especially fluid, by an oral contrast agent such as a barium suspension or water-soluble iodinated contrast material, is a promising method for differentiating residual feces from polyps and thus improving the accuracy in the detection of polyps

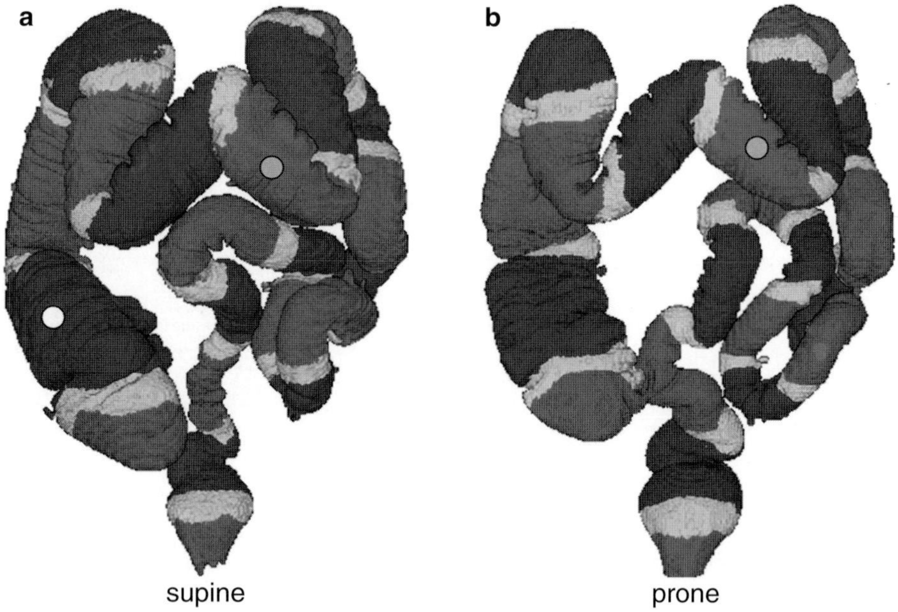

Fig. 14.9. (a, b) Region-based supine–prone correspondence method for reduction of false-positive detections (Reprint, with permission, from Yoshida and Dachman 2005)

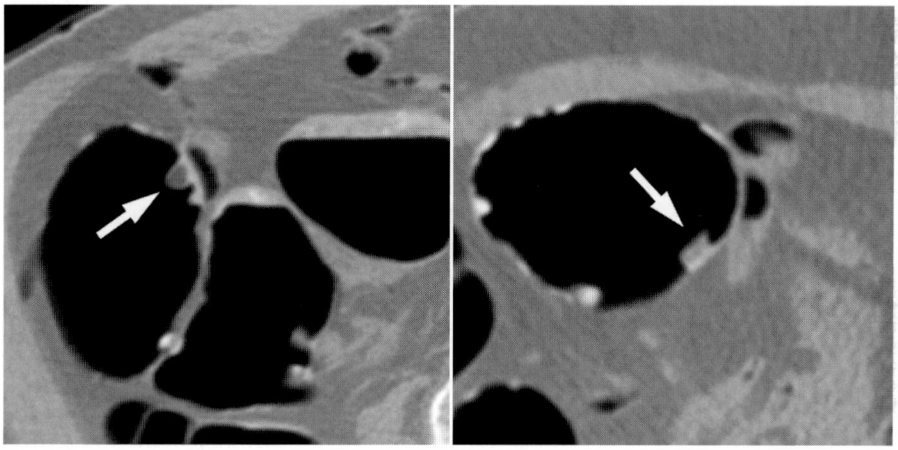

Fig. 14.10. Example of false-positives in CAD for fecal-tagging CTC (Courtesy of Lefere, Stedelijk Ziekenhuis, Roeselare, Belgium)

(Bielen et al. 2003; Lefere et al. 2002, 2004a, b; Pickhardt et al. 2003; Thomeer et al. 2003). Digital bowel cleansing is an emerging technology for removing the tagged stool and fluid, and thus it is useful for reducing bowel cleansing while maintaining the accuracy of human readers in detecting polyps (Pickhardt and Choi 2003; Zalis and Hahn 2001; Zalis et al. 2003, 2004b).

Tagging of feces introduces an additional challenge to CAD because reduced bowel cleansing tends to introduce a large amount of fecal residue, some of which may be tagged well, whereas some may not be tagged completely. Such a mixture of tagged and untagged stool can be a cause of false-positives in CAD (Yoshida et al. 2004a). Figure 14.10 shows examples of stool (arrows) adhering to the colonic wall that were not tagged by the barium-based tagging regimen and thus were erroneously detected as polyps by CAD.

Moreover, digital cleansing may introduce artifacts because of the partial volume effect and a suboptimal mucosal reconstruction method, especially at the interface of air and tagged fluid along the colonic wall or at the interface of air, fluid, and a fold (Zalis et al. 2004a). Digital cleansing may also create 3D artifacts that simulate polyps because incomplete cleansing due to suboptimal opacification of luminal fluid can result in artifacts that may have the appearance of polyposis (Pickhardt and Choi 2003), which can be a cause of false-positives in CAD.

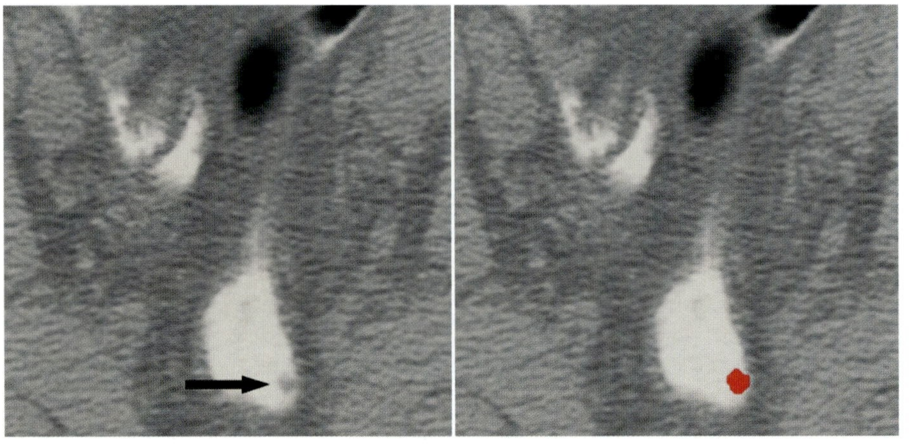

Fig. 14.11. Example of a true-positive in CAD for fecal-tagging CTC (Courtesy of Michael Zalis, Massachusetts General Hospital, Boston, MA)

Current investigations of CAD for fecal-tagging cases with cathartic preparation (Summers et al. 2005) and with reduced or minimum preparation (Yoshida et al. 2004a; Zalis et al. 2004a) are encouraging in that CAD showed the potential to detect polyps not only in the dry region of the colon, but also submerged in the tagged fluid. The left image in Fig. 14.11 shows an example of a polyp (black arrow) that was submerged in the tagged fluid; this polyp was correctly detected and segmented by CAD, as indicated by the black region in the right image.

Although encouraging, the results of these studies are very limited and are not conclusive; therefore, CAD for fecal-tagging CTC remains a subject for future research.

14.6.4 CAD for Rapid Interpretation: First Reader Paradigm

Some researchers proposed that CAD can reduce the interpretation time if radiologists focus on a small number of regions indicated by a CAD scheme. A reduction in time is most likely to occur when CAD is used as a first reader. Such a paradigm, often called "CAD as a first reader" (Evancho 2002; Mani et al. 2004), can possibly be used for separating out negative CTC cases even before radiologists read the cases. However, such a separation is likely to come with an increased number of missed abnormalities, because there is always a trade-off between sensitivity and specificity in CAD because the diagnostic performance of a CAD scheme is represented by a receiver-operating characteristic curve (Metz 2000). In other words, when a CAD scheme is set to yield a high true-negative rate (i.e., a high specificity), the price we need to pay is a high false-negative rate (i.e., a low sensitivity).

Thus far, no study has shown convincingly that CAD can shorten the interpretation time of CTC examinations, although some commercial CAD systems are advertised to be used in a similar manner to a first reader, and thus they imply that their CAD systems would reduce radiologists' interpretation time. In fact, conventional use of CAD as a second reader may increase the interpretation time, because additional time is needed for examining the possible lesions found by CAD but not by a human reader. However, such an increase in time is expected to be small, as demonstrated in CAD for mammography (Jiang et al. 1999), or the total reading time may be unchanged, as demonstrated by a recent observer study (Mani et al. 2004). Further studies need to be conducted for evaluation of the effect of CAD for rapid interpretation of CTC examinations as well as the efficacy of the use of CAD as a first reader.

14.7 Conclusion

CAD techniques for CTC have advanced substantially during the last several years. As a result, a fundamental CAD scheme for the detection of polyps has been established, and commercial products are now appearing. Thus far, CAD shows the potential for detecting polyps and cancers with high sensitivity and with a clinically acceptable low false-positive rate. However, CAD for CTC needs to be improved further for more accurate and reliable detection of polyps and cancers. There are a number of technical challenges that CAD must overcome, and the resulting CAD systems should be evaluated based on large-scale, multi-center, prospective clinical trials. If the assistance in interpretation offered by CAD is shown to improve the diagnostic performance substantially, CAD is likely to make CTC a cost-effective clinical procedure, especially in the screening setting.

In the future, no matter what types of visualization method (endoscopic, virtual dissection view, etc.) and reading method (2D primary or 3D primary reading) are widely used, it is expected that the detection of polyps by CTC will make use of some form of CAD. As the benefits of CAD are established, it will become more difficult to justify not using it, just as it would be difficult for a radiologist to justify not using a magnifying glass for reading mammographic films. CAD will be a powerful diagnostic tool that will provide radiologists with an opportunity to expand their sphere of influence by placing these CAD systems under their control, rather than losing procedures irretrievably to other specialists.

References

Acar B, Beaulieu CF, Gokturk SB et al (2002) Edge displacement field-based classification for improved detection of polyps in CT colonography. IEEE Trans Med Imaging 21:1461–1467

Astley SM, Gilbert FJ (2004) Computer-aided detection in mammography. Clin Radiol 59:390–399

Beaulieu CF, Jeffrey RB Jr, Karadi C et al (1999) Display modes for CT colonography. Part II. Blinded comparison of axial CT and virtual endoscopic and panoramic endoscopic volume-rendered studies. Radiology 212:203–212

Bielen D, Thomeer M, Vanbeckevoort D et al (2003) Dry preparation for virtual CT colonography with fecal tagging using water-soluble contrast medium: initial results. Eur Radiol 13:453–458

Bodily KD, Fletcher JG, Engelby T et al (2005) Nonradiologists as second readers for intraluminal findings at CT colonography. Acad Radiol 12:67–73

Chen D, Liang Z, Wax MR et al (2000) A novel approach to extract colon lumen from CT images for virtual colonoscopy. IEEE Trans Med Imaging 19:1220–1226

Chen SC, Lu DS, Hecht JR et al (1999) CT colonography: value of scanning in both the supine and prone positions. Am J Roentgenol 172:595–599

Cotton PB, Durkalski VL, Pineau BC et al (2004) Computed tomographic colonography (virtual colonoscopy): a multicenter comparison with standard colonoscopy for detection of colorectal neoplasia. JAMA 291:1713–1719

Dachman AH (2002) Diagnostic performance of virtual colonoscopy. Abdom Imaging 27:260–267

Dachman AH, Yoshida H (2003) Virtual colonoscopy: past, present, and future. Radiol Clin North Am 41:377–393

Dachman AH, Näppi J, Frimmel H, et al (2002) Sources of false positives in computerized detection of polyps in CT colonography. Radiology 225(P):303

Dachman AH, Yoshida H, Parsad N et al (2004) Observer performance study for evaluation of the effect of computer-aided detection of polyps in CT colonography. Am J Roentgenol 182:76

Doi K (2004) Overview on research and development of computer-aided diagnostic schemes. Semin Ultrasound CT MR 25:404–410

Evancho AM (2002) Computer-aided diagnosis: blessing or curse? Radiology 225:606; author reply 606–607

Fletcher JG, Johnson CD, MacCarty RL et al (1999) CT colonography: potential pitfalls and problem-solving techniques. Am J Roentgenol 172:1271–1278

Fletcher JG, Booya F, Johnson CD et al (2005) CT colonography: unraveling the twists and turns. Curr Opin Gastroenterol 21:90–98

Gluecker TM, Johnson CD, Harmsen WS et al (2003) Colorectal cancer screening with CT colonography, colonoscopy, and double-contrast barium enema examination: prospective assessment of patient perceptions and preferences. Radiology 227:378–384

Gokturk SB, Tomasi C, Acar B et al (2001) A statistical 3-D pattern processing method for computer-aided detection of polyps in CT colonography. IEEE Trans Med Imaging 20:1251–1260

Iordanescu G, Summers RM (2003) Automated centerline for computed tomography colonography. Acad Radiol 10: 1291–1301

Iordanescu G, Pickhardt PJ, Choi JR et al (2005) Automated seed placement for colon segmentation in computed tomography colonography. Acad Radiol 12:182–190

Jerebko AK, Malley JD, Franaszek M et al (2003a) Multiple neural network classification scheme for detection of colonic polyps in CT colonography data sets. Acad Radiol 10: 154–160

Jerebko AK, Summers RM, Malley JD et al (2003b) Computer-assisted detection of colonic polyps with CT colonography using neural networks and binary classification trees. Med Phys 30:52–60

Jiang Y, Nishikawa RM, Schmidt RA et al (1999) Improving breast cancer diagnosis with computer-aided diagnosis. Acad Radiol 6:22–33

Jiang Y, Nishikawa RM, Schmidt RA et al (2001) Potential of computer-aided diagnosis to reduce variability in radiologists' interpretations of mammograms depicting microcalcifications. Radiology 220:787–794

Johnson CD, Dachman AH (2000) CT colonography: the next colon screening examination? Radiology 216:331–341

Johnson CD, Harmsen WS, Wilson LA et al (2003a) Prospective blinded evaluation of computed tomographic colonography for screen detection of colorectal polyps. Gastroenterology 125:311–319

Johnson CD, Toledano AY, Herman BA et al (2003b) Computerized tomographic colonography: performance evaluation in a retrospective multicenter setting. Gastroenterology 125:688–695

Karadi C, Beaulieu CF, Jeffrey RB Jr et al (1999) Display modes for CT colonography. Part I. Synthesis and insertion of polyps into patient CT data. Radiology 212:195–201

Kiss G, Van Cleynenbreugel J, Thomeer M et al (2002) Computer-aided diagnosis in virtual colonography via combination of

surface normal and sphere fitting methods. Eur Radiol 12:77–81
Kobayashi T, Xu XW, MacMahon H et al (1996) Effect of a computer-aided diagnosis scheme on radiologists' performance in detection of lung nodules on radiographs. Radiology 199:843–848
Lefere PA, Gryspeerdt SS, Dewyspelaere J et al (2002) Dietary fecal tagging as a cleansing method before CT colonography: initial results–polyp detection and patient acceptance. Radiology 224:393–403
Lefere PA, Gryspeerdt SS, Baekelandt M et al (2004a) Laxative-free CT colonography. Am J Roentgenol 183:945–948
Lefere PA, Gryspeerdt SS, Baekelandt M et al (2004b) CT colonography after fecal tagging with a reduced cathartic cleansing and a small volume of barium. Am J Roentgenol 182:75–76
Li P, Napel S, Acar B et al (2004) Registration of central paths and colonic polyps between supine and prone scans in computed tomography colonography: pilot study. Med Phys 31:2912–2923
Mani A, Napel S, Paik DS et al (2004) Computed tomography colonography: feasibility of computer-aided polyp detection in a "first reader" paradigm. J Comput Assist Tomogr 28:318–326
Masutani Y, Yoshida H, MacEneaney PM et al (2001) Automated segmentation of colonic walls for computerized detection of polyps in CT colonography. J Comput Assist Tomogr 25:629–638
McFarland EG (2002) Reader strategies for CT colonography. Abdom Imaging 27:275–283
Metz CE (2000) Fundamental ROC analysis. In: Beutel J, Kundel HL, Metter RLV (eds) Handbook of medical imaging. SPIE, Bellingham, WA, pp 751–770
Morrin M, Sosna J, Kruskal J, et al (2003) Diagnostic performance of radiologists with differing levels of expertise in the evaluation of CT colonography. Radiology 226(P):365
Morrin MM, Farrell RJ, Keogan MT et al (2002) CT colonography: colonic distention improved by dual positioning but not intravenous glucagon. Eur Radiol 12:525–530
Mulhall BP, Veerappan GR, Jackson JL (2005) Meta-analysis: computed tomographic colonography. Ann Intern Med 142:635–650
Nain D, Haker S, Eric W et al (2002) Intra-patient prone to supine colon registration for synchronized virtual colonoscopy. In: Dohi T, Kikins R (eds) Lecture notes in computer science. Springer, Berlin, pp 573–580
Näppi J, Yoshida H (2002) Automated detection of polyps with CT colonography: evaluation of volumetric features for reduction of false-positive findings. Acad Radiol 9:386–397
Näppi J, Yoshida H (2003) Feature-guided analysis for reduction of false positives in CAD of polyps for computed tomographic colonography. Med Phys 30:1592–1601
Näppi J, Dachman AH, MacEneaney P et al (2002a) Automated knowledge-guided segmentation of colonic walls for computerized detection of polyps in CT colonography. J Comput Assist Tomogr 26:493–504
Näppi J, Frimmel H, Dachman AH, et al (2002b) Computer aided detection of masses in CT colonography: techniques and evaluation. Radiology 225(P):406
Näppi J, Frimmel H, Dachman AH et al (2004a) Computerized detection of colorectal masses in CT colonography based on fuzzy merging and wall-thickening analysis. Med Phys 31:860–872
Näppi J, Frimmel H, Dachman AH, et al (2004b) A new high-performance CAD scheme for the detection of polyps in CT colonography. In: Sonka M, Fitzpatrick JM (eds) Medical imaging 2004: image processing. SPIE, pp 839–848
Näppi J, Okamura A, Frimmel H et al (2005a) Region-based supine-prone correspondence for reduction of false positive CAD polyp candidates in CT colonography. Acad Radiol 12(6):695–707
Näppi J, Frimmel H, Yoshida H (2005b) Virtual endoscopic visualization of the colon by shape-scale signatures. IEEE Trans Inf Technol Biomed 9:120–131
Okamura A, Dachman AH, Parsad N et al (2004) Evaluation of the effect of CAD on observers' performance in detection of polyps in CT colonography. In: Lemke HU, Vannier MW, Inamura K, Farman AG, Doi K, Reiber JHC (eds) CARS–computer assisted radiology and surgery. Elsevier, Chicago, pp 989–992
Paik DS, Beaulieu CF, Rubin GD et al (2004) Surface normal overlap: a computer-aided detection algorithm with application to colonic polyps and lung nodules in helical CT. IEEE Trans Med Imaging 23:661–675
Pickhardt PJ (2005) CT colonography (virtual colonoscopy) for primary colorectal screening: challenges facing clinical implementation. Abdom Imaging 30:1–4
Pickhardt PJ, Choi JH (2003) Electronic cleansing and stool tagging in CT colonography: advantages and pitfalls with primary three-dimensional evaluation. Am J Roentgenol 181:799–805
Pickhardt PJ, Choi JR, Hwang I et al (2003) Computed tomographic virtual colonoscopy to screen for colorectal neoplasia in asymptomatic adults. N Engl J Med 349: 2191–2200
Ristvedt SL, McFarland EG, Weinstock LB et al (2003) Patient preferences for CT colonography, conventional colonoscopy, and bowel preparation. Am J Gastroenterol 98:578–585
Rockey DC, Paulson E, Niedzwiecki D et al (2005) Analysis of air contrast barium enema, computed tomographic colonography, and colonoscopy: prospective comparison. Lancet 365:305–311
Summers R, Yoshida H (2003) Future directions of CT colonography: computer-aided diagnosis. In: Dachman AH (ed) Atlas of virtual colonoscopy. Springer, Berlin, pp 55–62
Summers RM (2002) Challenges for computer-aided diagnosis for CT colonography. Abdom Imaging 27:268–274
Summers RM, Beaulieu CF, Pusanik LM et al (2000) Automated polyp detector for CT colonography: feasibility study. Radiology 216:284–290
Summers RM, Johnson CD, Pusanik LM et al (2001) Automated polyp detection at CT colonography: feasibility assessment in a human population. Radiology 219:51–59
Summers RM, Jerebko AK, Franaszek M et al (2002) Colonic polyps: complementary role of computer-aided detection in CT colonography. Radiology 225:391–399
Summers RM, Yao J, Johnson CD (2004) CT colonography with computer-aided detection: automated recognition of ileocecal valve to reduce number of false-positive detections. Radiology 233:266–272
Summers RM, Franaszek M, Miller MT et al (2005) Computer-aided detection of polyps on oral contrast-enhanced CT colonography. Am J Roentgenol 184:105–108
Thomeer M, Carbone I, Bosmans H et al (2003) Stool tagging applied in thin-slice multidetector computed tomography colonography. J Comput Assist Tomogr 27:132–139

van Gelder RE, Florie J, Stoker J (2005) Colorectal cancer screening and surveillance with CT colonography: current controversies and obstacles. Abdom Imaging 30:5–12

Wyatt CL, Ge Y, Vining DJ (2000) Automatic segmentation of the colon for virtual colonoscopy. Comput Med Imaging Graph 24:1–9

Yao J, Miller M, Franaszek M et al (2004) Colonic polyp segmentation in CT colonography based on fuzzy clustering and deformable models. IEEE Trans Med Imaging 23: 1344–1352

Yoshida H, Dachman AH (2004) Computer-aided diagnosis for CT colonography. Semin Ultrasound CT MR 25:419–431

Yoshida H, Dachman AH (2005) CAD techniques, challenges, and controversies in computed tomographic colonography. Abdom Imaging 30:26–41

Yoshida H, Näppi J (2001) Three-dimensional computer-aided diagnosis scheme for detection of colonic polyps. IEEE Trans Med Imaging 20:1261–1274

Yoshida H, Masutani Y, MacEneaney P et al (2002a) Computerized detection of colonic polyps at CT colonography on the basis of volumetric features: pilot study. Radiology 222:327–336

Yoshida H, Näppi J, MacEneaney P et al (2002b) Computer-aided diagnosis scheme for detection of polyps at CT colonography. Radiographics 22:963–979

Yoshida H, Lefere P, Näppi J, et al (2004a) Computer-aided detection of polyp in CT colonography with dietary fecal tagging: pilot assessment of performance. Radiology 227(P):577

Yoshida H, Näppi J, Parsad N et al (2004b) ColonChecker: a state-of-the-art CAD workstation for detection of polyps in CT colonography. Radiology 227(P):809

Zalis M, Yoshida H, Näppi J, et al (2004a) Evaluation of false positive detections in combined computer-aided polyp detection and minimal preparation/digital subtraction CT colonography (CTC). Radiology 227(P):578

Zalis ME, Hahn PF (2001) Digital subtraction bowel cleansing in CT colonography. Am J Roentgenol 176:646–648

Zalis ME, Perumpillichira J, Del Frate C et al (2003) CT colonography: digital subtraction bowel cleansing with mucosal reconstruction: initial observations. Radiology 226: 911–917

Zalis ME, Perumpillichira J, Hahn PF (2004b) Digital subtraction bowel cleansing for CT colonography using morphological and linear filtration methods. IEEE Trans Med Imaging 23:1335–1343

Quality and Consistency in Reporting CT Colonography

ABRAHAM H. DACHMAN, PIOTR R. OBARA, and MICHAEL E. ZALIS

CONTENTS

ABRAHAM H. DACHMAN, MD, FACR
PIOTR R. OBARA, MD
Department of Radiology, The University of Chicago, 5841 South Maryland Avenue, Chicago, IL, 60645, USA
MICHAEL E. ZALIS, MD
Department of Radiology, Massachusetts General Hospital, 55 Fruit Street Boston, MA 02114, USA

15.1 Introduction

Consistent and quality reporting of computer tomography colonography (CTC) results enables better evaluation of performance in both research and clinical settings. A thorough description of research methodologies and results allows the synthesis of data to create meta-analyses. Quality clinical reports not only provide useful information for the clinicians, but also enable retrospective analysis for internal audit and quality control purposes. In the near future, programs performing CTC may be subject to performance-based evaluations for accreditation purposes; standardized clinical reporting based on data-supported and expert guidelines will likely facilitate this process. Clinicians and authors should report information regarding the following categories: patient cohort and relevant history, bowel preparation and performance of the examination, examination interpretation, lesion characteristics (size, location, morphology, histology), and diagnostic performance. This chapter will discuss guidelines and factors regarding all these categories that hopefully will lead to better and more uniform CTC reporting.

15.2 Patient Cohort

Differences in risk and prevalence of lesions between patient populations may affect performance results. For example, the sensitivity of polyp detection may be lower in an average-risk population with few positive findings (SWETS 1992). The number of positive patient examinations will also determine the endoscopy referral rate, which is an important factor in assessing the cost-effectiveness of CTC. For these reasons, every patient examination report and research study should specify the patient's risk. Average-risk patients only have one risk factor, that is, being 50 years of age or older. Patients with moderate risk for colorectal cancer (CRC) will have one or more of the following: a personal history of adenomatous polyps or CRC, a family history of CRC, or symptoms indicating colonic abnormality (blood in stool, anemia, etc.). Patients considered at high risk for CRC, such as those with known polyposis syndrome or inflammatory bowel disease, are generally screened with optical colonoscopy instead of CTC because of the higher likelihood that they might harbor colonic neoplasia.

In addition to specifying symptoms and risk factors, each patient's report should include any conditions associated with CRC, such as ovarian or endometrial cancer. Any history of failed endoscopy or CTC should be specified to better characterize each patient. Research studies should present all the above-mentioned information in the patient characteristics section.

15.3 Patient Preparation

A well-prepped colon that is clear of particulate stool and excess fluid will undoubtedly lead to better CTC performance. Particulate stool can mimic or hide lesions and decrease the specificity or sensitivity. Certain preparation protocols, such as the polyethylene glycol lavage preferred by endoscopists, can leave behind significant amounts of excess fluid. The radiologist should still theoretically be able to observe all colonic surfaces by shifting fluid in varying patient positions (supine and prone). However, this may prevent the confirmation of a lesion on multiple views and decrease the radiologist's confidence. Differences in colon preparation can lead to varying performance results, and, therefore, the particular protocol used should be detailed in each patient report and research study. Additionally, any stool- and fluid-tagging methods or minimal colon preparation options used should be reported and the patients undergoing these regimens should be analyzed separately.

15.4 Spasmolytics and Insufflation Method

Spasmolytic drugs decrease the smooth muscle tone and are sometimes used during CTC to enhance the patient's comfort and colonic distension. However, spasmolytics may occasionally worsen colonic distension if the ileocecal valve becomes incompetent and starts leaking gas into the small bowel. In this case, an automated mechanical insufflation method may be able to better compensate for the lost gas than a manual pump. The quality of colonic distension can affect the ability to detect intraluminal lesions. Therefore, the method of insufflation and use of spasmolytics (including dose, route, and timing) should be included in all patient reports and studies.

15.5 CT Parameters

Image quality and resolution play a vital part in a radiologist's ability to detect and characterize colonic lesions. The factors that determine image quality should be reported and must include the following: scanner type, collimation, pitch, detector array for volume scanner, gantry rotation time, kVp, mA, mAs, radiation dose modulation, reconstruction kernel, pixel size, and reconstruction slice thickness and interval. Most studies now use "low radiation dose" scanning protocols that take advantage of the high contrast between colonic mucosa soft tissue and intraluminal air (Macari et al. 2002). However, there is currently no universal definition of what exactly a "low-dose" CTC protocol is; hence, all factors pertaining to the radiation dose should be reported. Detailed scanning parameters are a vital part of every clinical and research report, and will enable grouping of methodologically similar studies for review and meta-analysis purposes.

15.6 Examination Interpretation

15.6.1 Interpretation Factors

While continuous improvements in CTC software provide radiologists with more options for examination interpretation, they may also lead to an increased variability and complexity of the methods used in clinical practice and research. Each examination and study report should include not only the vendor and version of the platform used, but also the factors descriptive of the software that will make comparison with future versions possible. Descriptors of the interpretation method should include: single vs. dual monitor reading, mouse vs. button control of navigation, automated vs. manual fly-through, field of view, opacity, threshold, window and grayscale level, and contrast and lighting setting for surface-rendered displays. The primary interpretation method (2D, endoluminal fly-through, or "virtual dissection") should be described in detail. The ideal primary reading method is still under debate and may simply depend on the reader's preference; however, further data can be used for retrospective analyses and may help clarify this topic. The use of electronic "fluid cleansing" should be indicated if it was used. It is useful to know the reading time for cost-analysis studies, and hence the actual interpretation time should be recorded and specified separately from additional time needed to report findings and fill out forms. Additionally, the hardware and processor utilized may affect the reading time and should also be included.

15.6.2 Use of Computer-aided Detection

Developments in computer-aided detection (CAD) research are leading to an increased number of studies that include this detection tool in performance analysis. The CAD vendor and model should be included, and data using CAD should be reported separately. It is recommended that CAD be considered as a "second opinion" when comparing it with human-reader studies.

15.6.3 Readers' Experience

Studies involving multiple readers should include each reader's experience with the particular software and interpretation method used (i.e., the number of verified cases read). Different experience levels may significantly affect sensitivity and specificity rates and should be strongly considered when evaluating and comparing studies. Performance data for each reader should be analyzed and presented separately. Additionally, the report should indicate whether the decision about the presence of a lesion was made independently by each reader or as a group consensus.

15.6.4 Confidence Scales

Examination interpretation may often be hindered by visual obstacles, such as diverticula, excess stool, or colonic collapse. These factors may affect performance and should be specified in each patient report. Some studies have used confidence scales to rate factors that could potentially affect the quality of interpretation. If they are used, scales should be based on at least a 5-point scale, with a precise verbal description of each point. Some categories of examination quality that may be rated in this manner include (1) lumen distension, (2) residual fluid, (3) residual stool, and (4) presence of a polyp. While this rating system may make quality assessment more objective, it also introduces further variability that may make grouping and comparison of studies more difficult (Pickhardt et al. 2004a).

15.7 Lesion Size

15.7.1 CTC Measurement

Size remains the most important measure to assess the malignant potential, and consequently, the appropriate management, of a polyp. Therefore, it is critical that polyp measurements be precise, accurate, and consistent in methodology throughout a study. The report should at least indicate whether two-dimensional (2D) or three-dimensional (3D) views were used, and specify the window/level settings for 2D measurements. The authors recommend using lung window settings and reporting the largest polyp dimension (excluding stalk) in either 2D or 3D views. An estimated stalk length and diameter should be recorded for pedunculated polyps. Similar to the primary method of interpretation, the advantage of 2D vs. 3D measurement also remains an area of debate, and further data on this topic may help to determine the superior method (Pickhardt et al. 2005; Park et al. 2007). If any automated measurement software is utilized in a study, the software vendor and version should be specified, as the algorithms and results of these software packages differ according to vendor.

15.7.2 Size Categories

Polyp-size categories are an additional tool that can help standardize reporting and ease grouping and comparison of data from multiple studies. In 2005, the Boston Working Group on Virtual Colonoscopy published guidelines for describing lesion features (Table 15.1) and the C-RADS criteria (Table 15.2) for

Table 15.1. Feature descriptors of colonic lesions

Lesion size (mm) – for lesions 6 mm or larger, single largest dimension of polyp head (excluding stalk if present) in either 2D or 3D views. The type of view used for measurement should be stated
Location Refer to named standardized colonic segmental divisions: rectum, sigmoid, descending, transverse, ascending, and cecum
Morphology Sessile – broad-based lesion, the width of which is greater than the vertical height Pedunculated – polyp with stalk Flat – vertical height less than 3 mm above the surrounding normal colonic mucosa

Modified from ZALIS et al. 2005

Table 15.2. Classification of colonic findings and suggested follow-up

C0. Inadequate study/awaiting prior comparisons Inadequate colon preparation: cannot exclude lesions >10 mm due to excess fluid/feces Inadequate insufflation: one or more colonic segments collapsed on both views Awaiting prior colon studies for comparison
C1. Normal colon or benign lesion; continue routine screening every 5–10 years No visible abnormalities of the colon No polyps ≥6 mm Non-neoplastic findings, e.g., lipoma, diverticula
C2. Indeterminate lesion: surveillance recommended or endoscopy[a] Polyp 6–9 mm, <3 in number Findings indeterminate: cannot exclude polyps ≥6 mm
C3. Polyp, possibly advanced adenoma: follow-up colonoscopy recommended Polyp ≥10 mm ≥3 polyps, each 6–9 mm
C4. Colonic mass, likely malignant: surgical consultation recommended[b] Lesion compromises bowel lumen: demonstrates extracolonic invasion

Modified from ZALIS et al. 2005
[a]Evidence suggests surveillance can be delayed at least 3 years, subject to individual patient circumstance
[b]Communicate to referring physician as per accepted guidelines for communication, such as ACR Practice Guideline for Communication: Diagnostic Radiology. Subject to local practice, endoscopic biopsy may be indicated

classifying a patient examination based on the size and number of lesions found, with the appropriate treatment or follow-up indicated for each category (ZALIS et al. 2005). Clinicians and investigators are encouraged to use C-RADS to simplify CTC evaluation. Masses of 3 cm or larger should be analyzed separately from the polyps. In most patients, diminutive polyps that measure less than 6 mm do not have to be reported, because their very small risk of malignancy makes them clinically negligible (PICKHARDT et al. 2007; KIM et al. 2007). However, patients with inflammatory bowel disease or polyposis syndromes have higher risks of malignancy, and in these cases, all detected lesions must be included. It is important to make a distinction in reporting and analysis between 6 to 9 mm polyps and those 10 mm or larger; patients with one or two 6–9 mm polyps may be followed with additional CTC examinations while those with larger polyps require endoscopic removal (PICKHARDT et al. 2008; KIM et al. 2007). It may also be useful to report performance based on a 6-, 7-, 8-, and 9-mm cut-off size for detection. This additional data may help optimize protocols for excellent polyp detection using CTC while maintaining a small false-positive rate.

15.7.3 Endoscopic Measurement

To evaluate any virtual measurement method and validate polyps found on CTC, a high-quality strategy must be used to determine actual polyp size. An *in vivo* measurement during endoscopy using a caliper is the ideal method to obtain actual polyp size. However, the caliper is rarely used and size is most often estimated with an open forceps. If the forceps are used, they should be held as closely as possible to the polyp. The lesion may shrink if it is cut-off from blood supply or placed in formalin, and hence measurement of polyps prior to removal is most accurate. The method used to determine actual polyp size should be described in each study.

15.8 Lesion Location

15.8.1 CTC Location Reporting

The location of a lesion provides an intuitive reference for the endoscopist when trying to validate and remove a polyp detected by CTC. The six recommended colonic segments for reporting lesion location are listed in Table 15.1. The splenic and hepatic flexures do not have clear boundaries on endoscopy, and may not be very useful as segment descriptors when locating a polyp; therefore, their use is discouraged. The rectum is defined as part of the colon extending from the dentate line to the proximal valve of Houston. The proximal valve of Houston and the inferior aspect of the vertical descending colon border the sigmoid. The transverse segment spans the area between the cephalic most curvatures and the cecum lies inferiorly to the ileocecal valve. In addition to specifying the segment, it is useful for future reference to report the image numbers and views on which the polyp is visible. Descriptors of specific polyp locations, such as a fold or valve, and snapshot photos can also be included in each patient report to further enhance documentation and ease endoscopic validation.

15.8.2 Endoscopic Location Reporting

A thorough CTC description of a polyp's location is especially useful because the endoscopist lacks extraluminal reference, and pinpointing an exact location is difficult. Likewise, to improve the matching process, endoscopists should fully document their findings by including the following about each polyp: size, morphology (pedunculated, sessile, flat), distance from rectum, and its relationship to any nearby folds. An endoscopic video recording may be the best tool for matching lesions to CTC findings, although snapshots can also be used when video is not available. For patients with multiple polyps, a sequence of the polyps encountered is also helpful.

15.9 Lesion Morphology

CTC and endoscopy reports should include a descriptor of polyp morphology (sessile, pedunculated, and flat) to help with matching findings between the two methods (Table 15.1). Reporting polyp morphology will also help establish the prevalence and relative malignant potential of each type of polyp. Detailed reporting may be especially useful for flat lesions as their malignant potential and conspicuity remain less well defined, at least in part, due to the disparity of terms defining "flat" in the CTC and endoscopy literature (Soetikno et al. 2008; Park et al. 2005). On CTC, a flat lesion is defined as being 3 mm or less in vertical height above the surrounding normal colonic mucosa, and hence readers should measure the height dimension of any flat appearing lesion. The endoscopy literature employs the considerably more inclusive definition of "flat" as "height less than half of width," a definition that if applied to CTC includes many highly conspicuous sessile lesions (Soetikno et al. 2008). Reconciling the different definitions of "flat" is on-going at the time of this writing, and those interpreting CTC should at least be aware that the two non-concordant definitions are in use.

On CTC, the visibility of flat lesions may depend on the window/level used and the report should indicate whether only certain settings make identification possible. Flat lesions should also be separated into two subcategories: infiltrative ones that have no raised component and those that are raised and project into the lumen. CAD programs use these features for identification and additional data will help develop future CAD software. The clinical report description of every lesion should include its internal attenuation (soft-tissue polyp vs. fat-tissue lipoma). Lipomas are usually easily distinguished because of their lower attenuation, are not premalignant lesions, and should be excluded from any data analysis.

15.10 Lesion Histology

Research studies should group polyps by these histological categories when possible: adenomatous, hyperplastic, carcinomas, or normal mucosa. Histology data will help establish the prevalence and CTC performance differences for each type of lesion. While hyperplastic polyps may become flattened and more difficult to detect with greater colon distension, they are not premalignant and should be analyzed separately from adenomas and carcinomas (Fenlon et al. 1999; Dachman 2003). In addition, all polyp types should be analyzed in combination to enable comparison in performance to studies that do not consider histological data.

15.11 Definition of "Gold Standard"

The current best "gold standard" for verifying CTC performance is segmentally unblinded optical colonoscopy. Optical colonoscopy, uninformed of other results such as those from CTC, is not a perfect test and it may miss as many as 12% of lesions, most likely due to polyps hidden behind folds (Pickhardt et al. 2004b). Unblinding the colonoscopist to CTC findings segment by segment after an independent evaluation is made may be the best way to ensure that all polyps are found. This segmental unblinding method can also potentially reduce the CTC false-positive rate if it helps the endoscopist find polyps that were correctly detected with CTC (Pickhardt et al. 2003). Future colonic examinations such as barium enemas, endoscopies, or surgeries may identify additional polyps. These follow-up examinations should ideally be reviewed and performance data should be reported with and without this additional information. The endoscopic method used to verify CTC data should be specified and should follow the recommendations listed in the previous subsections (15.6.3 and 15.7.2) to improve the verification and polyp-matching process.

15.12 Diagnostic Performance

15.12.1 By-Patient Performance

Reporting performance based on patient data is most clinically useful and should include the sensitivity, specificity, and positive and negative predictive values. All statistics should be accompanied by their p values and confidence intervals. Performance statistics should be reported based on all patients combined and, if possible, separately for average-and above-average risk patient cohorts.

15.12.2 By-Polyp Performance

Performance statistics based on polyp data will vary from by-patient data with varying prevalence of synchronous polyps in the population and the diligence of the reader in searching for all polyps. For research purposes, a careful search for synchronous lesions should be performed because missing any will adversely affect by-polyp sensitivity. If possible, the number of patients with two or more polyps should be reported. Clinically, a careful search for synchronous lesions is essential; even though a single lesion may already qualify a patient for a full endoscopy, a synchronous lesion, if present, may be missed by endoscopy and could lead to devastating future consequences.

15.13 Conclusion

Standardized and thorough reporting of research methods and results will enable improved evaluation of CTC performance. Quality clinical reports serve as the starting point for excellence in research and allow for easier quality control and accreditation review processes. The authors hope that the information provided in this chapter will help improve research and clinical CTC reports and eventually lead to better patient care using CTC technology.

References

Dachman A (2003) Sessile polyps. In: Dachman A (ed) Atlas of virtual colonoscopy. Springer, New York, pp 109–110

Fenlon HM, Nunes DP, Schroy PC III et al (1999) A comparison of virtual and conventional colonoscopy for the detection of colorectal polyps. N Engl J Med 341:1496–1503

Kim DH, Pickhardt PJ, Taylor AJ (2007) Characteristics of advanced adenomas detected at CT colonographic screening: implications for appropriate polyp size thresholds for polypectomy versus surveillance. AJR 188:940–944

Macari M, Bini EJ, Xue X et al (2002) Colorectal neoplasms: prospective comparison of thin-section low-dose multi-detector row CT colonography and conventional colonoscopy for detection. Radiology 224:383–392

Park SH, Ha HK, Kim MJ et al (2005) False-negative results at multi-detector row CT colonography: multivariate analysis of causes for missed lesions. Radiology 235:495–502

Park SH, Choi EK, Lee SS et al (2007) Polyp measurement reliability, accuracy, and discrepancy: optical colonoscopy versus CT colonography with pig colonic specimens. Radiology 244:157–164

Pickhardt PJ, Choi JR, Hwang I et al (2003) Computed tomographic virtual colonoscopy to screen for colorectal neoplasia in asymptomatic adults. N Engl J Med 349:2191–2200

Pickhardt PJ, Choi JR, Nugent PA et al (2004a) The effect of diagnostic confidence on the probability of optical colonoscopic confirmation of potential polyps detected on CT colonography: prospective assessment in 1,339 asymptomatic adults. AJR Am J Roentgenol 183:1661–1665

Pickhardt PJ, Nugent PA, Mysliwiec PA et al (2004b) Location of adenomas missed by optical colonoscopy. Ann Intern Med 141:352–359

Pickhardt PJ, Lee AD, McFarland EG et al (2005) Linear polyp measurement at CT colonography: in vitro and in vivo comparison of two-dimensional and three-dimensional displays. Radiology 236:872–878

Pickhardt PJ, Hassan C, Laghi A et al (2007) Cost-effectiveness of colorectal cancer screening with computed tomography colonography: the impact of not reporting diminutive lesions. Cancer 109:2213–2221

Pickhardt PJ, Hassan C, Laghi A et al (2008) Small and diminutive polyps detected at screening CT colonography: a decision analysis for referral to colonoscopy. AJR Am J Roentgenol 190:136–144

Soetikno RM, Kaltenbach T, Rouse RV et al (2008) Prevalence of nonpolypoid (flat and depressed) colorectal neoplasms in asymptomatic and symptomatic adults. JAMA 299:1027–1035

Swets JA (1992) The science of choosing the right decision threshold in high-stakes diagnostics. Am Psychol 47: 522–532

Zalis ME, Barish MA, Choi JR, Working Group on Virtual Colonoscopy et al (2005) CT colonography reporting and data system: a consensus proposal. Radiology 236: 3–9

Virtual Colonoscopy: Beyond Polyp Detection

T. Mang, P. Pokieser, A. Maier, and W. Schima

CONTENTS

T. Mang, MD
W. Schima, MD, MSc
A. Maier, MD
P. Pokieser, MD
Department of Radiology, Medical University of Vienna, Waehringer Gürtel 18–20, 1090, Vienna, Austria

16.1 Introduction

Currently, there are two main indications for CT colonography (CTC). The first is polyp detection in patients who have an increased risk for colorectal cancer or for screening purposes in asymptomatic patients who are at average risk. The second common indication is incomplete or failed colonoscopy, where CTC is useful for complete colon visualization; for example, to detect additional lesions proximal to a stenotic cancer (Morrin et al. 1999; Macari et al. 1999; Copel et al. 2007). In addition to these main indications, there are several other situations where the role of CTC is not yet clearly defined. Some of these conditions may lead to colon obstruction, in which case, CTC is performed after incomplete colonoscopy. However, CTC may also be used for surveillance of these conditions, as an alternative to colonoscopy or barium enemas. Diverticular disease is the most common colonic disease in the Western world and often leads to diverticulitis. CTC is helpful in the assessment of not only the lumen, but also of any extramural changes (Table 16.1). Recent reports indicate a higher risk of colonic perforation in acute inflammatory conditions with CTC (Coady-Fariborzian et al. 2004; Burling et al. 2006; Triester et al. 2006; Wong et al. 2007). At chronic stages of inflammatory bowel disease (IBD), CTC can provide information about the extent of the disease, stenosis and pre-stenotic regions, as well as about the extracolonic extent and complications of the disease (Regge et al. 2009).

Although recent guidelines do not consider CTC as a surveillance option, a few recent studies have suggested its usefulness in post-surgical colorectal cancer surveillance (Fletcher et al. 2002; Laghi et al. 2003; Leonardou et al. 2006; You et al. 2006).

Table 16.1. CTC features of diverticular disease

Diverticula
Gas-filled outpouching of colon wall in 2D
Complete dark ring in 3D
Cave: *polypoid pseudolesion* in VE "*en face*"
Impacted diverticula
Polypoid pseudolesion in 3D
Incomplete ring shadowing in 3D
2D pathognomonic: filled with air, stool, retained barium, CM wall enhancement
Diverticulitis
Wall thickening with CM enhancement
Stenosis and pericolic fat stranding
VE: nonspecific

There is little experience about the feasibility of CTC in the evaluation of colonic lymphoma or post-interventional surveillance.

Although the primary target lesion for CTC is defined as the advanced adenoma, CTC is able to provide unique information about many other pathological conditions.

16.2 Diverticular Disease

Diverticular disease is the most common colonic disease in the Western world, affecting 10–30% of people at the age of 50 years and 30–60% at the age of 80. However, the disease is asymptomatic in the majority of patients. Together with aging, long-standing low fiber diet is the main predisposing factor for diverticular disease. Other etiological factors have been suggested, including increased consumption of red meat, fat, and salt.

The initial stage of the disease is the so-called pre-diverticulosis, which is characterized by thickening of the muscular layer, shortening of the taeniae, and luminal narrowing (Fig. 16.1a, b). With advancing disease, caliber and haustral abnormalities appear. This results in a continuous wall thickening of >4 mm, of long colonic segments with prominent semicircular folds, shortened interhaustral segments (concertina appearance), and a reduced colonic distensibility (Lefere et al. 2003) (Fig. 16.2a–d)

Histologically, most of the diverticula are pseudodiverticula, which are herniations of the mucosa and submucosa, through the circular muscularis propria layer at weak points in the colonic wall where nutrient arteries penetrate the muscularis propria. Rarely, true diverticula (most often at the proximal colon) are found, which are characterized by an outpouching of all wall layer (ie., mucosa, submucosa, and the muscularis propria). The radiological features of the two types of diverticula are not distinguishable. The CTC appearance of diverticula is easily recognized as air-filled outpouchings of the colonic wall on 2D images. On virtual endoscopic (VE) images, the diverticular orificium can be recognized as a complete dark circumferential ring when seen *en face*. Because of the complete dark ring, diverticula may simulate polyps when seen *en face* on VE images (Fenlon et al. 1998) (Fig. 16.3a, b).

Diagnostic problems can occur if a diverticulum inverts into the colonic lumen or is impacted with stool. A diverticulum may occasionally invert into the colonic lumen and produce a pseudopolypoid lesion on 2D and 3D images. The corresponding VE image is nonspecific and shows a polypoid lesion (Fig. 16.4a, b). The 2D images are pathognomonic to arrive at the correct diagnosis. Inverted diverticula with a pseudopolypoid shape sometimes contain fat

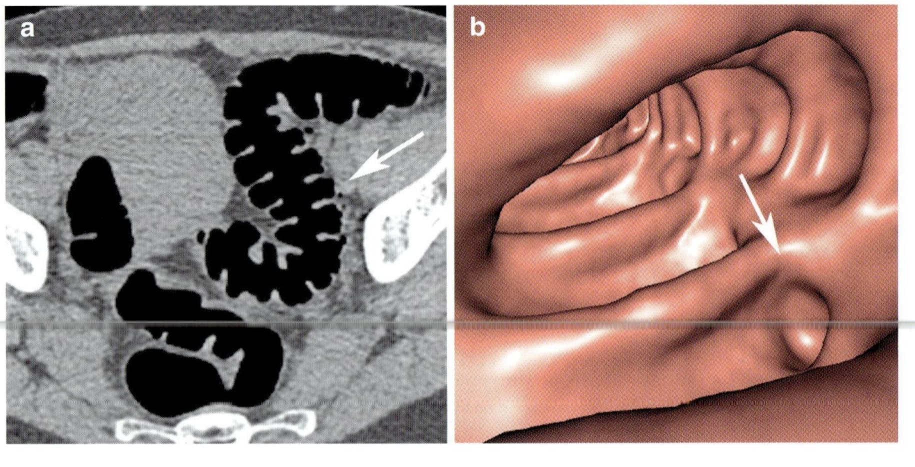

Fig. 16.1. Pre-diverticulosis. (**a**) Axial plane and (**b**) virtual endoscopic (VE) shows prominent semicircular folds, shortened interhaustral segments (concertina appearance), and a reduced distention of the sigmoid colon. (**b**) VE shows a single diverticulum (*arrow*)

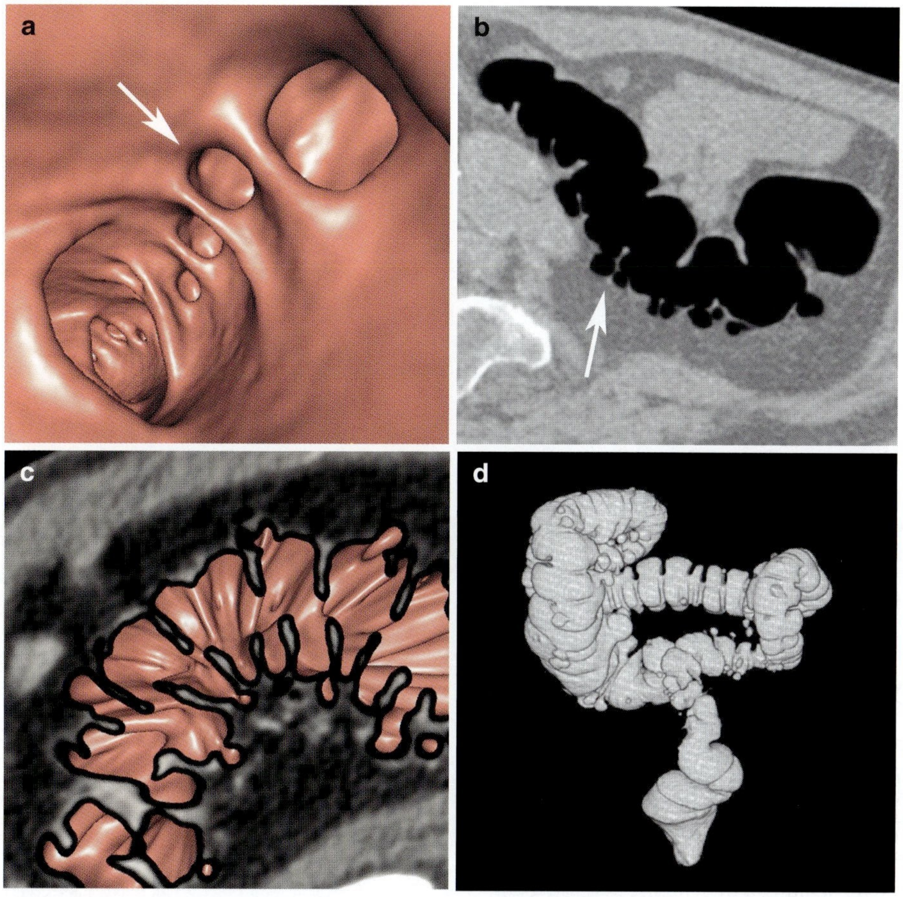

Fig. 16.2. Diverticulosis: VE shows multiple complete dark rings *(arrow)*, (**a**) finding that is typical for diverticula. (**b**) Curved planar reconstruction (CPR), and (**c**) combined 2D/3D view show multiple gas-filled outpouchings of colon wall in nearly all parts of the sigmoid colon (*arrows*); (**d**) global volume rendering views show the extent of the disease, with reduced colonic distension (concertina appearance), especially in the sigmoid colon (*arrow*)

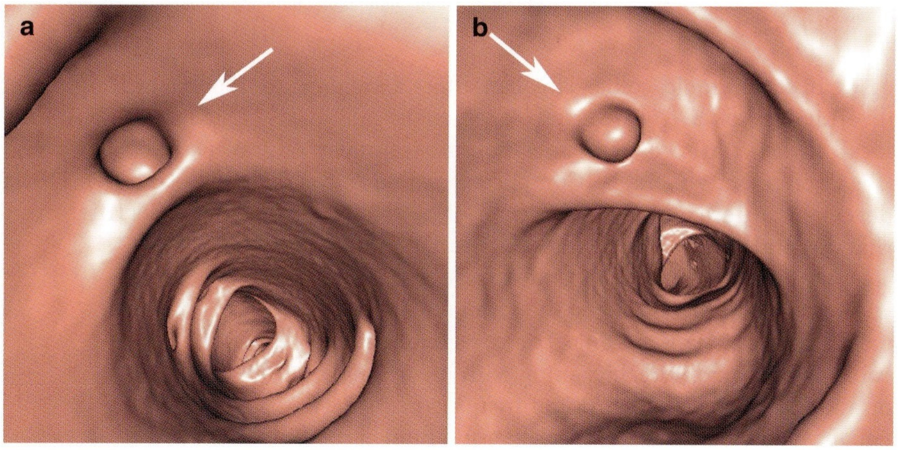

Fig. 16.3. Diverticulum vs. Polyp: (**a**) VE shows complete dark ring at the diverticulum (*arrow*); (**b**) incomplete ring shadowing at the polyp (*arrow*)

attenuation because of the inclusion of pericolic fat tissue (Fenlon 2002).

A more common finding than inverted diverticula are diverticula impacted with fecal material which may appear as a raised lesion and mimic polyps on VE images. On the 2D images, a hyperdense ring of encrusted fecal material with a hypodense center containing air or stool, or even retained barium from prior examinations, can be found in such a lesion (Hara et al. 1997) (Fig. 16.5a, b).

Inflammation of diverticula leads to symptomatic diverticulitis, which occurs in the vast majority of

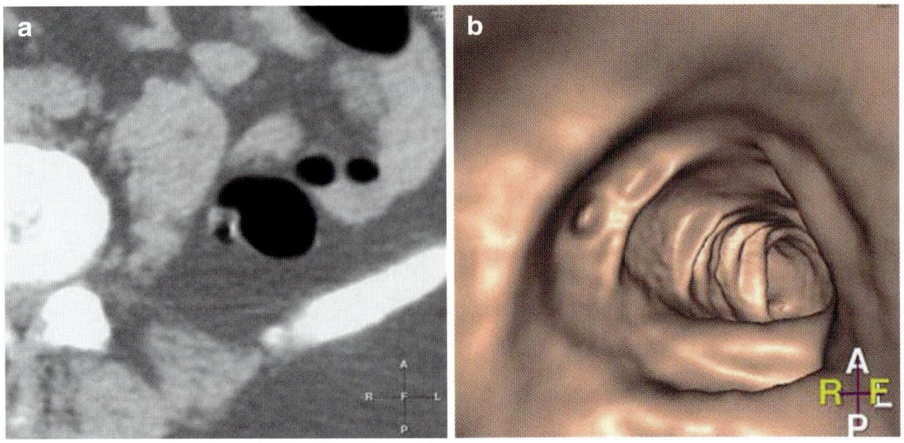

Fig. 16.4. **a,b** Inverted diverticulum: pseudo-polypoid shape on VE images. On 2D images, these lesions contain some air, residual stool, or fat attenuation because of a central umbilication in the inverted part of the diverticulum or because of the inclusion of perisigmoidal fat. (Used with permission of LEFERE et al. 2003)

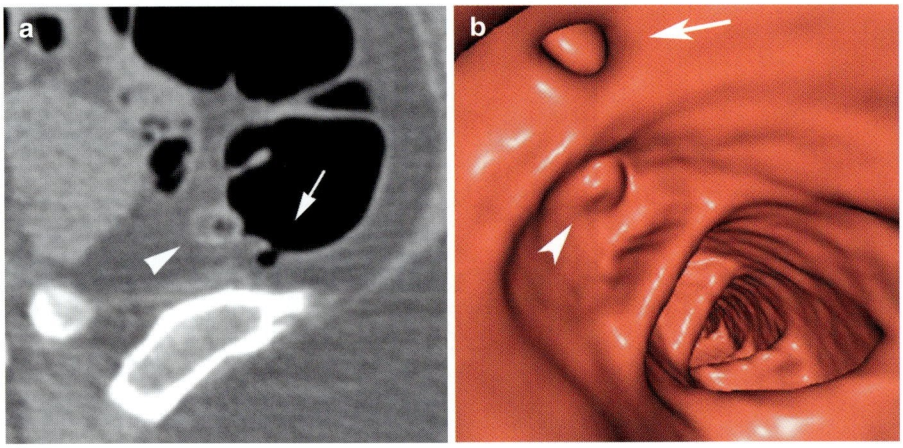

Fig. 16.5. Normal (*arrow*) and stool-impacted diverticulum (*arrowhead*). (**a**) VE shows complete dark ring at the normal diverticulum and incomplete ring shadowing at the impacted diverticulum, simulating a polypoid lesion. (**b**) On 2D images in the impacted diverticulum, a hyperdense ring with a hypodense center can be found

cases, in the sigmoid colon. This can affect a single diverticulum or a few diverticula, which is called focal diverticulitis, or a whole colonic segment (Figs. 16.6a–c and 17.7a, b). Complications that may develop are pericolic abscess, perforation, hemorrhage, fistula formation, and post-inflammatory stenosis. For diagnosis of acute diverticulitis, CT without colon distension is the primary imaging modality. Significant findings for diverticulitis are cone-shaped mild wall thickening with involvement of a long segment (>10 cm) and increased contrast enhancement, pericolic fat stranding, and fluid at the root of the mesentery (Fig. 16.7a, b). The most important differential diagnosis for diverticulitis is colon cancer. In contrast, extensive wall thickening with short extension (<5 cm), especially with shoulder formation and pericolonic lymph nodes, is suspicious for neoplasms (CHINTAPALLI et al. 1999).

Presently, CTC has no role in the diagnosis of acute diverticulitis, and, moreover, the distension of the colon may lead to perforation. Thus, diverticulitis is considered a contraindication for CTC by a majority of experts. However, in selected cases, CTC may help in the differential diagnosis between diverticulitis and cancer after the acute inflammatory episode has subsided.

16.3 Inflammatory Bowel Disease

Within the group of IBD, Crohn's disease (CD) and ulcerative colitis (UC) represent the most important conditions. The role of CTC in the evaluation of IBD is unclear and still a subject of discussion. CTC is currently not used routinely in patients with inflammatory bowel disease. Particularly in acute inflammatory conditions, colonic distention may increase the risk of perforation, and therefore, CTC may be

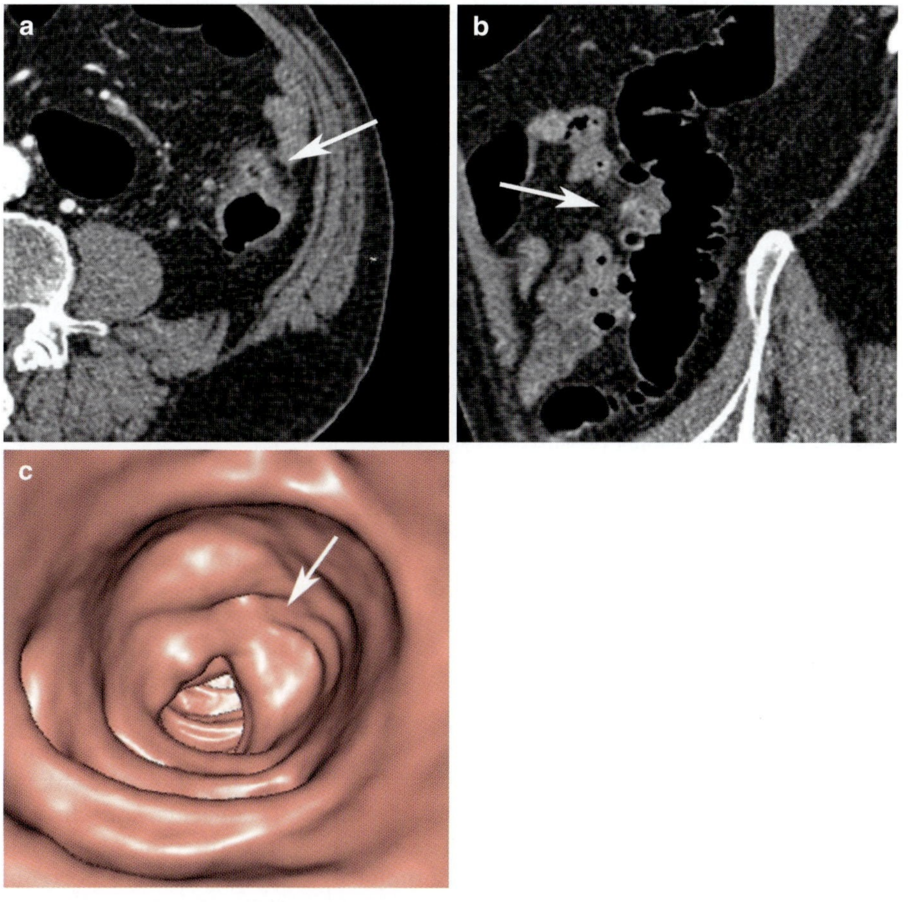

Fig. 16.6. Focal diverticulitis: (**a**) Axial plane shows focal semicircular wall thickening with increased CM enhancement in the area of a diverticulum in the descending colon (*arrow*). (**b**) Coronal plane shows that only one diverticulum is affected (*arrow*). (**c**) VE shows focal luminal narrowing that simulates a stenotic mass (*arrow*)

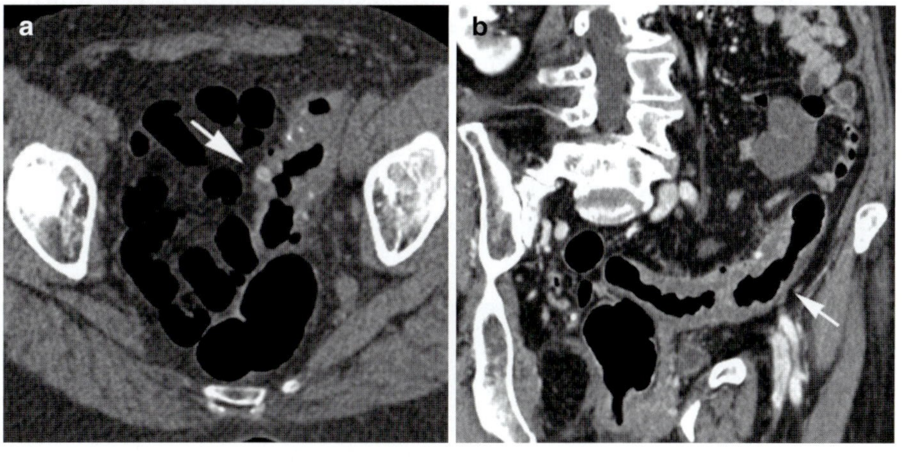

Fig. 16.7. Chronic diverticulitis on axial unenhanced (**a**) and contrast-enhanced CPR, (**b**) Wall thickening of a long segment (*arrow*) with CM enhancement, diverticula, stenosis, and fat stranding

contraindicated. However, in the chronic stages, CTC may help to assess the colon proximal to a stenosis, which cannot be passed with endoscopy (Ota et al. 2003) (Table 16.2). Furthermore, CTC is useful for evaluating the extracolonic extent and complications of the disease (Andersen et al. 2006). The i.v. administration of contrast is helpful for the evaluation of inflammatory wall changes (Harvey et al. 2001).

When evaluating patients with IBD, it is important to search for specific CT features and associated complications. The general CTC pattern of inflammatory bowel wall changes are wall thickening, increased CM enhancement, and pericolic inflammatory changes,

Table 16.2. CTC features of inflammatory bowel disease

Discrete irregular wall thickening (continuous vs. discontinuous)
Flattening or disappearance of haustra
Increased CM enhancement of wall
Stenosis
Pseudopolyps cobblestone pattern (Crohn)
Fibrofatty proliferation around colon (Crohn > UC)
Lymph nodes (Crohn > UC)
Abscess, fistula, pseudotumor (Crohn)
Cancer (UC >> Crohn)

such as fat stranding and fibrofatty proliferation (Fig. 16.8a, b).

16.3.1 Ulcerative Colitis

UC is an inflammatory bowel disease limited to the mucosa and submucosa of the colon. The disease typically begins in the rectum and continuously extends proximally to involve part of the colon or the entire colon (pancolitis). In 10–40% of cases, the distal ileum is also inflamed, which is referred to as backwash ileitis. The most severe complication is the toxic megacolon, which appears in up to 5% of cases and carries the risk of perforation and peritonitis (Fig. 16.9a, b).

There is still little experience in the evaluation of UC with CTC. The early subtle inflammatory mucosal changes, such as the granular pattern of the mucosa or tiny punctuate ulcers, known from double-contrast barium enemas, may be beyond the current spatial resolution of CTC.

Progression of the disease leads to hyperemia and submucosal edema, which then results in thickening of the wall, and is accompanied by increased paracolic vascularity. Increased ulceration and pseudopolyps appear and the mucosa becomes friable. Lymph node enlargement is only slight. The appearance of abscess or fistula formation is uncommon. In these acute stages, the diagnostic value of CTC, in contrast to conventional colonoscopy, seems to be questionable. Toxic megacolon represents an absolute contraindication to insufflation of air because of the extreme risk of perforation. In case of acute colitis without signs of toxic megacolon, CTC should be avoided. There are only a few reports about colonic perforations caused by CTC (Sosna et al. 2006; Burling et al. 2006). However, in most cases stenotic or otherwise diseased colons were affected and UC has been reported as one of these predisposing conditions (Coady-Fariborzian et al. 2004). The air distension of the colon may lead to intramural laceration or frank perforation (Fig. 16.10a, b.).

Subacute and chronic forms lead to thickening and stiffening of the wall. Narrowing of the colonic lumen and foreshortening of the colon may occur (Macari and Balthazar 2001). The bowel loses its haustral pattern, which can result in a tubular "lead pipe" appearance. Post-inflammatory pseudo polyps may be present. As a result of inflammation, there may be proliferation of the pericolic fat (Fig. 16.11a–c.), resulting in widening of the presacral space.

The risk of development of colorectal cancer increases with the extent and the duration of the disease. Focal wall thickening, shoulder formation, or

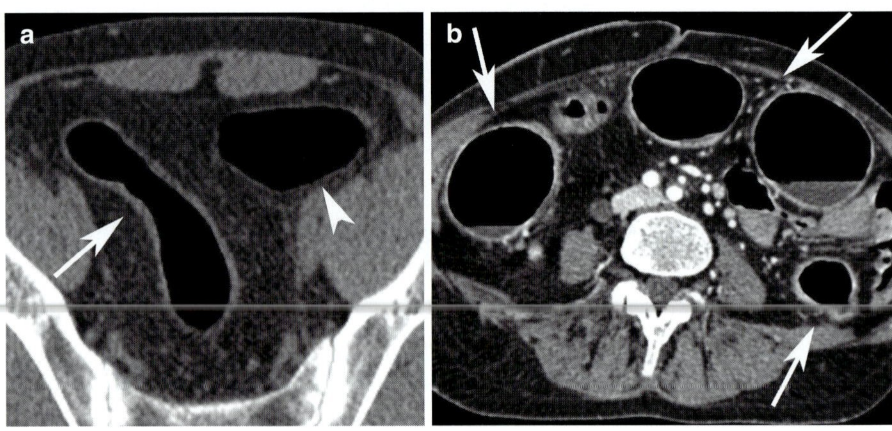

Fig. 16.8. Inflammatory wall thickening at CT colonography: (**a**) Axial unenhanced view shows mild wall thickening and fibrofatty proliferation of the rectum (*arrow*). Compare to normal wall thickness of the sigmoid colon (*arrowhead*). (**b**) Axial contrast-enhanced CT image shows wall thickening and increased CM enhancement of the colon (*arrow*)

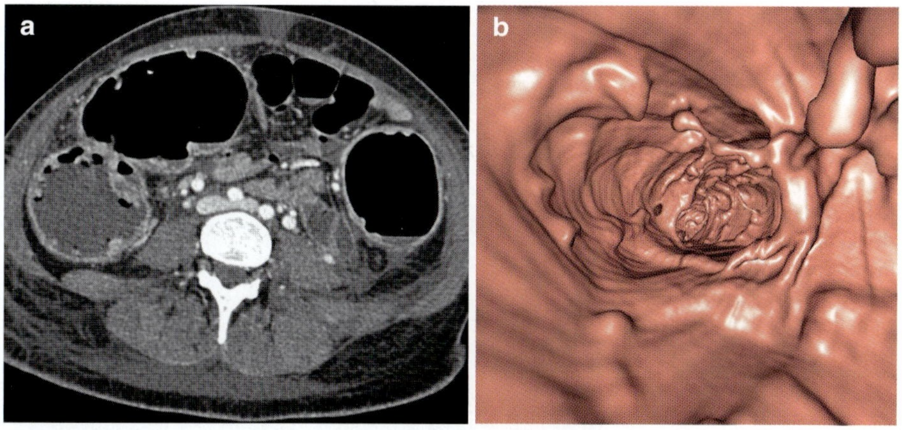

Fig. 16.9. Toxic megacolon: Colonic dilatation (without air insufflation!) with intraluminal air and fluid (**a**). The luminal contour is distorted and anhaustral. Diffuse slight wall thickening with increased CM enhancement of the whole colon and ill-defined nodular/pseudopolypoid surface (**b**)

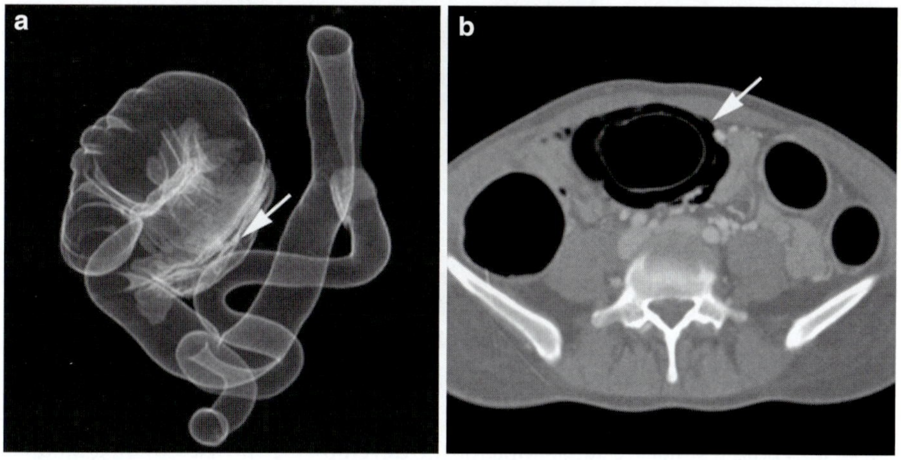

Fig. 16.10. Acute ulcerative colitis with perforation because of air insufflation: (**a**) Surface-rendered 3D view shows total flattening and disappearance of the haustra, a sign of colitis. (**b**) Focal paracolic air formations around the transverse colon are a sign of perforation (*arrow*)

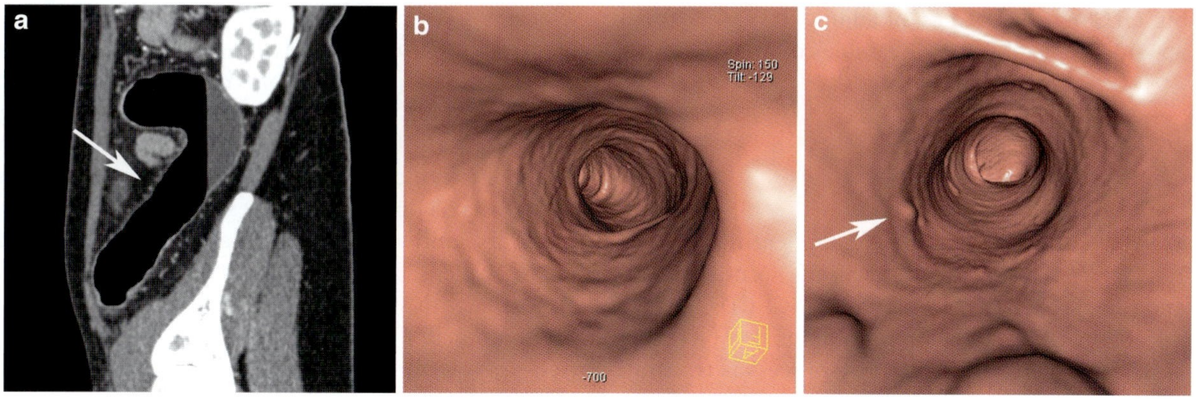

Fig. 16.11. Chronic ulcerative colitis: (**a**, **b**) narrowing of the colonic lumen and foreshortening of the colon with total flattening and disappearance of the haustra, leading to tubular appearance ("lead pipe") of the colon (*arrow*); (**c**) pseudopolyps (*arrow*)

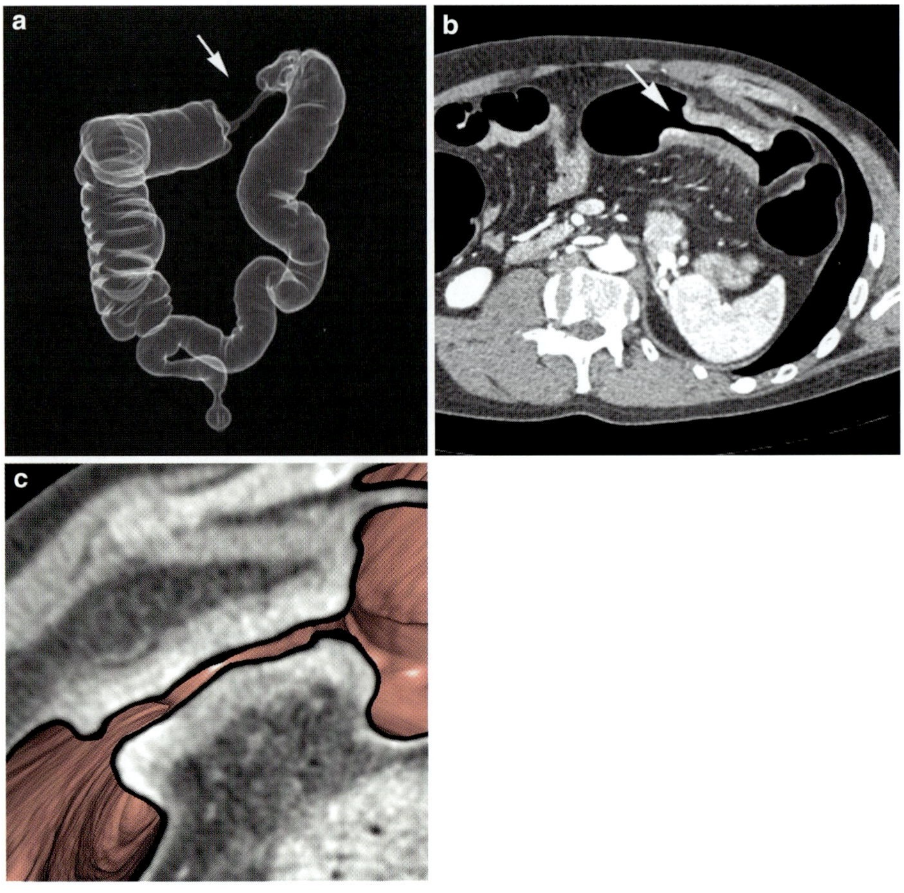

Fig. 16.12. Ulcerative colitis with stenotic cancer in the transverse colon (*arrow*): (**a**) local flattening and disappearance of the haustra in the sigmoid and descending colon. (**b**) Stenotic, circular wall thickening with shoulder formation in the transverse colon, soft tissue attenuation, and CM enhancement. (**c**) Combined 2D + 3D view of the stenotic cancer

large polypoid lesions are suspicious for the development of colorectal cancer (Fig. 16.12a–c). Differentiation between an inflammatory stenosis in UC and cancer is the domain of endoscopy with biopsy, but CTC may be used as an adjunct in patients with an endoscopically non-accessable colon.

16.3.2 Crohn's Disease

CD may involve segments of the entire GI tract. However, CD most often affects the terminal ileum and the proximal colon. Unlike UC, CD typically affects the GI tract in a discontinuous way (so-called skip lesions). The inflammatory process is transmural in nature.

CT usually misses the early stages of CD (Biancone et al. 2003). With progression of the disease, mural thickening and luminal narrowing occur. The outer contour of the colon wall is irregular. The degree of contrast enhancement of the bowel wall correlates with the severity of the disease (Gore et al. 1996). As a result of the hyperemia from the inflammatory process, the local mesenteric vessels are dilated and widely spaced, which has been described as the "comb sign." A progressive increase in pericolic fat is called fibrofatty proliferation. It is an attempt of the body to contain the inflammatory process, resulting in separation of the bowel loops. Usually, multiple mesenteric lymph nodes, rarely exeeding 10 mm in the short axis diameter, are present. Extensive, linear, transverse and longitudinal ulcerations can result in the so called "cobblestone pattern," which can be evaluated with VE images (Tarjan et al. 2000). With progression of the disease, the transmural inflammation is accompanied by irreversible fibrosis. (Fig. 16.13a–c)

Frequent complications are fistula, abscesses, adhesions, and stenosis, leading to bowel obstruction. Fistula can appear as ill-defined soft tissue bands extending into the paraintestinal fat. After

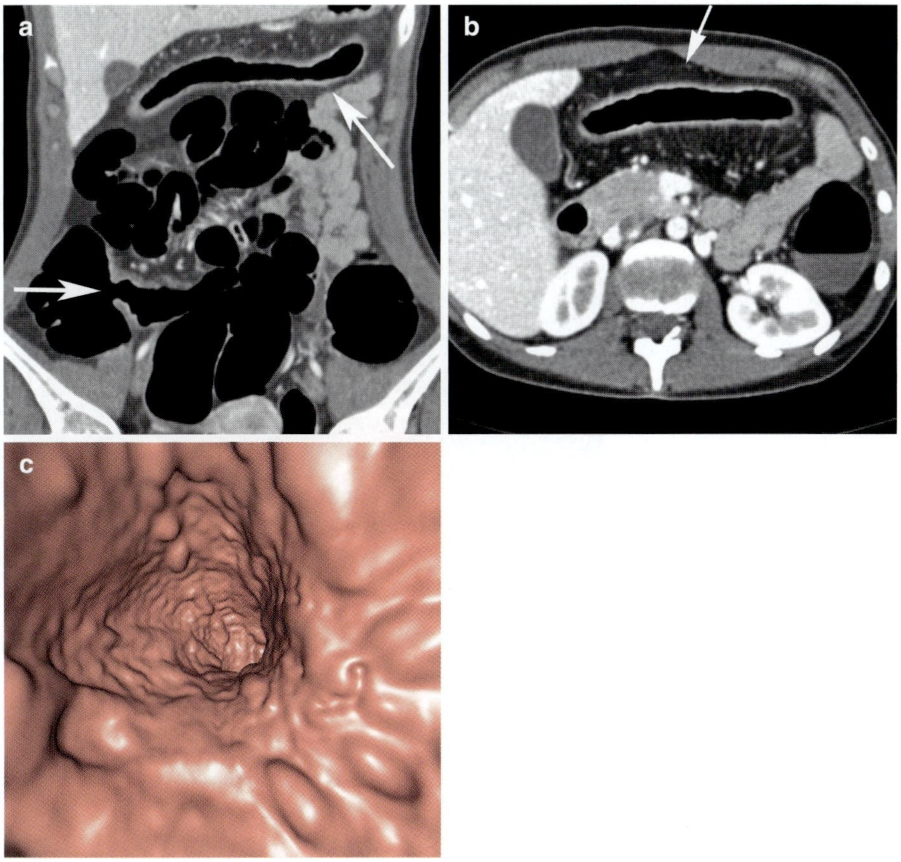

Fig. 16.13. Crohn's disease: (**a**) Skip lesions (*arrow*) in the terminal ileum and the transverse colon. (**b**) Irregular wall thickening and stenosis of the transverse colon, with pericolic fat stranding and flattening and disappearance of the haustra (*arrow*). (**c**) Virtual colonoscopy shows luminal narrowing and cobblestone pattern

colonic air insufflation, the presence of small amounts of air in the fistulas is pathognomonic (Tarjan et al. 2000). On endoluminal views, the fistula opening is sometimes depicted (Fig. 16.14b). A fistula opening may be seen at the top of a pseudopolypoid lesion of granulation tissue formation. In these cases, the combination of 3D and 2D images may provide sufficient information for complex disease. Abscesses are most frequently associated with small bowel disease or ileo-colitis and may extend into adjacent tissues, bowel loops, or organs. Stenosis in CD shows, in many cases, circular cone-shaped wall thickening with increased CM enhancement and involvement of a longer segment. In other cases, short stenoses with wall thickening and abrupt shoulders at the proximal and distal end occur, which makes differentiation from malignant stenosis impossible (Figs. 16.14a and 16.15a–c). Perforations are uncommon and usually contained (Triester et al. 2006; Wong et al. 2007). Conglomerate masses are present if there is an involvement of multiple bowel segments or a large bowel segment with fistulation and abscess formation (Fig. 16.14c).

There is a slightly increased risk of developing colorectal cancer and lymphoma as a complication of the disease. These neoplasms mostly affect the small bowel. The presence of lymph node enlargement >10 mm in the short axis diameter should raise the suspicion of malignancy.

For evaluation of the small bowel involvement, CT enteroclysis is the preferred technique. There is little experience about the feasibility of CTC in CD. Published results indicate that CTC can be helpful in the evaluation of colonic involvement, especially if conventional colonoscopy is incomplete (Biancone et al. 2003). In addition, the extracolonic extent and complications of the disease can be evaluated.

16.4 Colorectal Carcinoma

Adenocarcinomas are the most common colonic primary malignancies. The peak incidence is between 50 and 70 years of age. Approximately 90% arise from

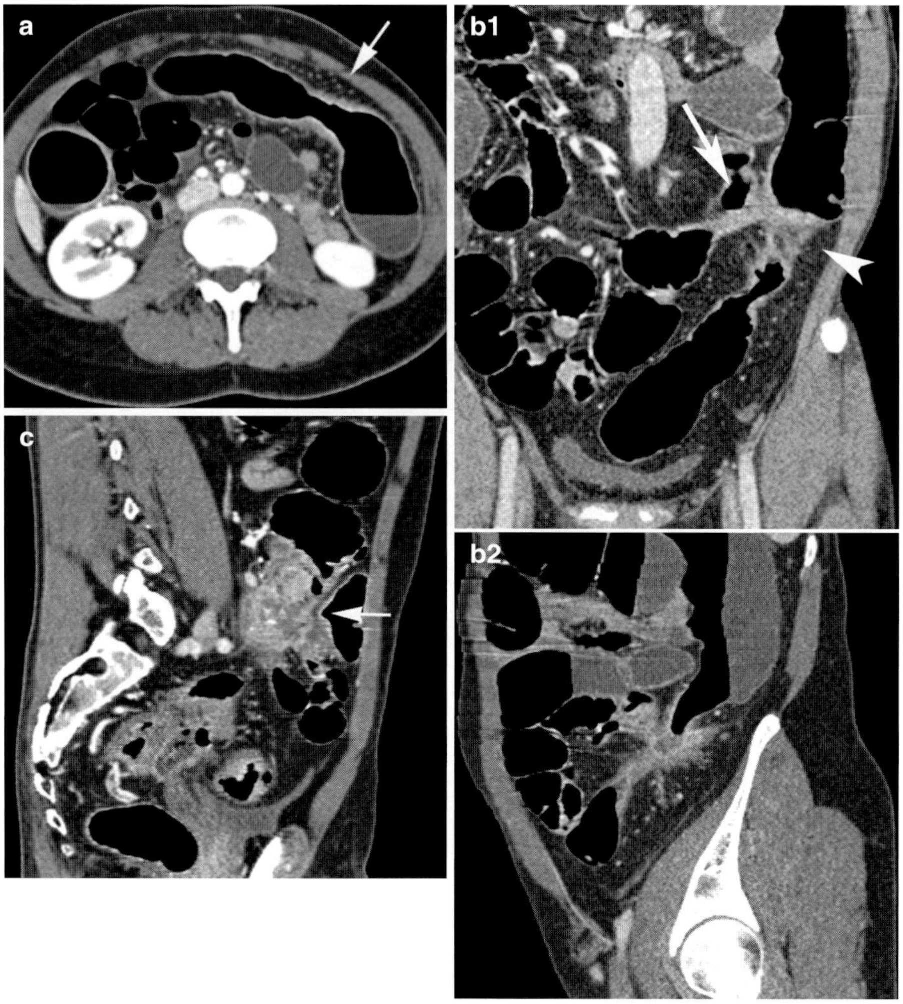

Fig. 16.14. Crohn's disease in three different patients: (**a**) stenosis in the transverse colon (*arrow*); (**b**) stenosis in the descending colon (arrowhead) with fistula to the sigmoid colon (*arrow*). (**c**) Conglomerate mass between cecum and small bowel loops (*arrow*)

benign adenomatous polyps. Most carcinomas show an exophytic, polypoid type of growth with frequent central necrosis or ulceration. Adenocarcinomas tend to infiltrate the bowel wall circumferentially and 50% are found in the rectum, and 25% in the sigmoid. In up to 5% of cases, a second colon carcinoma is present (synchroneous cancer) (Fig. 16.22a, b).

In cases of stenotic cancer, conventional colonoscopy may not pass the stenosis and, therefore, may be incomplete. The main indication for CTC in colorectal cancer is the evaluation of the colon proximal to the stenosis to detect additional tumors or polyps (Fenlon et al. 1999; Morrin et al. 2000a; Neri et al. 2002; Schima and Mang 2004) (Table 16.3). CTC also provides information about local tumor invasion, lymph nodes, and distant metastases (Filippone et al. 2004; Chung et al. 2005; Iannaccone et al. 2005). For this purpose, the i.v. administration of contrast media is indicated (Morrin et al. 2000b).

Table 16.3. CTC features of colorectal carcinoma

Focal, asymmetric, or circular wall thickening
Annular stricture
Wall irregularity
CM enhancement
Pericolic invasion (pericolic soft tissue stranding)
Local lymphadenopathy
Metastases
T Staging
T1: invasion of the mucosa and submucosa
T2: infiltration of the muscularis propria
T3: infiltration of pericolic fat
T4: invasion of adjacent organs
N Staging
N0: no local lymph nodes present
N1: ≤3 pericolic lymph nodes present
N2: >3 pericolic lymph nodes present

Reliable differentiation between mucosal /submucosal invasion (T1) and infiltration of the muscularis propria (T2) with CT is still not possible

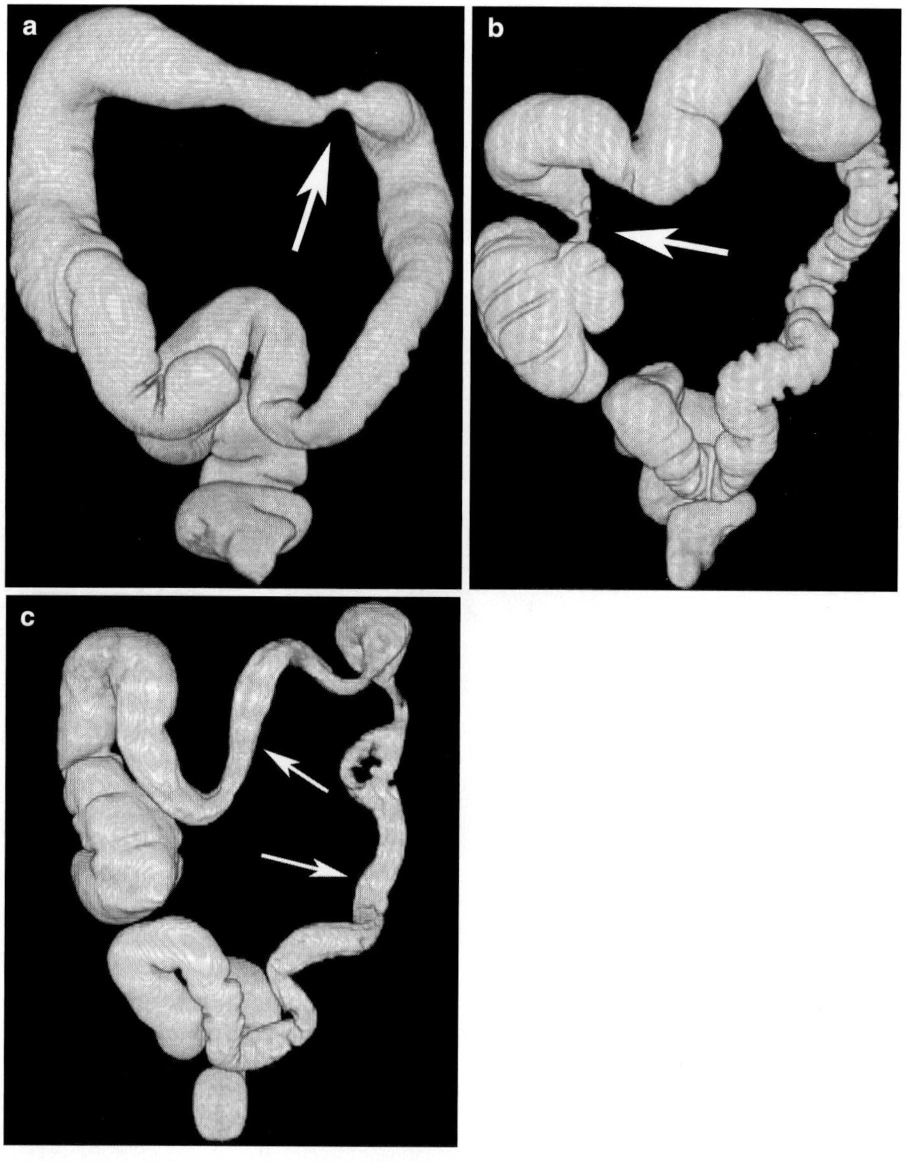

Fig. 16.15. Crohn's disease: various forms of stenoses (*arrow*) and disappearance of the haustra in three different patients. (**a**) Cone-shaped stenosis of the transverse colon. (**b**) Stenosis with extension into the ascending colon. (**c**) Long-segment stenosis of the transverse and descending colon

The role of CTC for T staging of known colorectal cancer is still a matter of discussion because primary tumors are resected, even if metastases are present, to prevent bowel obstruction. Less invasive surgical approaches, such as local tumor resection (mucosal resection) in early cancer, may indicate the need for re-evaluation of the role of CTC in T-staging.

Unlike polypoid lesions, which are more easily detected on 3D endoluminal views, invasive mass lesions are better depicted on 2D images, which allow mural and extramural evaluation (Pickhardt 2004).

Colorectal cancer typically shows extensive focal polypoid, asymmetric, or circular wall thickening with short extension (<5 cm), especially with shoulder formation (Fenlon et al. 1998; Taylor et al. 2003a). Colorectal carcinomas show moderate enhancement with intravenous contrast (Oto et al. 2003; Sosna et al. 2003) (Fig. 16.16a, b). CT differentiation between stage T1 (invasion of mucosa and/or submucosa) and T2 (invasion of the muscularis propria) is not feasible. However, tumor extension beyond the colon wall (T3), characterized by stranding, an indistinct boundary, and nodular protrusions into pericolic fat tissue, is readily appreciated by CT (Fig. 16.17a, b). Tumor infiltration to adjacent organs (T4) is most likely if the carcinoma shows a broad-based contact, no intervening fat planes, and indistinct boundaries to other organs (Fig. 16.18a, b).

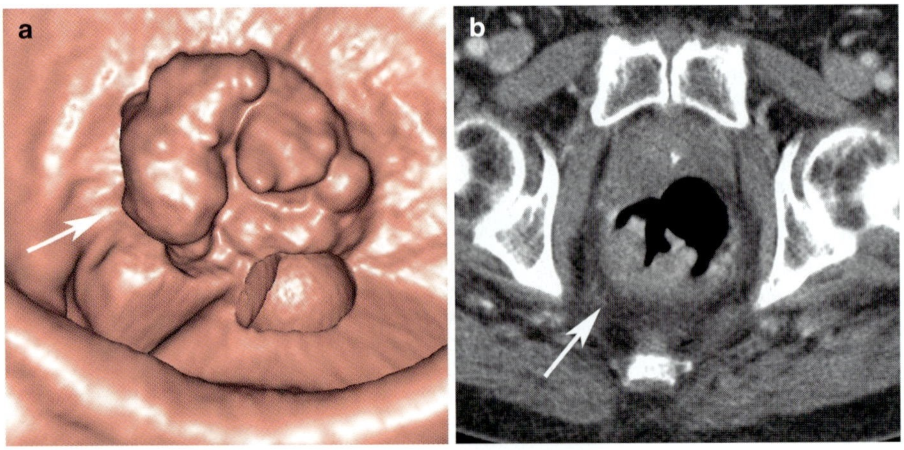

Fig. 16.16. Polypoid rectal cancer (*arrow*): large polypoid, lobulated mass in the rectum (**a**). The lesion shows soft tissue attenuation and CM enhancement (**b**)

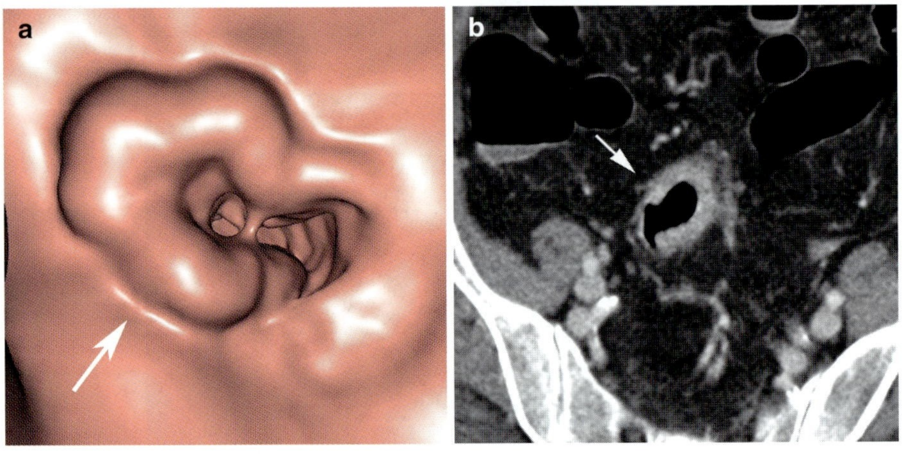

Fig. 16.17. Semicircular sigmoid carcinoma (*arrow*): focal, asymmetric, semicircular wall thickening with shoulder formation in the sigmoid colon (**a**). The lesion shows CM enhancement and pericolic soft tissue stranding (**b**)

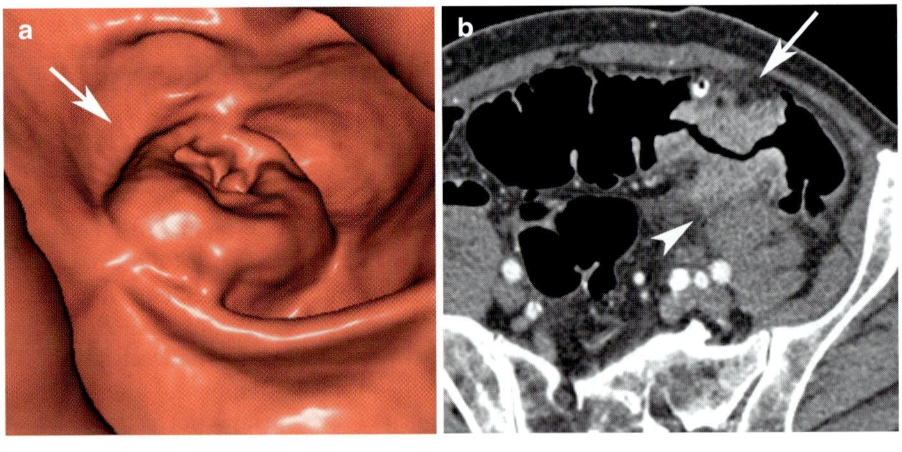

Fig. 16.18. Circular sigmoid carcinoma T4 (*arrow*): focal, symmetric, circular wall thickening with shoulder formation and pericolic soft tissue stranding in the sigmoid colon (**a**). The lesion shows a broad-based contact, no intervening fat planes, and indistinct boundaries to the psoas muscle (*arrowhead*), indicative of infiltration (**b**)

Pericolonic lymph nodes and distant metastasis are signs of progression of the disease and can be evaluated on 2D planes.

Lymph node enlargement >10 mm in the short axis diameter, and a shape that is more round than oval, are CT signs of lymph node metastasis. However, micrometastasis may be present in lymph nodes with a normal size and shape. Depending on the number of local lymph nodes, stage N1 (≤3) and N2 (>3) can be differentiated.

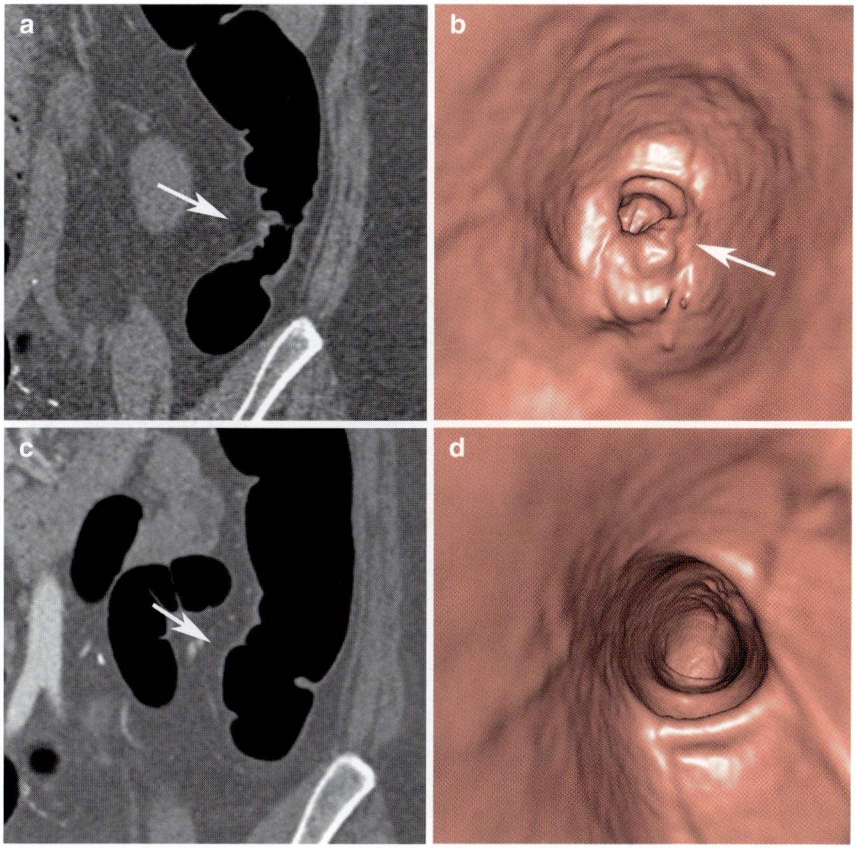

Fig. 16.19. Segmental colonic spasm in the descending colon (*arrow*): focal, irregular circular wall thickening with shoulder formation in the prone position (**a**, **b**). The lesion shows soft tissue attenuation (**a**). Normal colon wall without wall thickening or stenosis after changing the patient position to supine, and after intravenous administration of butylscopolamine (Buscopan) (**d**). It is important to identify the same segment as that seen in the supine position

The most common pitfalls is segmental luminal narrowing due to other causes, such as inflammatory stenosis or segmental colonic spasm (Mang et al. 2007). Inflammatory and post-inflammatory stenoses more often show cone-shaped mild wall thickening with involvement of a long segment (>10 cm) and pericolonic fat stranding. Sometimes, fluid is present at the root of the mesentery (Chintapalli et al. 1999) (compare Figs. 16.13b and 16.14a vs. 16.17 and 16.18).

Segmental colonic spasm is a physiological luminal narrowing due to peristaltic muscular contraction of the colon. The administration of antispasmotic drugs, such as butylscopolamine (Buscopan) and glucagon, improve colonic distension and, thus, reduce the appearance of spasms (Taylor et al. 2003b). Often, these pseudostenoses disappear during the examination when changing the patient's position from prone to supine or vice versa. In these cases, the evaluation of the second series is diagnostic to see that the pseudostenosis disappears when the spasm relaxes (Fig. 16.19a–d).

16.5 Colorectal Lymphoma

Lymphoma involves the colon either as a primary neoplasm or as a part of a disseminated disease. In contrast to the small bowel, where lymphomas are the most frequent primary tumor, lymphomas in the colon are rare. In secondary colonic lymphoma, the involvement of the gastrointestinal tract follows a previously diagnosed extra-abdominal lymphoma (O'Connell and Thompson 1978; Megibow et al. 1983).

The primary colonic lymphoma is usually found in middle-aged or elderly people. Males are twice as often affected as females. Common symptoms include abdominal pain, weight loss, and changing bowel habits, with an average duration of about 4–6 months. Primary colonic lymphomas occur more frequently in the setting of inflammatory bowel disease and immunosuppression, and are found most commonly in the cecum or the rectum (Bruneton et al. 1983) (Fig. 16.20a–c).

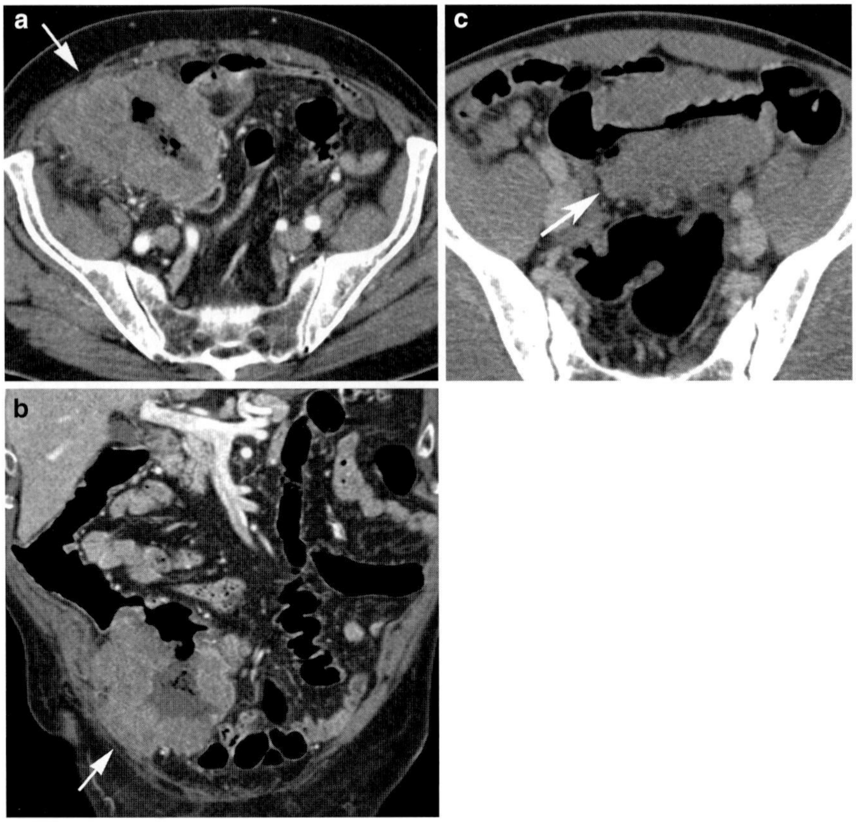

Fig. 16.20. Colorectal lymphoma in two patients. (**a**, **b**) Axial and coronal view show circumferential bowel wall thickening of the cecum with moderate CM enhancement (*arrow*). Focal wall defects as a sign of an early fistula. (**c**) Axial view shows circumferential wall thickening of the sigmoid colon with moderate CM enhancement (*arrow*) in a 36-year-old HIV-positive man

The radiological appearance can be classified as focal or diffuse. The most common focal type is the intraluminal mass (O'Connell and Thompson 1978). These polypoid lesions are lobulated, broad-based, and sessile, with or without central ulcerations and only slight CM enhancement. They are often morphologically indistinguishable from adenomatous polyps.

The focal appearance can also consist of an infiltration that results in pronounced eccentric or circumferential bowel wall thickening. As a consequence, the intestinal lumen may be narrowed. However, unlike colon cancer, lymphoma can also show a dilated caliber in the form of an "aneurysmal" dilatation due to infiltration and destruction of the myenteric plexus (Montgomery and Chew 1997). Ulcerations, necrosis, and fistulae between adjacent bowel loops may appear. Regional, mesenteric, and retroperitoneal lymphadenopathy may be present. Another focal form of lymphoma is the endo-eccentric mass with large ulcerations involving adjacent bowel loops where fistulae can appear (O'Connell and Thompson 1978).

The diffuse form presents with multiple polypoid lesions and is called diffuse mucosal nodularity or malignant lymphomatous polyposis (O'Connell and Thompson 1978; Callaway et al. 1997). The polyps appear smooth and sessile, but can also be irregular or pedunculated. Often, the entire colon or a long segment is involved.

Table 16.4. CTC features of colorectal lymphoma

Common in cecum and rectum (primary/secondary)
Focal, asymmetric, or circular wall thickening, lymphomatid polyposis
Lumen dilated or stenotic
Slight CM enhancement
Ulceration, necrosis, fistula
Pericolic invasion (pericolic soft tissue stranding)
Pericolic lymphadenopathy

The radiologic patterns of primary colonic lymphoma, such as intraluminal masses, polyps, stenosis, and polyposis, are often quite similar to those of carcinomatous stenosis, adenomatous polyps, and familial polyposis, and can also be evaluated by CTC (Table 16.4). The possibility of lymphoma should be considered when cecal tumors involve the terminal ileum, when tumors do not invade the pericolonic fat or adjacent structures, and when there are secondary findings, such as splenomegaly or bulky abdominal lymph node enlargement (WYATT et al. 1994). However, in most cases, a reliable radiological differentiation is not possible and the specific diagnosis is only possible with histology. In cases of stenosis or incomplete colonoscopy, CTC could be helpful in the evaluation of the prestenotic colon. Extracolonic involvement, fistulae, and lymphadenopathy can easily be evaluated with planar images.

16.6 Surveillance Post-Surgery or Post-Intervention

With regard to post-surgical conditions in the colon, there is no general agreement about the use of CTC. Contrast-enhanced CTC has the potential to detect local recurrence, metachronous disease, and distant metastases in patients with a history of invasive colorectal cancer (FLETCHER et al. 2002; LAGHI et al. 2003; NERI et al. 2005).

Currently, endoscopy or barium enemas are performed, in many cases, after colonic surgery for routine surveillance, to detect tumor recurrence, or to discover a metachronous cancer. Particularly after partial colonic resection, some of these follow-up examinations could be replaced by contrast-enhanced CTC. In most cases, CTC allows visualization of the entire colon, which is important for demonstrating the post-surgical anatomic conditions. 2D views are superior to 3D views, offering information about the wall morphology of the anastomosis and the extraluminal soft tissues. This is important because the majority of local recurrences are extraluminal and, therefore, endoscopically occult. Only one-third to one-half of local recurrences have an intraluminal component (BARKIN et al. 1988; WANEBO et al. 1989).

Colonic or ileocolic anastomoses can be made in an end-to-end or end-to-side fashion by manually suturing or by using a surgical stapler. A normal anastomosis typically presents as a smooth, circumferential ridge on CTC. The anastomotic edge may appear sharp or blunted. On 2D images, surgical sutures can be recognized as a hyperdense ring structure (CHOI et al. 2007). The bowel wall in the area of the anostomosis is of normal thickness. The border to the pericolic fat tissue is smooth (Fig. 16.21a–e). Most colonic anastomoses at CTC will not demonstrate an excess of soft tissue. However, benign findings, such as polypoid granulation tissue or benign nodularity, can be seen frequently endoscopically and at CTC.

Polypoid filling defects and enhancing mucosal soft tissue at a colonic anastomosis are nonspecific findings on CTC in patients with a history of colorectal cancer, and can represent granulation tissue, inflammation, or recurrent or metachronous disease.

Therefore, differentiation between granulation tissue, inflammatory stenosis, and cancer recurrence is the domain of endoscopy with biopsy. If possible, pericolonic lymph nodes and distant metastasis can be evaluated on 2D planes.

Anastomotic or local tumor recurrences present more often as extraluminal lesions rather than as intraluminal lesions. Intraluminal recurrent carcinomas appear as ulcerated lesions, strictures with friable mucosa, bulky luminal masses, or polypoid lesions on CTC and on optical colonoscopy. Planar 2D images demonstrate focal or circular wall thickening, increased CM enhancement, and pericolic fat stranding (Fig. 16.22a, b and 16.23a, b).

Extraluminal recurrences present on CT as enhancing extra-colonic masses adjacent to the anastomosis, or as colonic wall thickening at the anastomotic site that may be accompanied by pericolic infiltration (CHOI et al. 2007).

Treatment of large bowel obstruction using self-expanding metal stents is now well-established and a routine procedure in many institutions. Stenting is used in patients with incurable disease for definitive palliation, or, preoperatively, for patients where curative resection is possible (CAMUNEZ et al. 2000).

Follow-up of the location and the lumen of a stent may be feasible with CTC if stents cannot be passed by conventional colonoscopy, In theese cases CTC may be preferable to contrast enemas. CTC provides additional information about the location and the lumen of the stent and the proximal colon (Fig. 16.24a, b). During the same procedure, the extracolonic conditions of the disease (metastases, lymph nodes) can be evaluated.

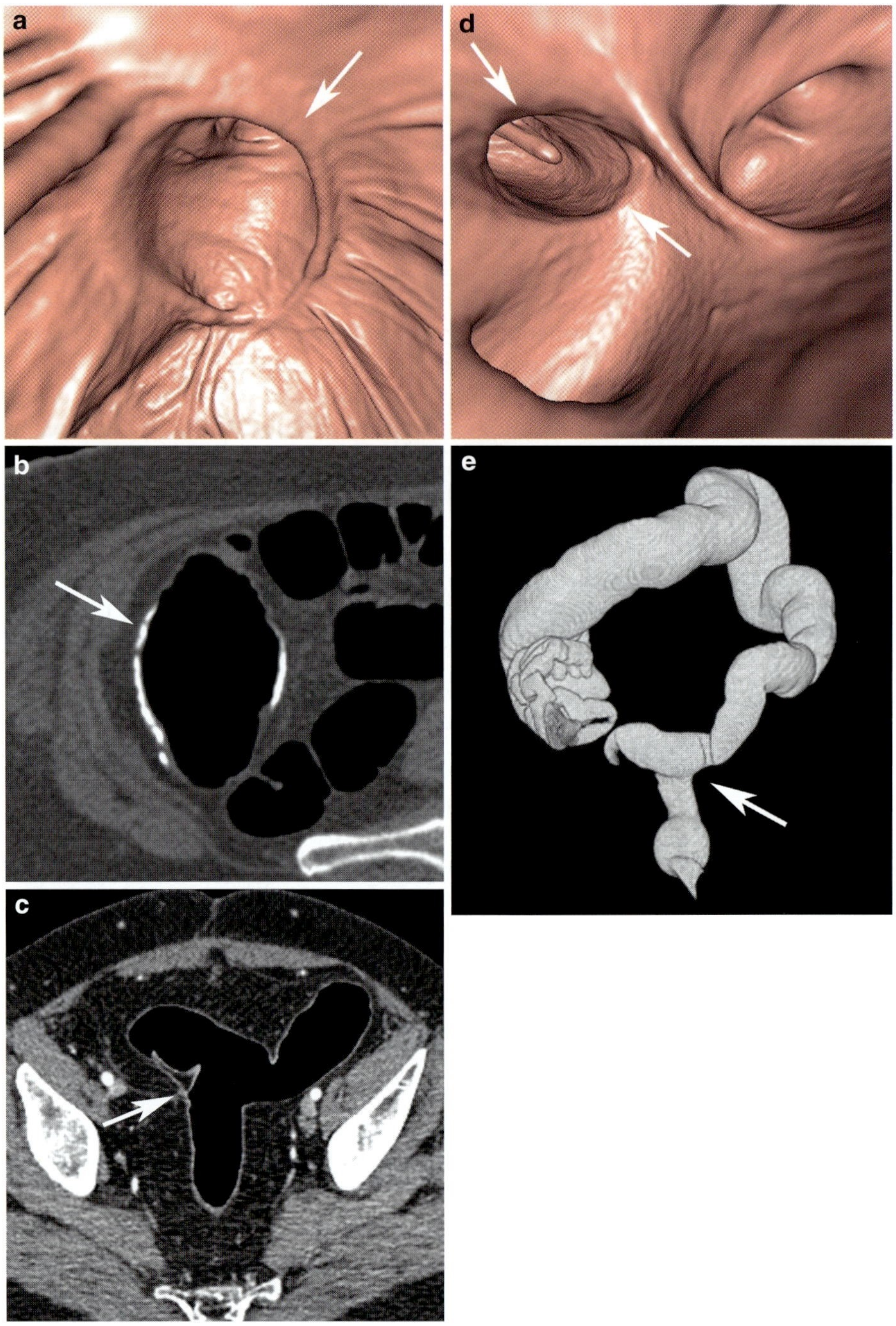

Fig. 16.21. Colonic anastomosis. (**a**, **b**) Regular entero-colic anastomosis after right hemicolectomy: (**a**) VE shows a smooth, circumferential ridge (*arrow*). (**b**) 2D curved multiplanar view shows surgical suture as a hyperdense ring structure (*arrow*). Note that the bowel wall is of normal thickness with a smooth border to the pericolic fat tissue. (**c**–**e**) Regular end-to-side colorectal anastomosis after low anterior resection (*arrow*)

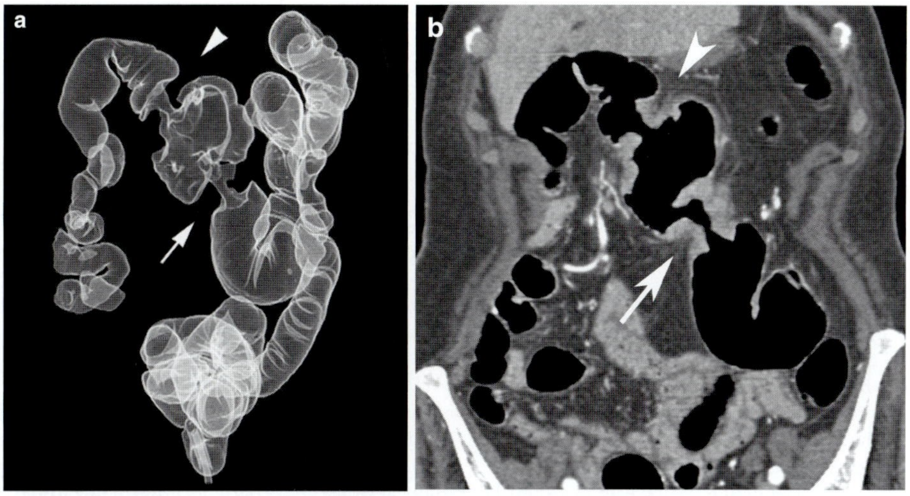

Fig. 16.22. (**a**, **b**) Right hemicolectomy: CT colonography reveals a second (metachronous) cancer in the transverse colon (*arrow*) and a cancer recurrence at the entero-colic anastomosis (*arrowhead*), which was not diagnosed by endoscopy

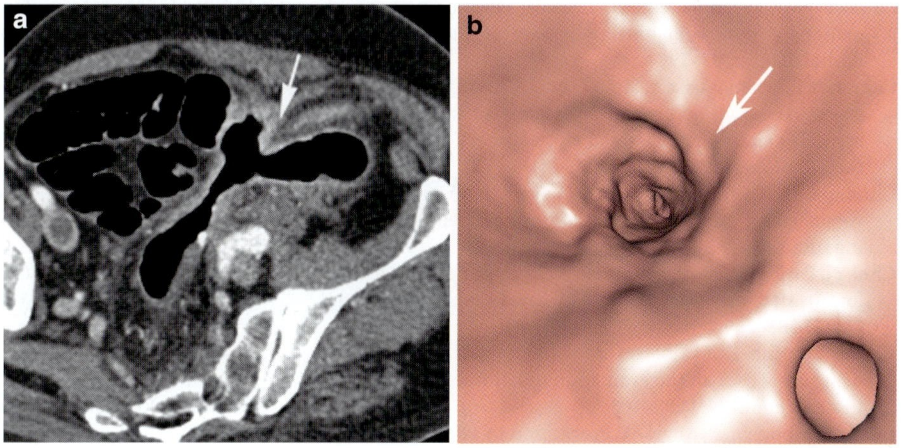

Fig. 16.23. (**a**, **b**) Inflammatory stenosis at the anastomosis after colonic resection: Mild wall thickening with stenosis and periocolic fat stranding (*arrow*). Virtual colonoscopy shows luminal narrowing (*arrow*) and diverticula

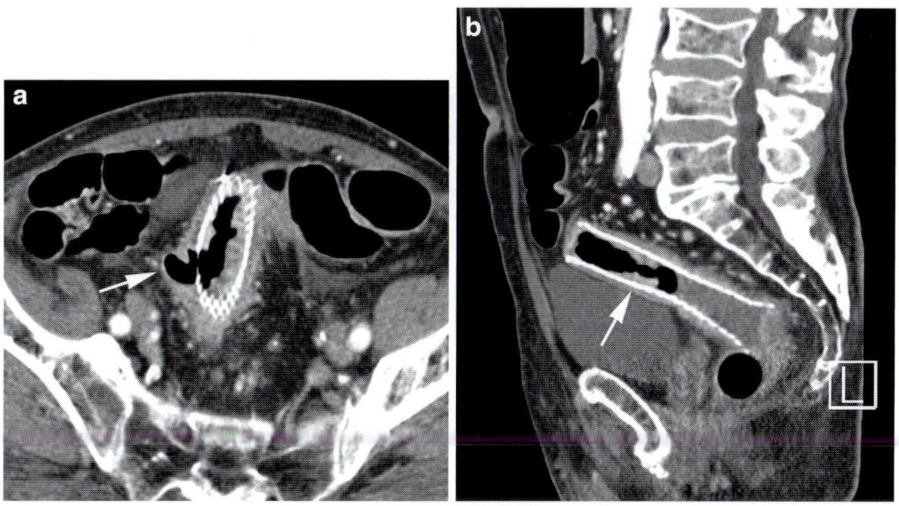

Fig. 16.24. Rectal cancer with rectal stent for palliation, on axial, coronal, and sagittal views: (**a**) Stent fracture (*arrow*) with air leakage. (**b**) Beginning tumor invasion (*arrow*) into the stent graft

References

Andersen K, Vogt C, Blondin D et al (2006) Multi-detector CT-colonography in inflammatory bowel disease: prospective analysis of CT-findings to high-resolution video colonoscopy. Eur J Radiol 58(1):140–146

Barkin JS, Cohen ME, Flaxman M et al (1988) Value of a routine follow-up endoscopy program for the detection of recurrent colorectal carcinoma. Am J Gastroenterol 83(12): 1355–1360

Biancone L, Fiori R, Tosti C et al (2003) Virtual colonoscopy compared with conventional colonoscopy for stricturing postoperative recurrence in Crohn's disease. Inflamm Bowel Dis 9(6):343–350

Bruneton JN, Thyss A, Bourry J et al (1983) Colonic and rectal lymphomas. A report of six cases and review of the literature. Rofo 138(3):283–287

Burling D, Halligan S, Slater A et al (2006) Potentially serious adverse events at CT colonography in symptomatic patients: national survey of the United Kingdom. Radiology 239(2): 464–471

Callaway MP, O'Donovan DG, Lee SH (1997) Case report: malignant lymphomatous polyposis of the colon. Clin Radiol 52(10):797–798

Camunez F, Echenagusia A, Simo G et al (2000) Malignant colorectal obstruction treated by means of self-expanding metallic stents: effectiveness before surgery and in palliation. Radiology 216(2):492–497

Chintapalli KN, Chopra S, Ghiatas AA et al (1999) Diverticulitis versus colon cancer: differentiation with helical CT findings. Radiology 210(2):429–435

Choi YJ, Park SH, Lee SS et al (2007) CT colonography for follow up after surgery for colorectal cancer. Am J Roentgenol 189(2):283–289

Chung DJ, Huh KC, Choi WJ et al (2005) CT colonography using 16-MDCT in the evaluation of colorectal cancer. Am J Roentgenol 184(1):98–103

Coady-Fariborzian L, Angel LP, Procaccino JA (2004) Perforated colon secondary to virtual colonoscopy: report of a case. Dis Colon Rectum 47(7):1247–1249

Copel L, Sosna J, Kruskal JB et al (2007) CT colonography in 546 patients with incomplete colonoscopy. Radiology 244(2): 471–478

Fenlon HM (2002) CT colonography: pitfalls and interpretation. Abdom Imaging 27(3):284–291

Fenlon HM, Clarke PD, Ferrucci JT (1998) Virtual colonoscopy: imaging features with colonoscopic correlation. Am J Roentgenol 170(5):1303–1309

Fenlon HM, McAneny DB, Nunes DP et al (1999) Occlusive colon carcinoma: virtual colonoscopy in the preoperative evaluation of the proximal colon. Radiology 210(2): 423–428

Filippone A, Ambrosini R, Fuschi M et al (2004) Preoperative T and N staging of colorectal cancer: accuracy of contrast-enhanced multi-detector row CT colonography–initial experience. Radiology 231(1):83–90

Fletcher JG, Johnson CD, Krueger WR et al (2002) Contrast enhanced CT colonography in recurrent colorectal carcinoma: feasibility of simultaneous evaluation for metastatic disease, local recurrence, and metachronous neoplasia in colorectal carcinoma. Am J Roentgenol 178(2):283–290

Gore RM, Balthazar EJ, Ghahremani GG et al (1996) CT features of ulcerative colitis and Crohn's disease. Am J Roentgenol 167(1):3–15

Hara AK, Johnson CD, Reed JE (1997) Colorectal lesions: evaluation with CT colonography. Radiographics 17(5):1157–1167

Harvey CJ, Renfrew I, Taylor S et al (2001) Spiral CT pneumocolon: applications, status and limitations. Eur Radiol 11(9):1612–1625

Iannaccone R, Laghi A, Passariello R (2005) Colorectal carcinoma: detection and staging with multislice CT (MSCT) colonography. Abdom Imaging 30(1):13–19

Laghi A, Iannaccone R, Bria E et al (2003) Contrast-enhanced computed tomographic colonography in the follow-up of colorectal cancer patients: a feasibility study. Eur Radiol 13(4):883–889

Lefere P, Gryspeerdt S, Baekelandt M et al (2003) Diverticular disease in CT colonography. Eur Radiol 13(Suppl 4):L62–L74

Leonardou P, Striggaris K, Pappas P et al (2006) Screening of patients after colectomy: virtual colonography. Abdom Imaging 31(5):521–528

Macari M, Balthazar EJ (2001) CT of bowel wall thickening: significance and pitfalls of interpretation. Am J Roentgenol 176(5):1105–1116

Macari M, Berman P, Dicker M et al (1999) Usefulness of CT colonography in patients with incomplete colonoscopy. Am J Roentgenol 173(3):561–564

Mang T, Maier A, Plank C et al (2007) Pitfalls in multi-detector row CT colonography: a systematic approach. Radiographics 27(2):431–454

Megibow AJ, Balthazar EJ, Naidich DP et al (1983) Computed tomography of gastrointestinal lymphoma. Am J Roentgenol 141(3):541–547

Montgomery M, Chew FS (1997) Primary lymphoma of the colon. Am J Roentgenol 168(3):688

Morrin MM, Farrell RJ, Raptopoulos V et al (2000a) Role of virtual computed tomographic colonography in patients with colorectal cancers and obstructing colorectal lesions. Dis Colon Rectum 43(3):303–311

Morrin MM, Farrell RJ, Kruskal JB et al (2000b) Utility of intravenously administered contrast material at CT colonography. Radiology 217(3):765–771

Neri E, Giusti P, Battolla L et al (2002) Colorectal cancer: role of CT colonography in preoperative evaluation after incomplete colonoscopy. Radiology 223(3):615–619

Neri E, Vagli P, Picchietti S et al (2005) CT Colonography in the follow up of patients with partial colectomy. Eur Radiol 15(3):164

O'Connell DJ, Thompson AJ (1978) Lymphoma of the colon: the spectrum of radiologic changes. Gastrointest Radiol 2(4):377–385

Ota Y, Matsui T, Ono H et al (2003) Value of virtual computed tomographic colonography for Crohn's colitis: comparison with endoscopy and barium enema. Abdom Imaging 28(6): 778–783

Oto A, Gelebek V, Oguz BS et al (2003) CT attenuation of colorectal polypoid lesions: evaluation of contrast enhancement in CT colonography. Eur Radiol 13(7):1657–1663

Pickhardt PJ (2004) Differential diagnosis of polypoid lesions seen at CT colonography (virtual colonoscopy). Radiographics 24(6):1535–1556

Regge D, Neri E, Turini F et al (2009) Role of CT colonography in inflammatory bowel disease. Eur J Radiol 69(3):404–408

Schima W, Mang T (2004) CT colonography in cancer detection: methods and results. Cancer Imaging 4:33–41
Sosna J, Morrin MM, Kruskal JB et al (2003) Colorectal neoplasms: role of intravenous contrast-enhanced CT colonography. Radiology 228(1):152–156
Sosna J, Blachar A, Amitai M et al (2006) Colonic perforation at CT colonography: assessment of risk in a multicenter large cohort. Radiology 239(2):457–463
Tarjan Z, Zagoni T, Gyorke T et al (2000) Spiral CT colonography in inflammatory bowel disease. Eur J Radiol 35(3):193–198
Taylor SA, Halligan S, Bartram CI (2003a) CT colonography: methods, pathology and pitfalls. Clin Radiol 58(3):179–190
Taylor SA, Halligan S, Goh V et al (2003b) Optimizing colonic distention for multi-detector row CT colonography: effect of hyoscine butylbromide and rectal balloon catheter. Radiology 229(1):99–108
Triester SL, Hara AK, Young-Fadok TM et al (2006) Colonic perforation after computed tomographic colonography in a patient with fibrostenosing Crohn's disease. Am J Gastroenterol 101(1):189–192
Wanebo HJ, Llaneras M, Martin T et al (1989) Prospective monitoring trial for carcinoma of colon and rectum after surgical resection. Surg Gynecol Obstet 169(6):479–487
Wong SH, Wong VW, Sung JJ (2007) Virtual colonoscopy-induced perforation in a patient with Crohn's disease. World J Gastroenterol 13(6):978–979
Wyatt SH, Fishman EK, Hruban RH et al (1994) CT of primary colonic lymphoma. Clin Imaging 18(2):131–141
You YT, Chang Chien CR, Wang JY et al (2006) Evaluation of contrast-enhanced computed tomographic colonography in detection of local recurrent colorectal cancer. World J Gastroenterol 12(1):123–126

Pictorial Overview of Normal Anatomy, Mimics of Disease, and Neoplasia Using CT Colonography

J. G. Fletcher, Fargol Booya, and Luis S. Guimaraes

CONTENTS

J. G. Fletcher, MD
Department of Radiology, Mayo Clinic Rochester, 200 First Street, SW, Rochester, MN, 55905, USA
Fargol Booya, MD
Department of Radiology, Mayo Clinic Rochester, 100 First Street, SW, Rochester, Minnesota, 55905, USA
Luis S. Guimaraes, MD
Department of Radiology, Hospital de São Teotónio, Avenida Rei D. Duarte, 3504-509, Viseu, Portugal

17.1 Introduction

Interpretation of computer tomography (CT) colonography data requires a radiologist to interactively interrogate a high spatial resolution, three-dimensional (3D) dataset of the air-filled human colon. Optimal scanning and interpretive techniques can yield diagnostic results on par with optical colonoscopy (Yee et al. 2001; Pickhartdt 2003; Macari et al. 2004, Johnson et al. 2007, 2008; Graser et al. 2008). While colonic neoplasia can have a variety of appearances at CT colonography, the spectrum of neoplastic disease within the colorectum and the methods used to examine the CT dataset are well defined. The purpose of this chapter is to pictorially review the spectrum of normal and pathological findings within the human colon using CT colonography.

Examination of CT colonography datasets generally involves two steps: (1) screening the colorectum for suspicious abnormalities and (2) problem-solving to determine if suspicious abnormalities represent neoplasia or benign or normal findings. Preliminary screening of the colorectum for suspicious lesions may be performed using either two-dimensional (2D) axial and 2D multiplanar reformatted images (Dachman et al. 1998; Macari et al. 2000), or reviewing the 3D endoluminal surface of the colon (Pickhartdt 2003), with the optimal approach incorporating both 2D and 3D search. Primary 2D search involves panning through enlarged 2D images from anus to cecum using lung or "colon" window settings (e.g., window 2000, level 0) to detect intraluminal filling defects, often followed by reverse screening of the colon with narrower window settings, to detect focal regions of colonic wall thickening. 3D screening typically involves viewing forward and reverse endoluminal fly-throughs (i.e., perspective, volume renderings) of the colorectum from anus to cecum, but can also rely upon other 3D endoluminal renderings of the human colon (Fletcher et al. 2000). The aim of both these screening techniques is to quickly identify all potential lesions, which can then be interrogated electronically using the computer workstation, by employing well-established problem-solving techniques.

Standard problem-solving techniques are employed once suspicious filling defects are identified using 2D or 3D screening methods. First, the morphology of the filling defects is examined using 2D multiplanar and 3D endoluminal images. Most polyps possess a typical polypoid morphology on both 2D and 3D images. If a filling defect remains suspicious, the internal attenuation and textural features are subsequently displayed by changing the CT window settings. Stool will often contain internal locules of air or be labeled with barium or iodine (if fecal tagging was employed), while lipomas possess internal fat attenuation. Neoplasms possess soft-tissue attenuation in the absence of partial volume effects. Finally, the appearance of suspicious lesions is compared between supine and prone datasets (Fletcher et al. 2000). While stool will generally change positions with gravity (Fletcher et al. 2000), most lesions can be seen in both positions. Rarely, additional scanning with intravenous contrast or repositioning with reinflation of the colon is used (Morrin et al. 2000). By investigating the colon systematically using these techniques, questionable filling defects can be confidently diagnosed as intraluminal neoplasms or benign findings.

The purpose of this chapter is to elucidate the spectrum of findings that radiologists may encounter within the colon at CT colonography. Illustrations are generously employed to expand the visual understanding of the spectrum of normality (Fletcher et al. 1999; Macari and Megibow 2001; Macari et al. 2003, Silva et al. 2006, 2007), with only a brief review of the appearances of neoplasia (Hara et al. 1997; Halligan et al. 2005), which are highlighted elsewhere in the text. In this chapter, we first examine the intrinsic features of the normal colon, followed by common benign findings encountered during CT colonography. Intraluminal and extra colonic processes that may simulate disease may juxtapose to the common appearance of colonic neoplasia found in CT colonography. The spectrum of findings associated with neoplasia will subsequently be summarized.

17.2 Intrinsic Features of the Normal Colon

Unlike endoscopists, most radiologists examine the colon from the rectum to the cecum. The spectrum of normal findings within the colon is therefore discussed in this order.

17.2.1 Hemorrhoids

Internal hemorrhoids can be seen as smoothly marginated and curved filling defects that project into the rectal vault, lying adjacent to the rectal tube tip (Fig. 17.1). In contrast, low rectal cancers will normally have shouldering, and arise some distance from the anus itself. Physical examination usually confirms the presence of internal hemorrhoids. If the remainder of the colorectum has been cleared of significant lesions, a limited proctoscopic or sigmoidoscopic examination can be performed, if required.

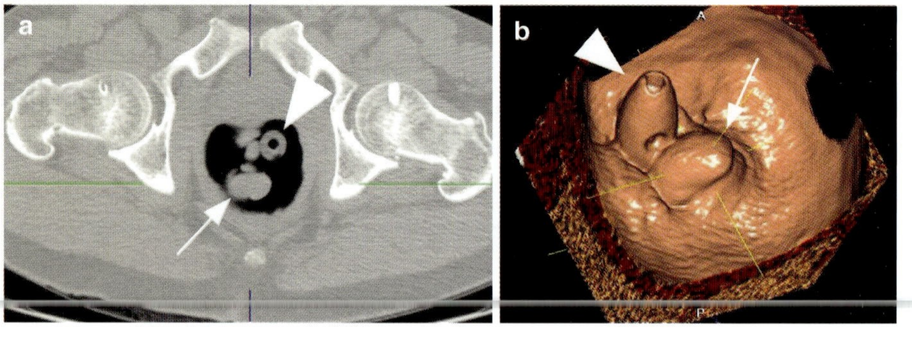

Fig. 17.1. Sixty-eight-year-old male with large internal hemorrhoids found by endoscopy. (**a**) axial CT image, (**b**) 3D endoluminal image at CT colonography. Note the smoothly marginated and curved filling defects (*arrow*) that project into the rectal vault, lying adjacent to the rectal tube tip (*arrowhead*).

17.2.2 Diverticulosis

Diverticular disease is exceedingly common, and is seen as focal outpouchings of the colonic lumina projecting beyond the colonic wall on 2D axial and 2D MPR images. 3D endoluminal images demonstrate the internal orifices projecting from the colonic lumen (Figs. 17.2 and 17.3). Occasionally, muscular hypertrophy of diverticulosis can cause colonic wall thickening, but in these segments, we usually observe diverticula interposed throughout the regions of

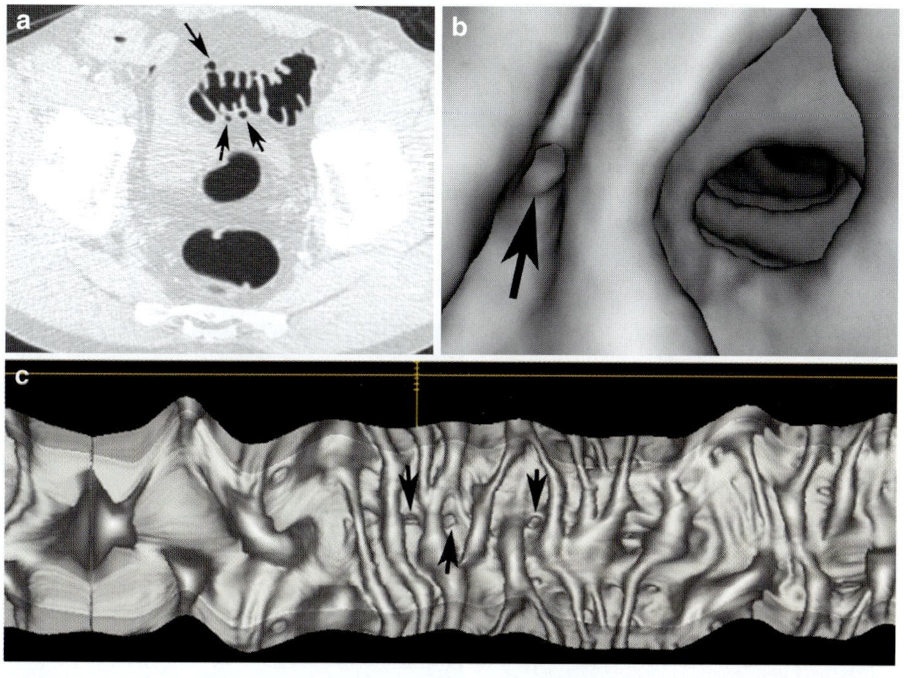

Fig. 17.2. Diverticulosis in a patient with normal colonoscopy. Note the focal outpouchings of the colonic lumina on 2D axial image (**a**). 3D endoluminal images (**b, c**) show diverticular orifices (*arrows*) projecting from the colonic lumen.

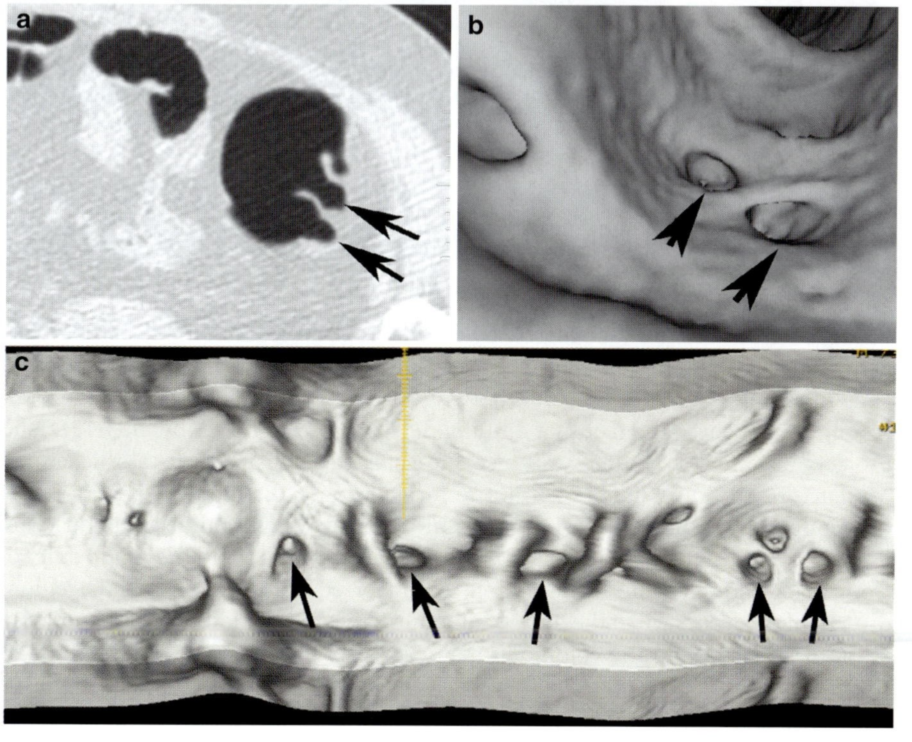

Fig. 17.3. Diverticulosis in a normal patient. Note the focal outpouchings of the colonic diverticula on 2D MPR images (*arrows*) (**a**), with diverticular orifices projecting from the colonic lumen on 3D endoluminal images (*arrows*, **b, c**).

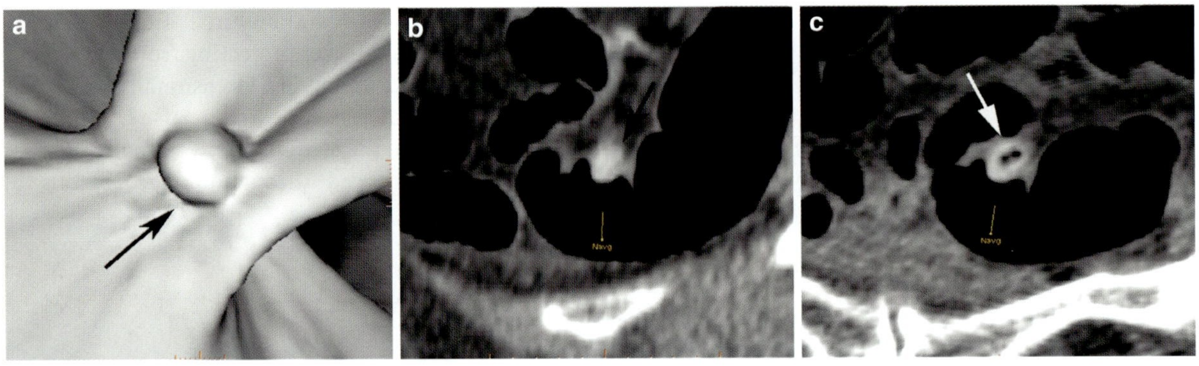

Fig. 17.4. 3D endoluminal image demonstrates a polypoid filling defect (**a**, arrow). 2D images with soft-tissue window settings show the filling defect to project beyond the colonic wall into the pericolonic fat (**b**) and contain barium and air (**c**, arrow), indicating that the defect is retained stool and barium within a diverticulum

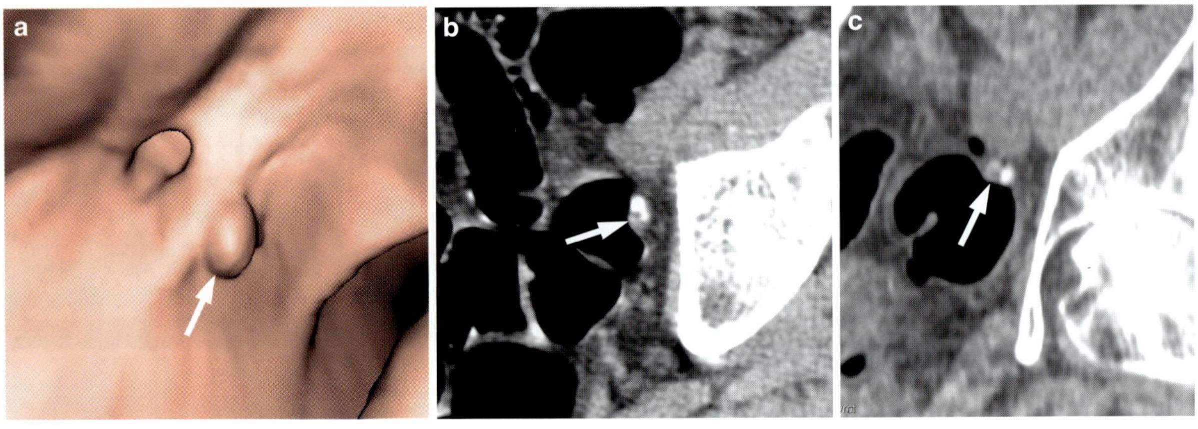

Fig. 17.5. 3D endoluminal image demonstrates a polypoid filling defect (**a**, arrow). 2D images with soft-tissue window settings show that a portion of the filling defect projects into the colonic lumen and contains pericolonic fat (**b**, arrow), indicating it is an inverted diverticulum, which lies adjacent to labeled stool (**c**, arrow)

colonic wall thickening. Filling defects can be associated with diverticular disease. The most common of these is the stool-containing diverticulum (Fig. 17.4). Untagged stool can be recognized by its heterogeneous internal attenuation characteristics, the presence of intralesional air, and pointed edges on 3D endoluminal views. The fact that a filling defect also projects beyond the colonic wall also indicates the presence of the diverticulum or intramural lesion (as opposed to the neoplastic mucosal lesions). Frequently, diverticula will have residual barium from prior radiographic examination. An inverted diverticulum occurs when the diverticular outpouching intussuscepts into the colonic lumen (Fig. 17.5). In such cases, the perienteric fat can be seen within the filling defect.

17.2.3 Folds

Colonic folds can be particularly complex, especially in the flexures and rectum. Fused folds are common in these locations (Fig. 17.6). Fused folds are simply recognized by their 3D shape. Occasionally, one may visualize focal thickening within a fold. Folds can be distinguished from polyps by the obtuse margins, internal attenuation (which will often contain some fat), and the nonfocality of the lesion. Thickened folds are usually seen in regions of suboptimal colonic distension; hence, comparison with the complementary dataset in a different position with improved distention will frequently assist in the identification of thickened folds (Fig. 17.7).

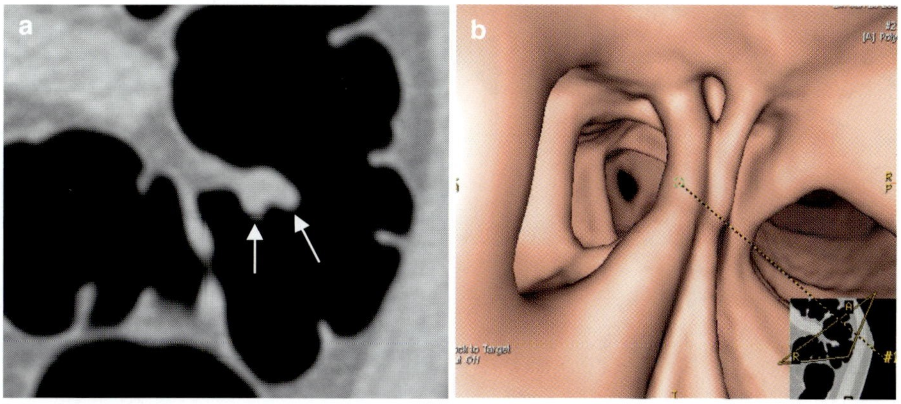

Fig. 17.6. Complex colonic folds can mimic polyps. These folds are particularly common in the colonic flexures. They can easily be recognized using 2D (**a**, *arrows*) and 3D (**b**, *arrows*) endoluminal images.

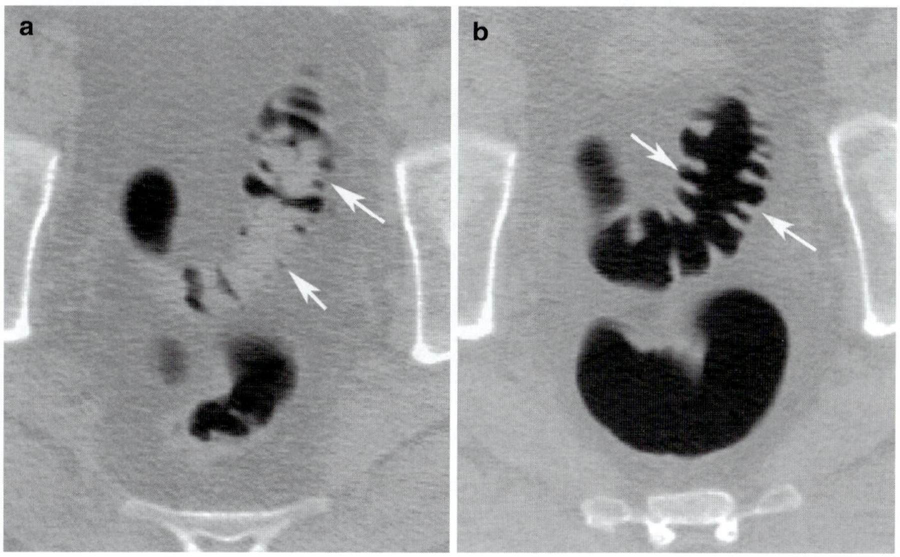

Fig. 17.7. (**a**) Thickened folds in a suboptimally distended sigmoid colon (*arrows*). (**b**) Repositioning distends the sigmoid colon to easily allow for the recognition of colonic folds.

17.2.4 Collapse and Contraction

Luminal collapse can be confused with malignant scirrhous tumors by radiologists learning CT colonography. Imaging patients in two positions has been shown by multiple observers to result in complementary distension and can be employed to distend collapsed bowel (Chen et al. 1999; Fletcher et al. 2000; Yee 2003). In general, the patient should be rolled such that the collapsed bowel loop is in the most nondependent location (Fig. 17.8) (Gryspeerdt et al. 2004). Contraction often appears as a focal area of wall thickening which can mimic an anular-constricting lesion (Fig. 17.9). Delayed imaging in another position usually will relax the colonic bowel segment (Figs. 17.10 and 17.11). Alternatively, glucagon can be given as a spasmolytic when contraction is suspected.

In our experience, the most common type of annular constricting neoplasms are scirrhous tumors, which (in contradistinction) have well-defined soft-tissue shoulders (Fig. 17.12). These lesions will retain the marked colonic wall thickening and irregularity to the intraluminal margins of the mass, potentially extending into the pericolonic tissues (if invasive), as other large carcinomas, and cause persistent luminal narrowing despite inflation maneuvers.

17.2.5 Ileocecal Valve

The ileocecal valve is the entry point for the enteric contents from the small bowel as they dump into the cecum. It is important to understand that the ileocecal valve is located within a fold within the cecum.

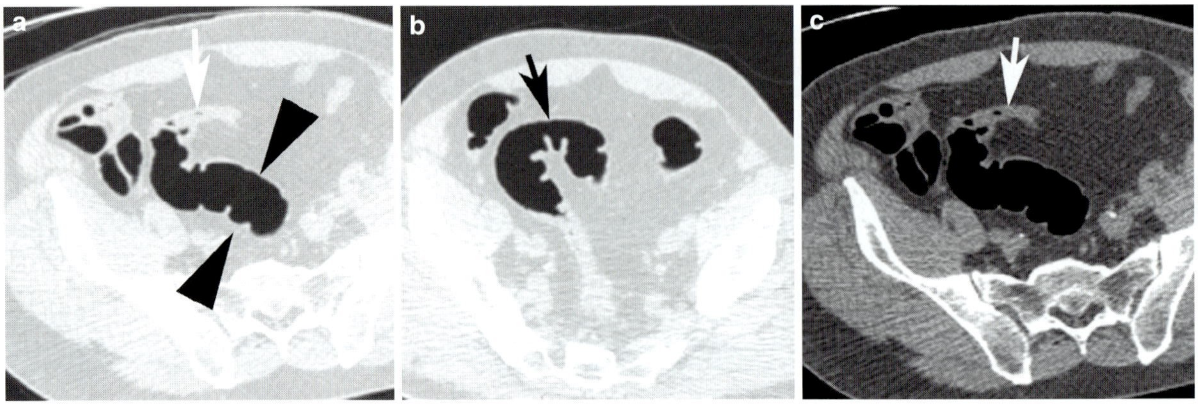

Fig. 17.8. A collapsed sigmoid loop (**a**, *white arrow*) demonstrates a smooth transition to distal distention (*black arrowheads*), as well as inflation in the complimentary position (**b**, *black arrows*). Soft-tissue window shows the collapsed segment. There is a smooth transition in the colonic wall thickening from the distended to the collapsed sigmoid colon (**c**, *white arrow*).

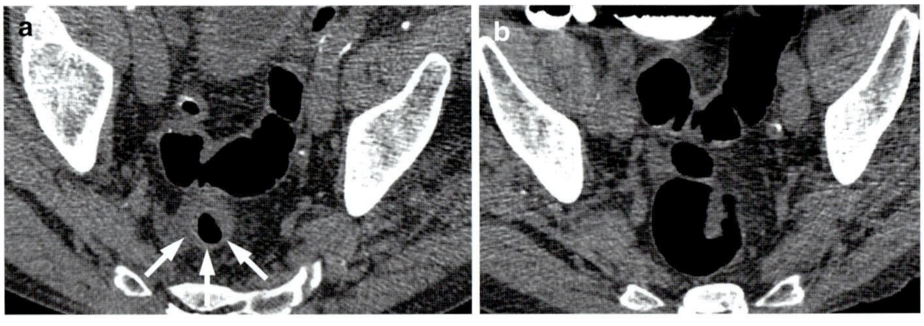

Fig. 17.9. Rectal contraction seen in the supine position (arrows) may be indistinguishable from a scirrhous cancer. Figure B, achieved with the patient in a complimentary position and the rectum in a nondependent position, demonstrates excellent rectal distension, eliminating the possibility of a cancer at this location.

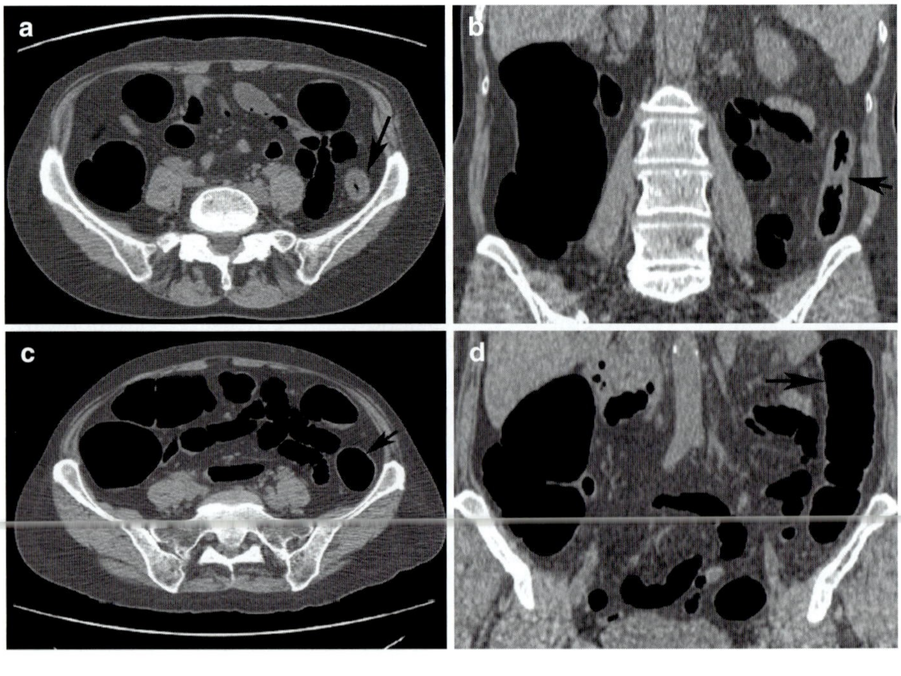

Fig. 17.10. Colonic contraction in the descending colon (*arrow*, **a**, **b**) causes focal wall thickening. Delayed imaging in a complimentary position shows inflation of previously contracted descending colon (**c**, **d**, *arrows*).

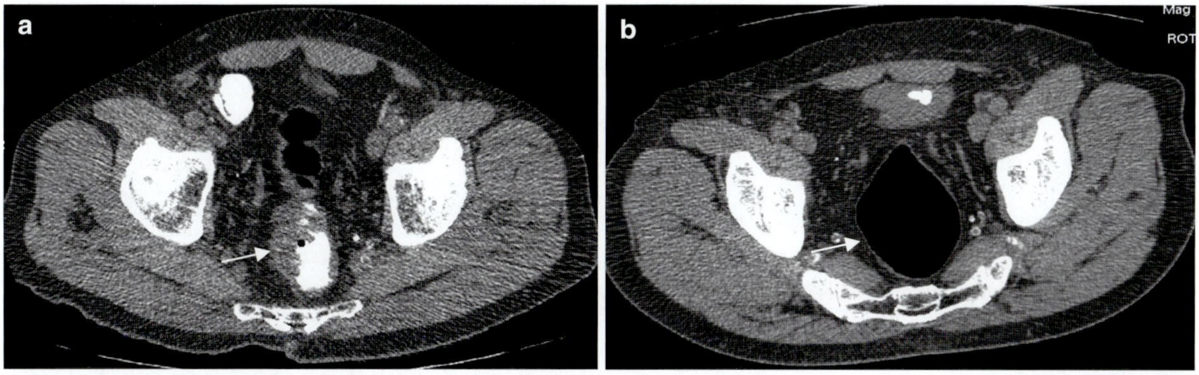

Fig. 17.11. Rectal contraction (*arrow*, **a**) also can cause focal wall thickening. (**b**) Delayed imaging in a complimentary position again shows inflation of previously contracted segment.

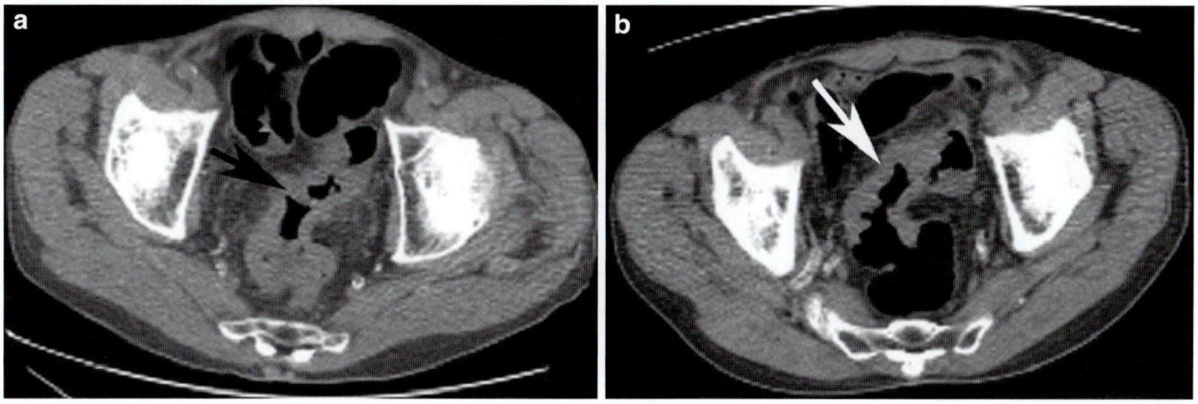

Fig. 17.12. Annular constricting cancers should not be confused with collapse. Colonic wall thickening and intraluminal irregularity observed in these types of lesion are persistent in complimentary positions. Note the persistent nondistension and segmental sigmoid wall thickening that is present in both supine (**a**) and prone (**b**) images.

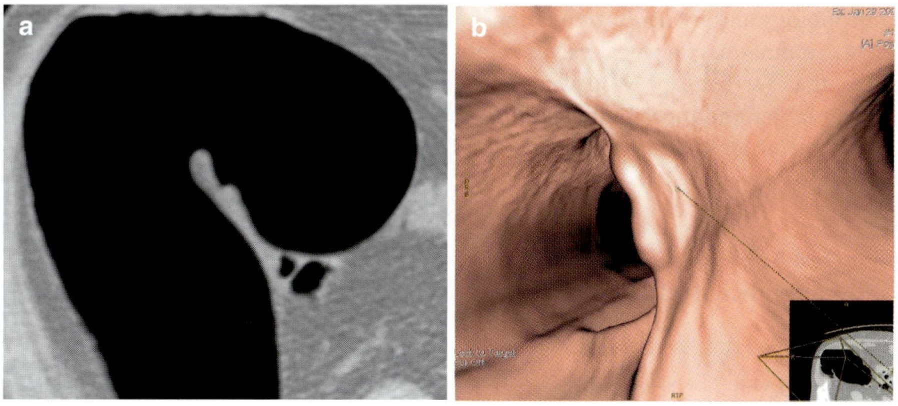

Fig. 17.13. Normal ileocecal valve. The valve should be symmetric with respect to the valve orifice on 2D and 3D views (**a, b**). By narrowing the window and level settings to soft-tissue settings, one can visualize the internal fatty attenuation of the valve and its associated fold (**a**).

The valve should be symmetric with respect to the valve orifice on 2D and 3D views. By narrowing the window and level settings to soft-tissue settings, one can visualize the internal fatty attenuation of the valve and its associated fold, and distinguish this from suspicious filling defects (Figs. 17.13 and 17.14). Several normal variants of ileocecal valve morphology have been described (Macari and Megibow 2001,

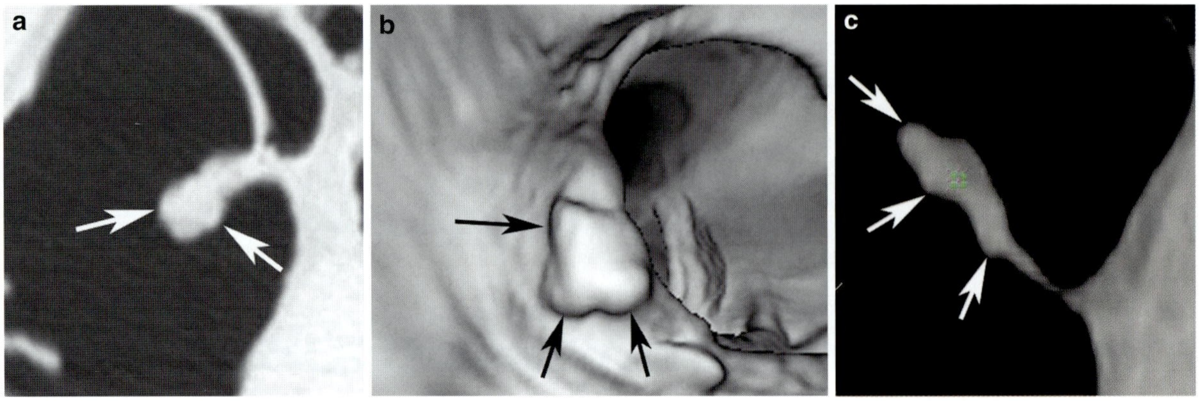

Fig. 17.14. Ileocecal valve with lobulated polypoid filling defects on 2D and 3D views (*arrows* (**a**, **b**)) without symmetry with respect to the valve orifice. Soft-tissue windows revealed internal soft-tissue attenuation (*arrow*, **c**). Endoscopy demonstrated an adenoma on the ileocecal valve.

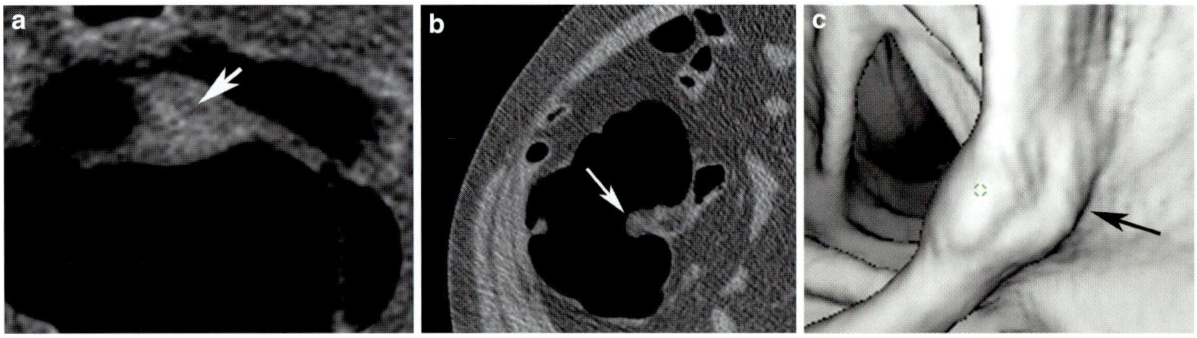

Fig. 17.15. Lipomatous ileocecal valves retain benign features, only appearing more bulbous. They possess homogenous fatty internal attenuation (**a**, prone image) and appear smoothly marginated without focal lesions on 3D endoluminal views (**b**, **c**, supine images)

Silva et al. 2007), but an assessment of the 2D and 3D morphology and internal attenuation is usually sufficient. Lipomatous ileocecal valves retain benign features that we have previously described, and only appear larger and more bulbous, with a homogenous fatty internal attenuation (Fig. 17.15).

17.2.6 Inverted Appendiceal Stump and Appendiceal Intussusception

An inverted appendiceal stump can appear identical to a polyp (Fig. 17.16), and is located at the site of prior appendectomy. Both the appendiceal stump and intraluminal neoplasm will enhance with intravenous contrast. When such a filling defect is encountered in a patient with a prior appendectomy, endoscopic correlation is required. Appendiceal intussusception can also occur. Barium enema has the advantage of being able to cause reduction in the intussusception manually, so that the filling defect disappears during reduction. In CT colonography, this is usually not the case, and such filling defects require further endoscopic or fluoroscopic evaluation.

17.3 Benign Findings

17.3.1 Lipomas

Lipomas are the most common submucosal tumor of the colon and are visualized frequently. Large lipomas may bleed, and heterogeneity within a lipoma is thought to correlate with internal hemorrhage. Lipomas are smoothly marginated filling defects within the colon with internal fatty attenuation (Fig. 17.17).

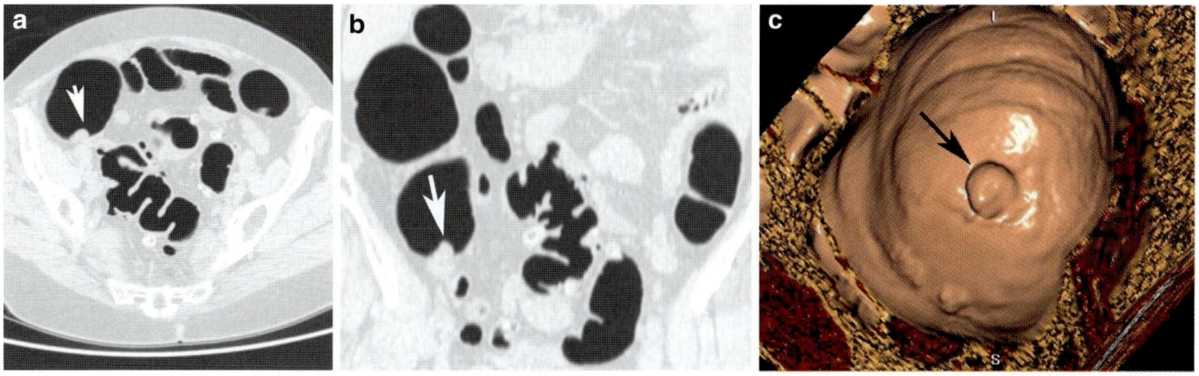

Fig. 17.16. An inverted appendiceal stump can appear identical to a polyp and is located at the site of prior appendectomy (arrows in **a**, **b**, **c**). Close correlation to patient's history of prior appendectomy and absence of appendix on 2D views are required under these circumstances.

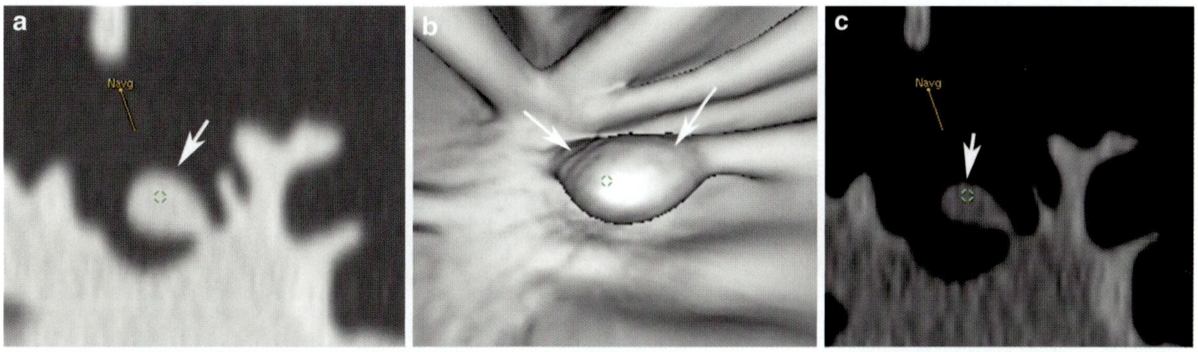

Fig. 17.17. Lipoma. Note the smoothly marginated filling defect (**a**, **b**, *arrows*) with internal fatty attenuation (**c**, *arrows*).

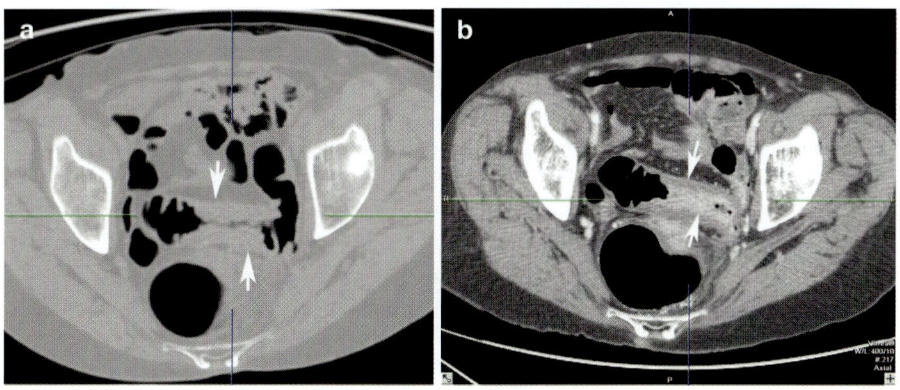

Fig. 17.18. Diverticulitis may mimic an annular constricting neoplasm when the majority of inflammation is intramural, rather than extending into the pericolonic tissues (**a**). Contrast enhancement may demonstrate mural stratification (**b**, *arrow*).

17.3.2 Diverticulitis

Diverticulitis may mimic an anular constricting neoplasm when the majority of inflammation is intramural, rather than extending into the pericolonic tissues. We have infrequently encountered this appearance. From our limited experience with this entity, we presume that contrast-enhancement may be helpful by demonstrating mural stratification and diverticula within the lesion (Fig. 17.18). Close correlation with clinical history and clinical follow-up, and reimaging or endoscopy after the episode has occurred, is prudent.

17.3.3
Pneumatosis Cystoides Coli

Pneumatosis cystoides coli (PCC) is a rare condition characterized pathologically by multiple thin-walled, noncommunicating, gas-filled cysts in the submucosal or subserosal layer of the colonic wall. Using lung window settings, CT colonography can easily demonstrate the air-filled cysts with a bubble-like appearance within the wall of the colon (Fig. 17.19) (Pickhardt et al. 2008). Optical colonoscopy reveals submucosal masses with normal mucosa overlying them, but these cannot be confirmed to be gas-containing intramural cysts without radiologic correlation.

17.4
Intracolonic and Extracolonic Processes Mimicking Disease

17.4.1
Stool

Stool is the most frequent cause of false-positive findings in CT colonography (Fletcher et al. 2000). There are several imaging characteristics that usually aid in the identification of stool. If fecal tagging has been used, stool appears as a bright hyperdense filling defect or mass in the colonic lumen with or without air inclusions (Fig. 17.20). If fecal tagging has not been used, stool will have heterogeneous internal attenuation, often with internal air, lacking a clear point of attachment to the colonic wall (Fig. 17.21). Additionally, stool particles usually lie along the dependent colonic

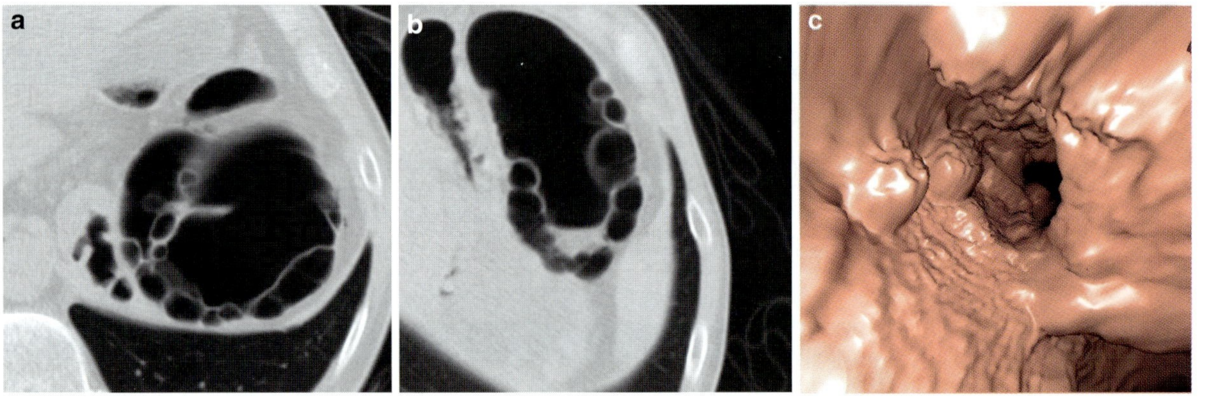

Fig. 17.19. Pneumatosis cystoides coli. Axial CT colonography images with lung window settings (**a, b**) shows air-filled cysts with a bubble-like appearance within the wall of the colon. Volume-rendered images demonstrate innumerable filling defects indistinguishable from stool or neoplasia without 2D images (**c**).

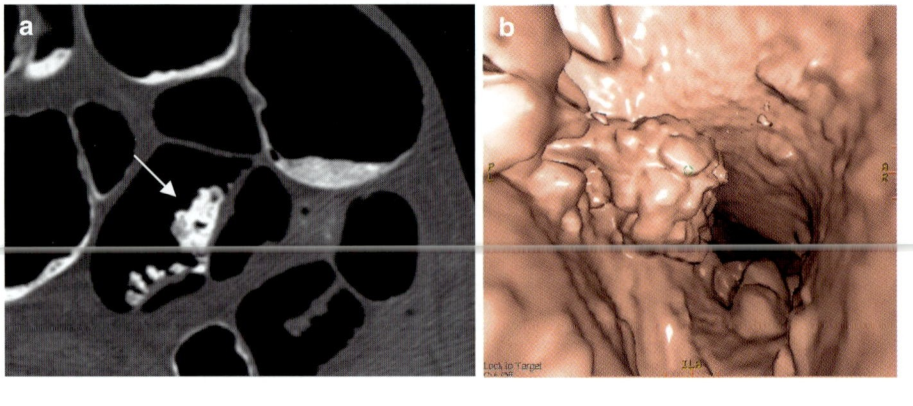

Fig. 17.20. With inhomogeneous fecal tagging, solid untagged stool is mixed with tagged stool, iodine, and barium (**a**, arrow). On 3D endoluminal images, stool often demonstrates sharp intraluminal projections (**b**).

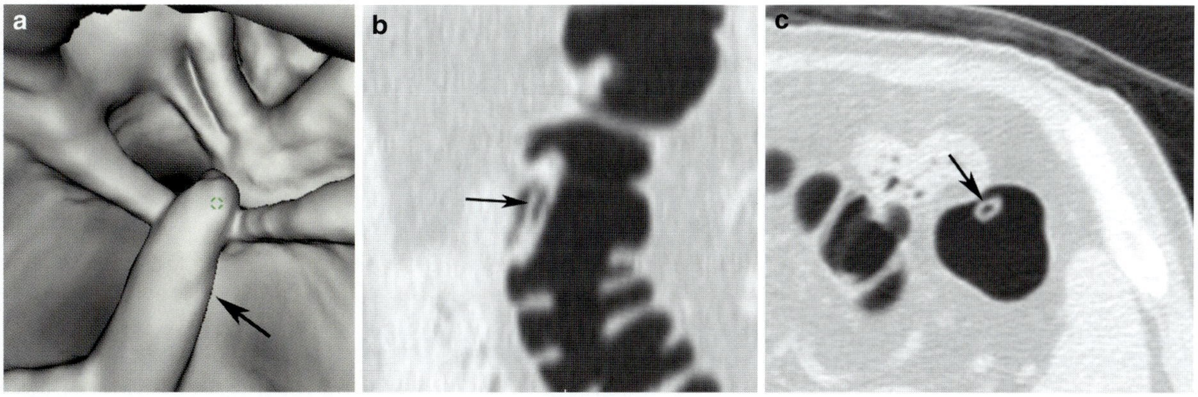

Fig. 17.21. Stool may mimic polyps (**a**). In this case, internal air and lack of a clear point of attachment to the wall (**b**, **c**, *arrows*) distinguishes stool from polyp.

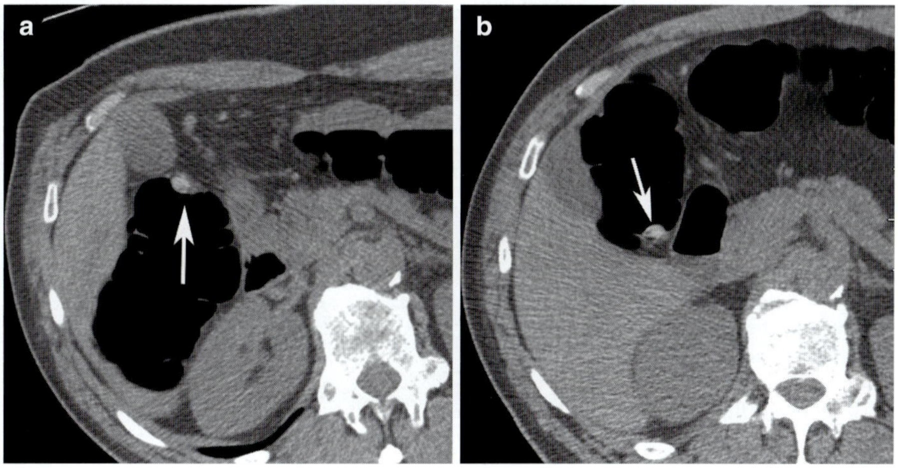

Fig. 17.22. (**a**, **b**) Stool particles generally change location with changes in the patient positioning, with stool particles usually located along the dependent wall (*arrows*).

wall and change location with changes in patient positioning (Fig. 17.22) (Fletcher et al. 2000). On 3D normal endoluminal images, stool often demonstrates sharp intraluminal projections (Fig. 17.23). Stool particles also demonstrate a lack of enhancement when intravenous contrast is given.

17.4.2 Fluid

Fluid redistributes between prone and supine imaging (Fig. 17.24). Bowel preparation using polyethylene glycol electrolyte solution typically results in more retained colonic fluid, compared with other bowel preparation regimens, but leaves less particulate stool matter in the colon. Fluid can also be seen in 3D endoluminal images (Fig. 17.25). When there is excessive fluid and fluid tagging has not been used, intravenous contrast can be used to enhance submerged lesions. Alternatively, fluid tagging can be used. Tagged fluid appears brightly hyperdense (Fig. 17.26) and permits the visualization of the colonic wall adjacent to the fluid on the 2D images, facilitating the detection of submerged lesions as negative filling defects in the fluid (Fig. 17.27).

17.4.3 Extrinsic Compression

Extrinsic compression on the colon can result from multiple structures, such as the iliac vessels, liver, renal masses, ribs, and stomach (Fig. 17.28), and can be dis-

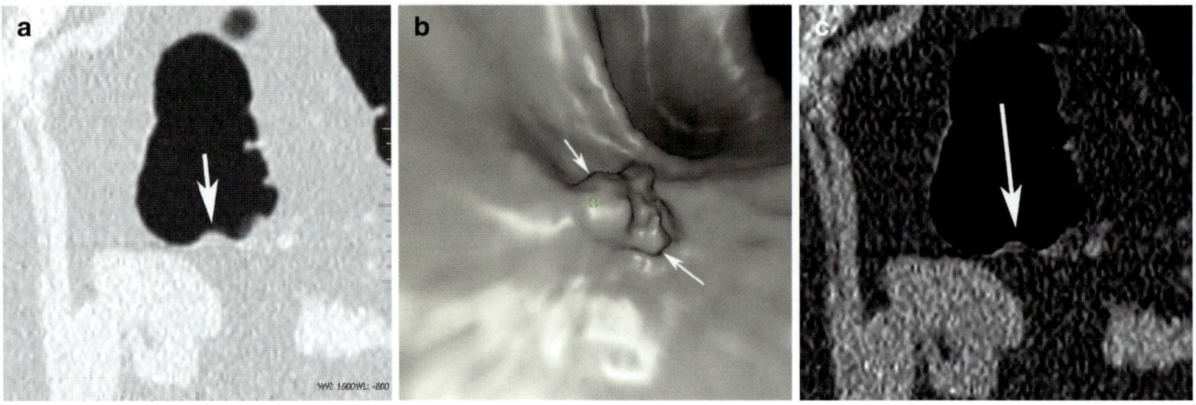

Fig. 17.23. A suspicious filling defect on 2D images (**a**, *arrow*) demonstrates sharp intraluminal projections on 3D endoluminal images (**b**) and is not of soft-tissue attenuation (**c**). These features indicate that the lesion represents stool.

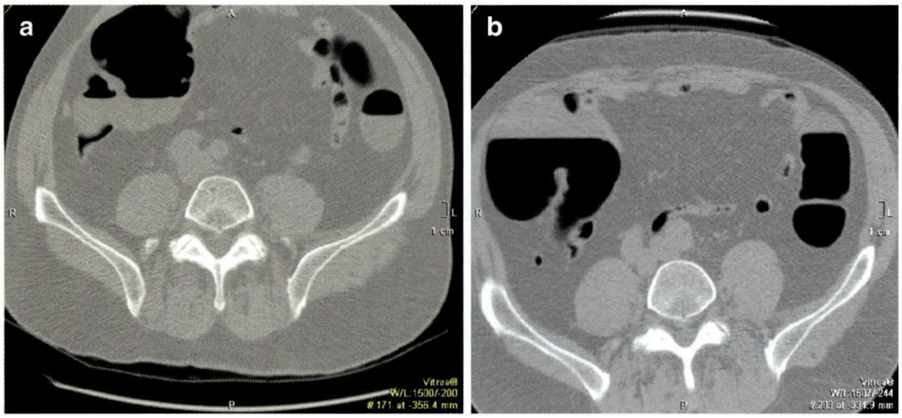

Fig. 17.24. (**a**, **b**) Cecal fluid redistributes between prone and supine imaging (*arrows*). When there is excessive fluid, intravenous contrast can be used to enhance submerged lesions. Note the dependent position of the fluid.

cerned by correlating 3D endoluminal filling defects with these structures in 2D images (Macari and Megibow 2001). Compression by one of the iliac arteries is a relatively common finding, and results in a linear extrinsic compression on the sigmoid colon (Fig. 17.29).

17.4.4 Technical Artifacts

Technical artifacts are easy to recognize. Breathhold and motion artifacts are usually best seen with sagittal or coronal oblique planes, which better display the motion along the *Z*-axis (Fig. 17.30). Higher slice multidetector row CT scanners permit significant increases in table speed resulting in faster scanning of the abdomen and pelvis and in the minimization of these artifacts (Hara et al. 2001). Metallic artifacts cause beam-hardening artifacts, and can obscure the colon lumen. Stairstep artifacts are usually not seen with thin slice thickness, but can be seen with thicker slice thicknesses (such as 5 mm) on 3D normal luminal images and 2D multiplanar reformatted images, most commonly within the rectum and cecum, where there are great changes in the luminal diameter along the *Z*-axis.

17.5 Colonic Neoplasia in CT Colonography

17.5.1 Polyps

Polyps may be sessile, pedunculated, or flat (alternatively defined as either the base measuring more than twice that of the height or a height of ≤ 2mm). Sessile

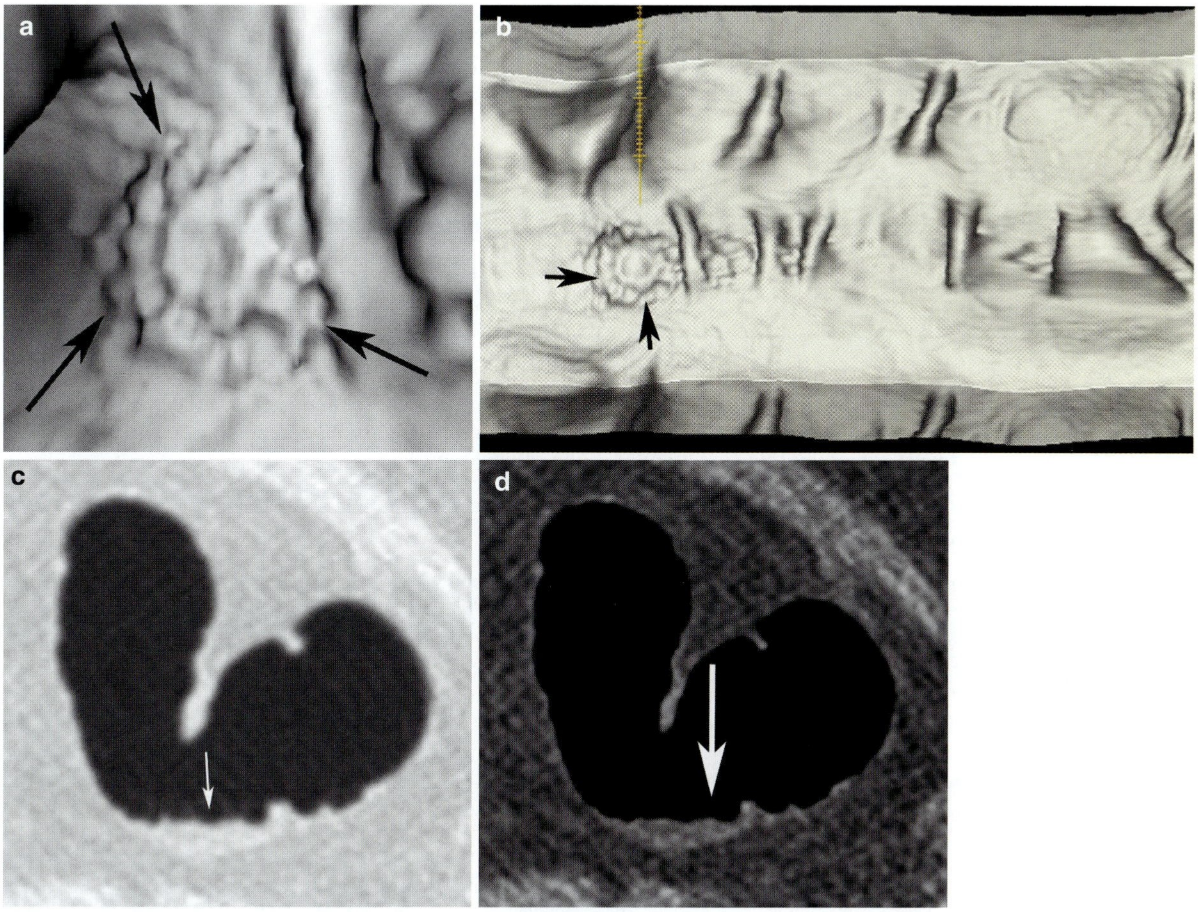

Fig. 17.25. Fluid can be seen on 3D endoluminal images (**a**, *arrow*) and on virtual pathology (**b**, *arrow*) as a filling defect. Axial 2D image shows the air-fluid level (**c**, *arrow*) and soft-tissue windows demonstrate that the lesion does not have soft-tissue attenuation (**d**, *arrow*).

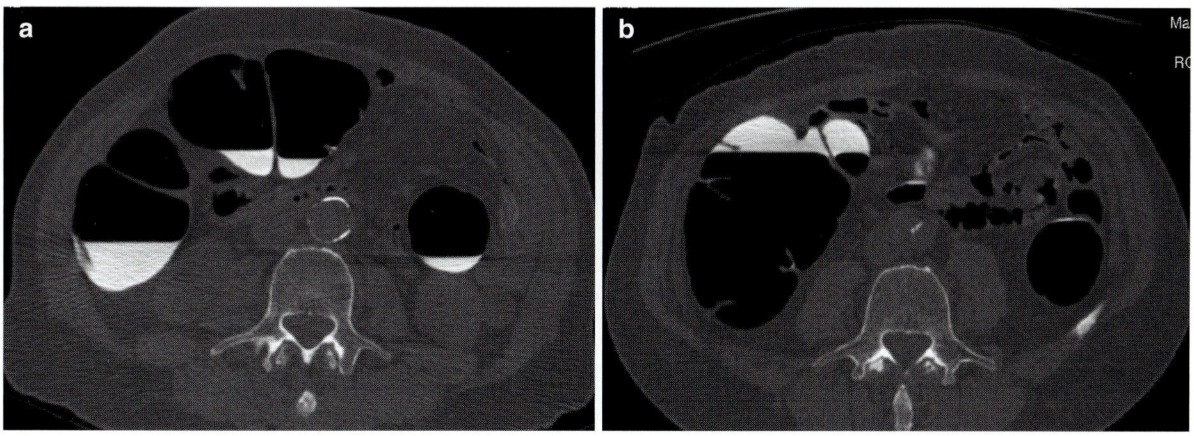

Fig. 17.26. (**a**, **b**) When fluid tagging is used, fluid appears brightly hyperdense, permitting visualization of the colonic wall adjacent to fluid.

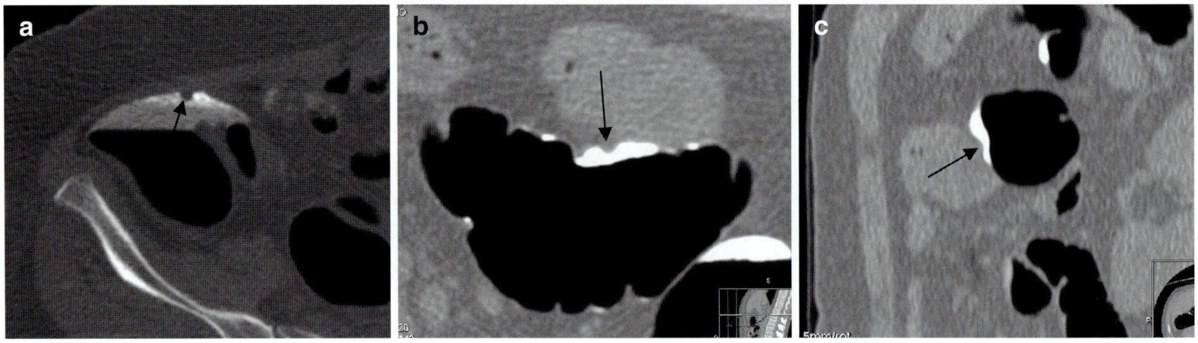

Fig. 17.27. Submerged sessile polyps in two patients, both seen as a negative filling defect in the midst of tagged fluid (*arrows*). (**a**) A submerged polyp in the cecum on prone axial CT colonography image corresponding to a tubular adenoma found at this location at endoscopy. (**b, c**) 2D supine and sagittal MPR images in another patient demonstrating a submerged tubular adenoma, later confirmed using colonoscopy.

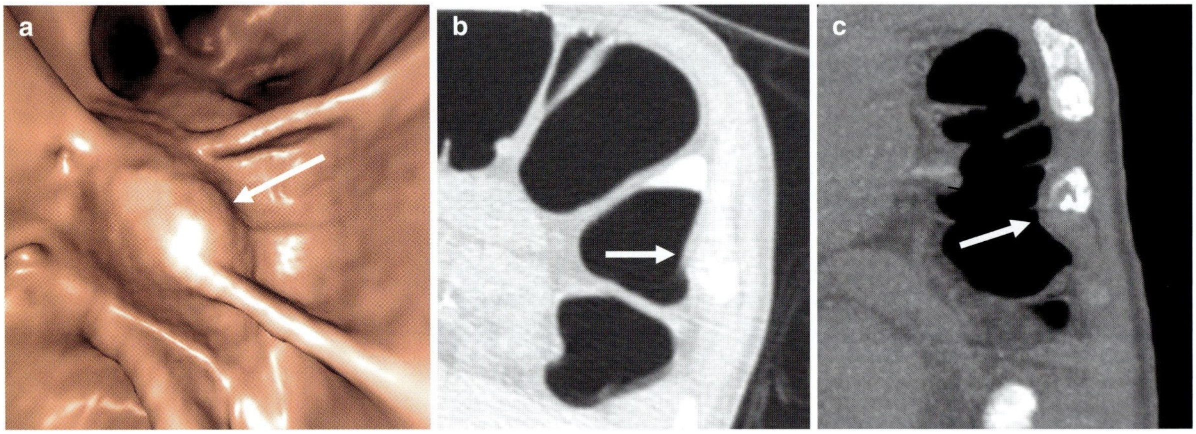

Fig. 17.28. A filling defect can be seen on the 3D endoluminal view (**a**) and 2D lung windows (**b**). Close correlation with the coronal 2D MPR image (**c**) shows the filling defect to correspond to extrinsic compression by a rib (arrows, b and c).

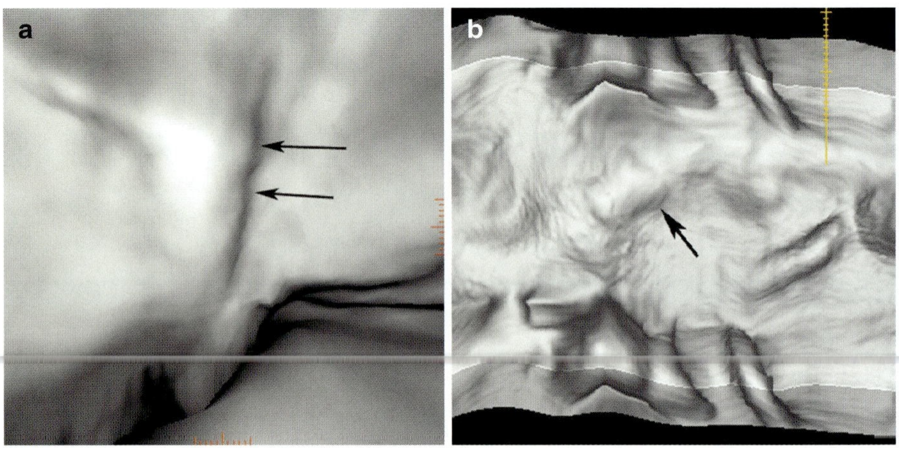

Fig. 17.29. Compression by one of the iliac arteries in this case has resulted in a linear extrinsic compression on the sigmoid colon that is well demonstrated on 3D endoluminal view (**a**, *arrows*) and virtual pathology (**b**, *arrow*). 2D axial images demonstrate the extrinsic nature of these lesions (**c**, **d**, *arrows*).

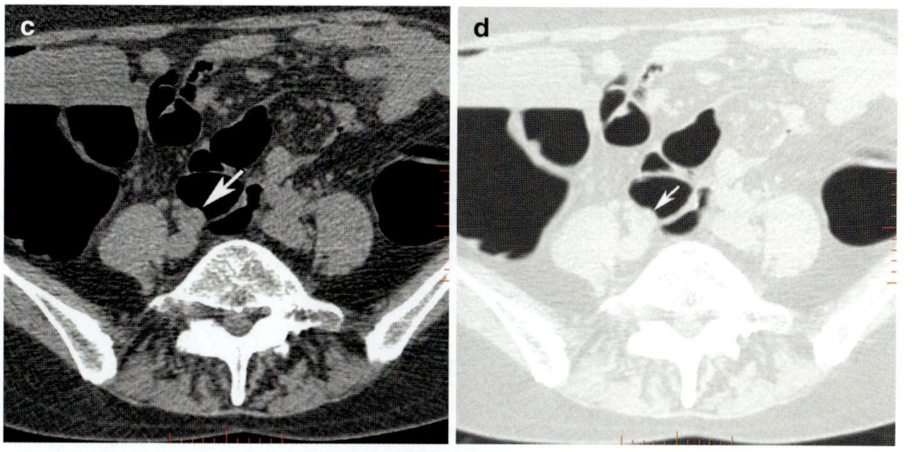

Fig. 17.29. (continued)

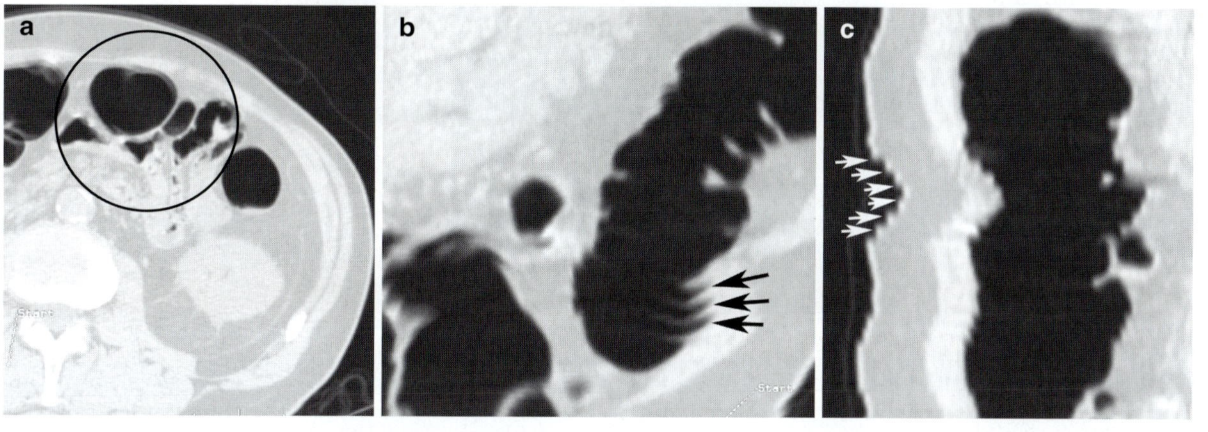

Fig. 17.30. Motion artifacts cause image blur on axial images (**a**, *circle*), but are best appreciated using 2D oblique coronal or sagittal images, which show luminal incongruity along the *Z*-axis of the colon and skin surface (*arrows* **b, c**).

polyps will possess polypoid morphology on axial, 2D multiplanar reformatted, and 3D endoluminal views (Fig. 17.31). When sessile polyps are of sufficient size (generally considered to be three times the slice thickness), they will also possess internal soft-tissue attenuation. Sessile polyps are generally seen on both supine and prone views, but about 10–15% of medium-sized polyps will be seen only in one view, owing to suboptimal distention, or stool or fluid in the same colonic segment in the complementary position. Lesions that appear as sessile polyps in one position should not be disregarded unless the same segment is optimally seen in the corresponding position. Enhancement after the administration of intravenous contrast material can help to differentiate polyps from stool or thickened folds (Fig. 17.32).

Pedunculated polyps possess a stalk and a head. They are best seen on 2D axial and 2D MPR images (Fig. 17.33). Using 3D endoluminal renderings, it has been observed that the stalk of a pedunculated polyp is often inseparable from the colonic wall. Polyps with long stalks maybe missed during CT colonography, as the larger filling defect representing the head of the polyp may appear to move between colonic segments (Fenlon et al. 1999). Careful interrogation of suspicious filling defects for a stalk connecting them to the colonic wall is imperative in diagnosing pedunculated polyps. We observed that pedunculated polyps can be found with a high degree of accuracy.

Flat lesions can be difficult to visualize both endoscopically and radiographically. On CT, flat lesions appear as focal regions of colonic wall thickening with soft-tissue attenuation. Flat lesions are often cigar-shaped, and are best seen on 2D axial and MPR images with narrow window settings (such as bone window settings) (Fidler et al. 2002). Perturbation in the

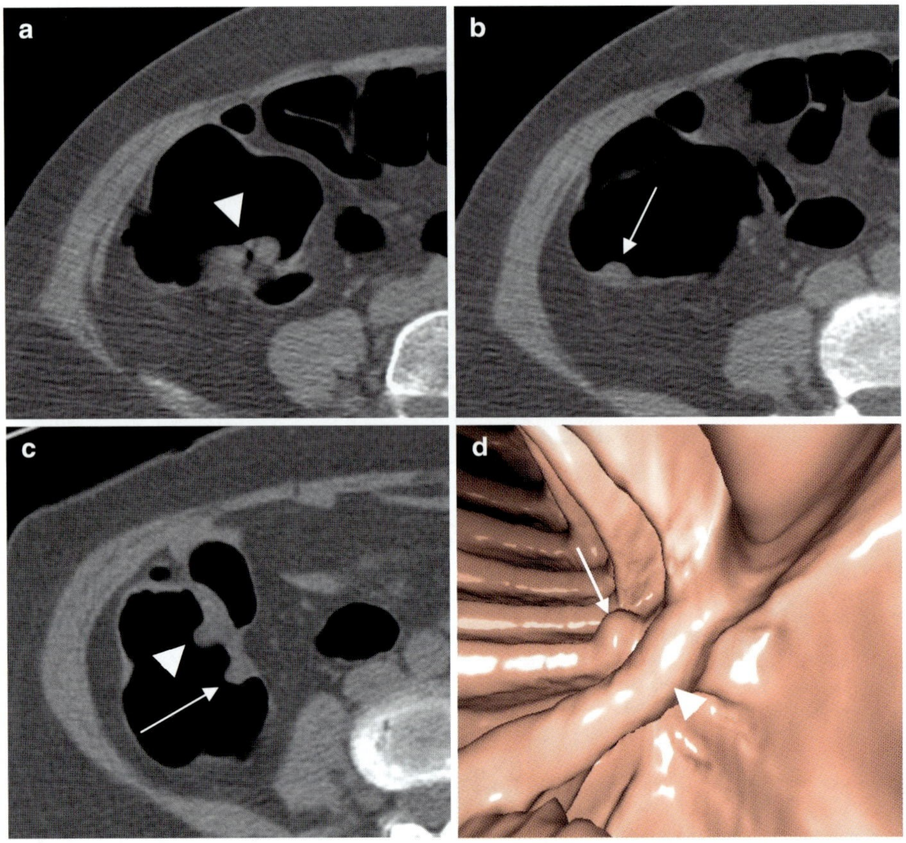

Fig. 17.31. Sessile adenomatous polyp and colonic rotation. (**a, b**) Supine axial images demonstrate a normal ileocecal valve (arrowhead, **a**) as well as a sessile polyp (arrow, **b**) along the posterior wall of the cecum and ascending colon. (**c**) Image acquired with the patient in prone position which again shows the ileocecal valve and the sessile polyp. Note the greater than 90° counter clockwise rotation of the cecum between the supine and prone position; however, the spatial relationship of the polyp to the ileocecal valve is preserved. Figures C and D demonstrate that the polyp (**c, d**, arrow) is of polypoid morphology on 2D and 3D views and demonstrates internal soft-tissue attenuation.

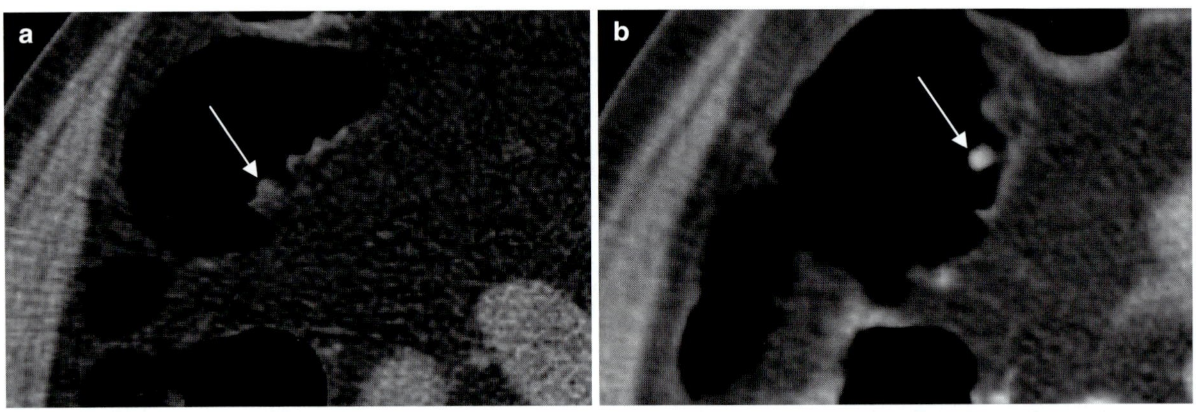

Fig. 17.32. Enhancing sub-centimeter polyp. In (**a**) (without intravenous contrast material), a suspicious filling defect is identified (*arrow*). After the administration of intravenous contrast, the filling defect enhances unequivocally (**b**, *arrow*), permitting confident diagnosis of a colonic polyp. Even small polyps can be seen to enhance following intravenous contrast administration.

colonic wall can be visualized when surveying the colon with 2D images using lung windows, and when these perturbations are discovered, interrogation of soft-tissue window settings is imperative (Figs. 17.34–17.36). Similar perturbations can often be seen on 3D endoluminal views, but can be occult. Like other polyps, flat lesions are usually seen in both the supine and prone views, unless the segment in which the

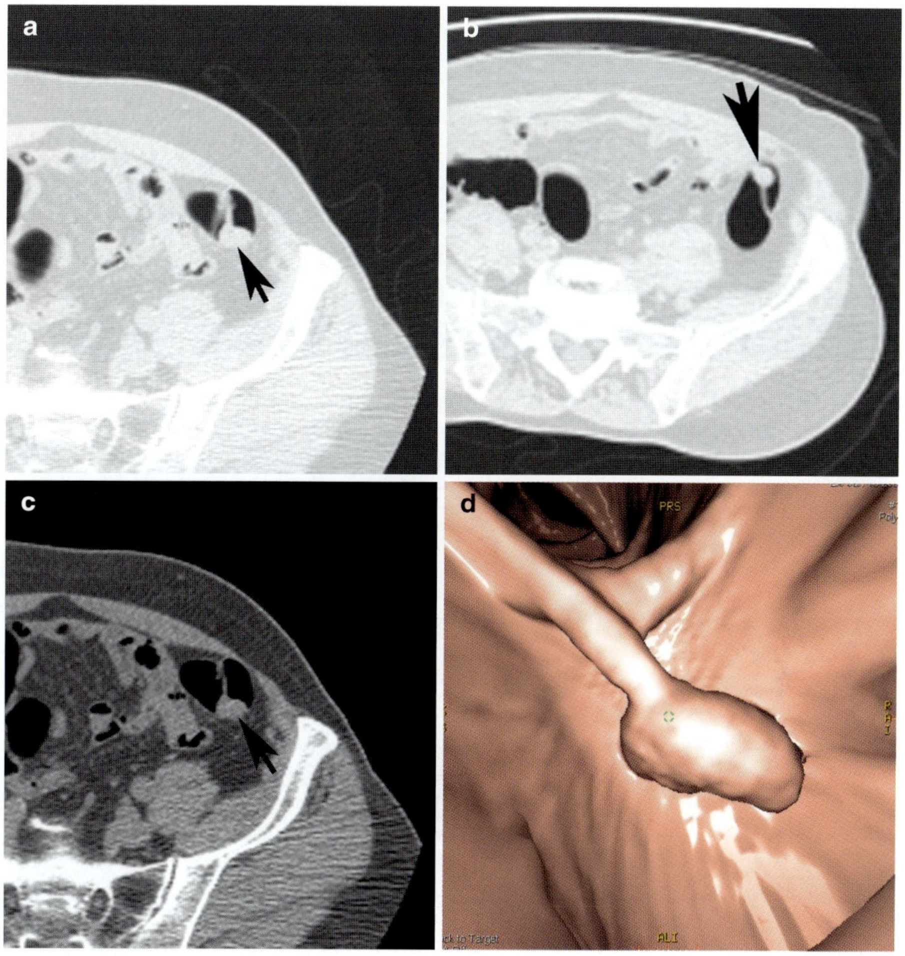

Fig. 17.33. Pedunculated polyp. Supine 2D axial image (**a**) and prone 2D axial image (**b**) show a polyp in the descending colon associated with a stalk (arrowhead). Note how the polyp head dangles toward the dependent surface. Soft-tissue window setting shows the lesion to have soft-tissue attenuation (**c**). Note that the lesion changes position to the dependent position owing to its long stalk. (**d**) Endoluminal view.

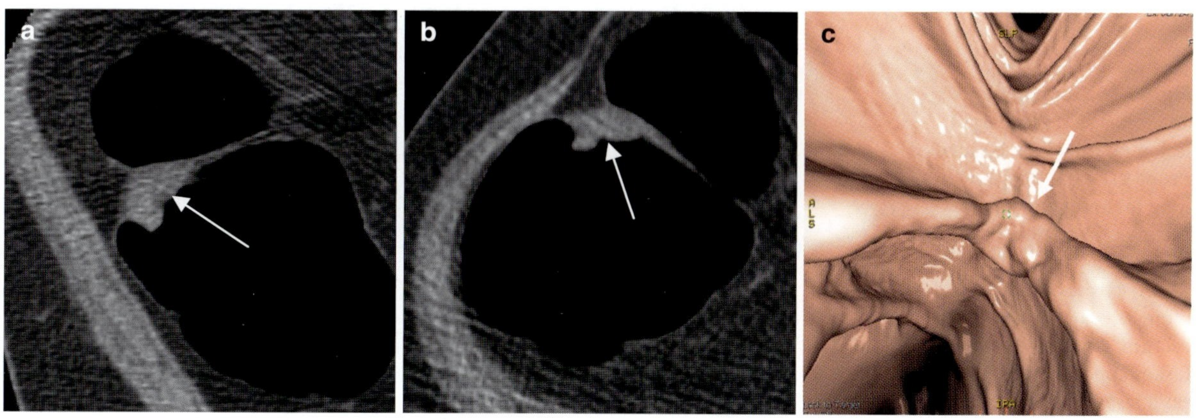

Fig. 17.34. Flat cancer. 2D axial prone (**a**) and supine (**b**) images show a focal flat region of soft-tissue thickening along the lateral aspect of the ascending colon (**a**, **b** *arrows*). On 3D endoluminal view, the lesion appears as a focal thickening along a haustral fold (**c**, *arrow*). Pathologic examination demonstrated an invasive adenocarcinoma, invading into muscularis propria but not the pericolonic fat.

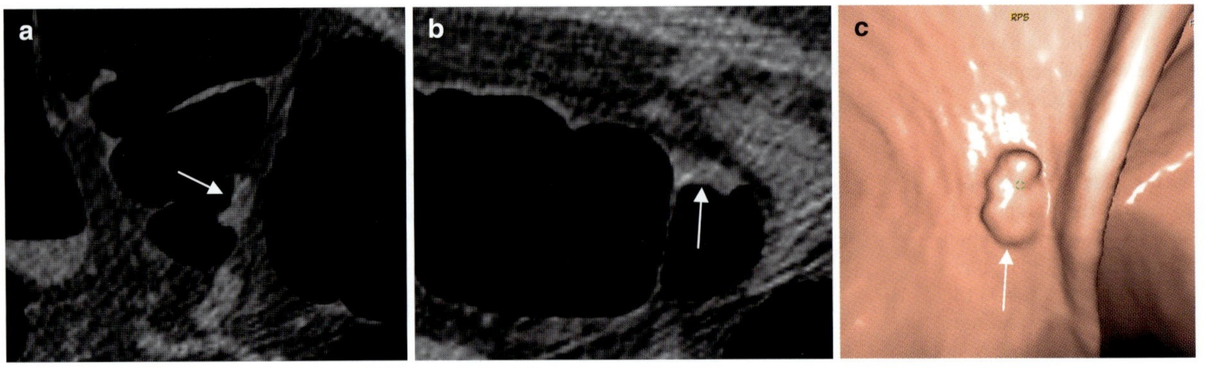

Fig. 17.35. Flat Tubular adenoma. 2D axial supine (**a**) and prone (**b**) images show a focal flat region of soft-tissue thickening along the lateral aspect of the descending colon (**a, b** *arrows*). On 3D views, the flat nature of the lesion can be appropriately appreciated (*arrow*). Pathologic examination revealed this lesion to be a tubular adenoma.

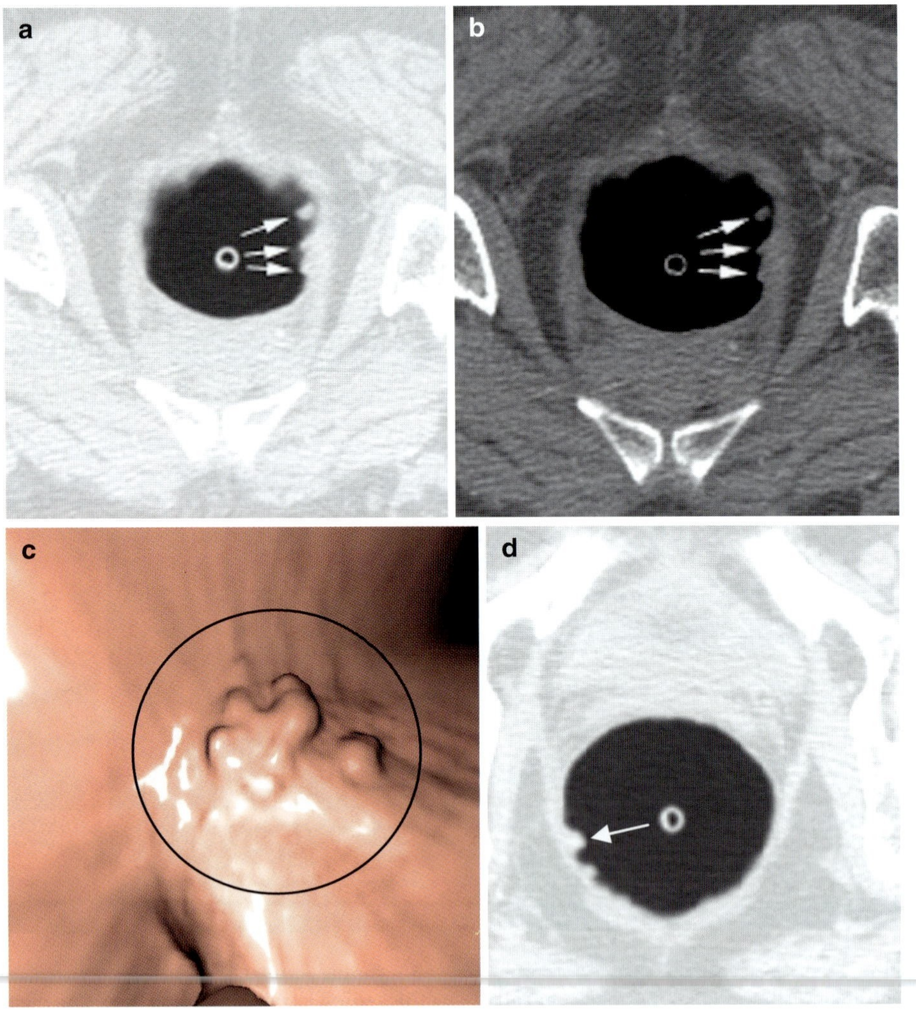

Fig. 17.36. Tubulovillous adenoma seen as a carpet lesion (arrows in **a**, **b** and **c**). Prone 2D axial image with lung (**a**) and bone window settings (**b**) demonstrate a focal, nodular region of soft-tissue thickening along the lateral wall of the rectum. On 3D views, the lesion appears as a polypoid lesion (**c**, circled), with the nodular filling defect appearing unchanged on the corresponding supine view (**d**).

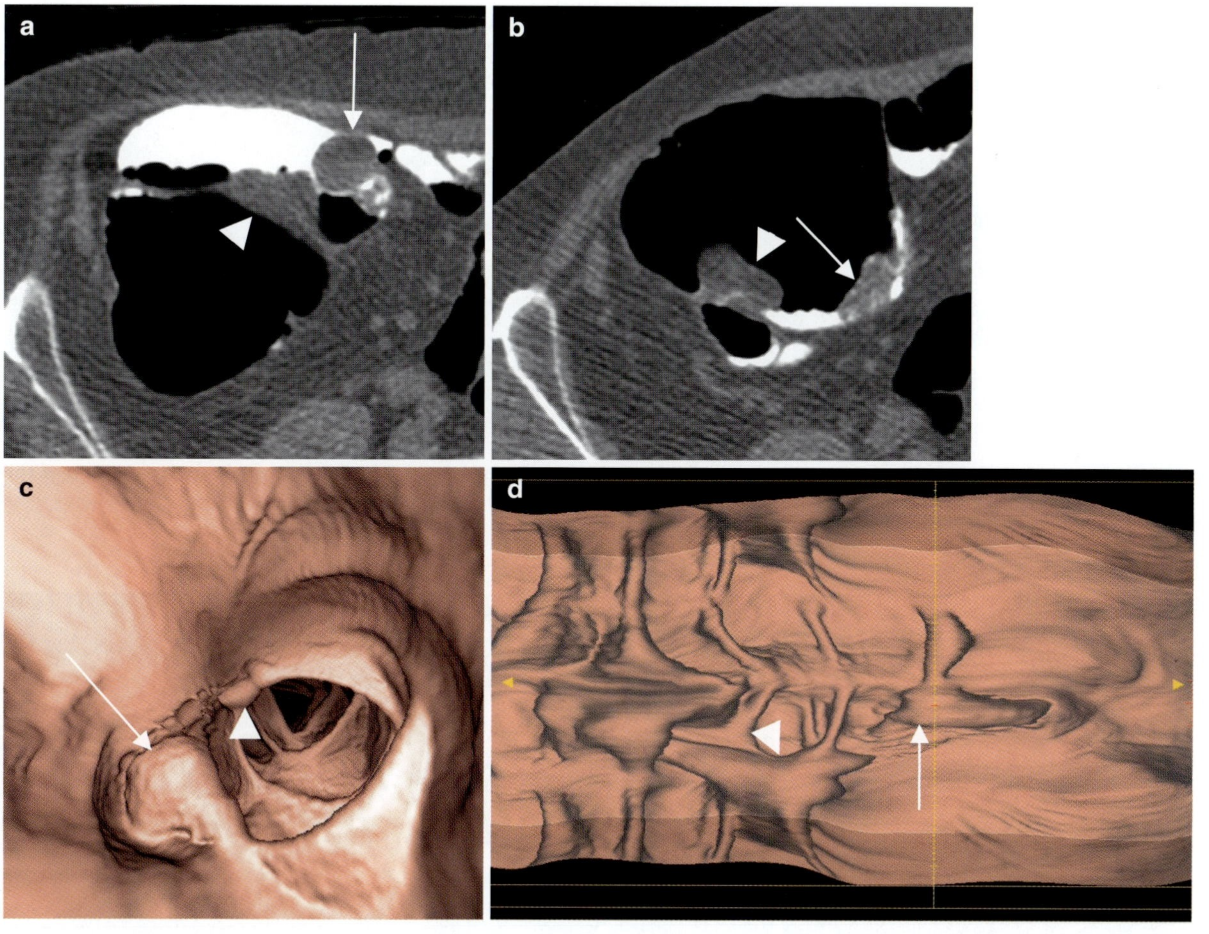

Fig. 17.37. Large sessile cecal tubulovillous adenoma located inferomedially to the ileocecal valve. Note that the lesion is submerged in the prone view (**a**), and surrounded by tagged fluid in the supine view (**b**), with some interstices being filled with fluid in both the views. (**c, d**) 3D endoluminal views demonstrating both the lesion surrounded by fluid (*arrow*) and the ileocecal valve (*arrowhead*).

lesion is located is suboptimally visualized in one of the views. Intravenous contrast can be useful in characterizing flat lesions. Flat lesions should not be confused with luminal collapse. The colonic wall does thicken as it collapses. The thickened colonic wall can be distinguished from the true flat lesion in that it is not well-defined, should be distended in the corresponding position, and have a smooth margin, as the colonic wall tapers to a normal thickness in the adjacent areas of appropriate distention (Fig. 17.7). The term "flat lesion" can represent a variety of pathologies, from flat adenomas to hyperplastic lesions to tubulovillous adenomas and flat carcinomas. In general, flat lesions tend to be more advanced lesions.

Villous lesions can appear as sessile polyps (Fig. 17.37) or carpet lesions (Fig. 17.36), seen as focal regions of colonic wall thickening (Galdino and Yee 2003). Similar to their fluoroscopic appearance, their surface has a cauliflower-appearing surface, with tagged barium often filling the interstices of the neoplasm (Fig. 17.37) (O'Connor et al. 2006). When villous morphology is discovered, it is imperative to describe it owing to the increased likelihood of malignancy (or progression to malignancy).

17.5.2 Carcinomas

Carcinomas can assume a variety of shapes. Smaller cancers may be identical to large polyps and flat lesions, while semi-annular and annular, and scirrhous cancers have a unique CT appearance. Semi-annular and annular cancers are seen as focal, segmental regions of luminal narrowing, accompanied by focal wall thickening, usually with proximal

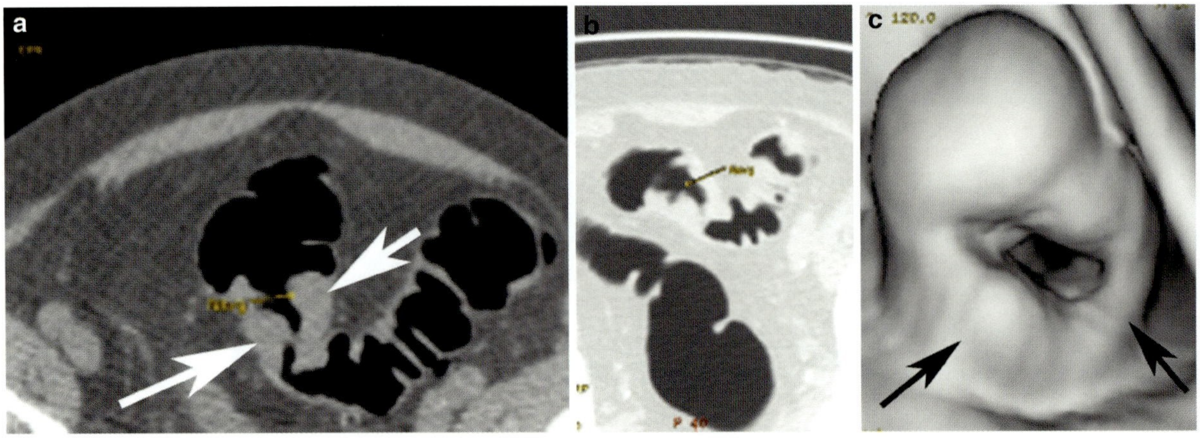

Fig. 17.38. Annular cancer. 2D axial images (**a**) and (**b**) soft-tissue window setting shows the soft-tissue attenuation of the lesion (**a**, *arrows*). Note the shape of the lesion on 3D views (**c**, *arrows*).

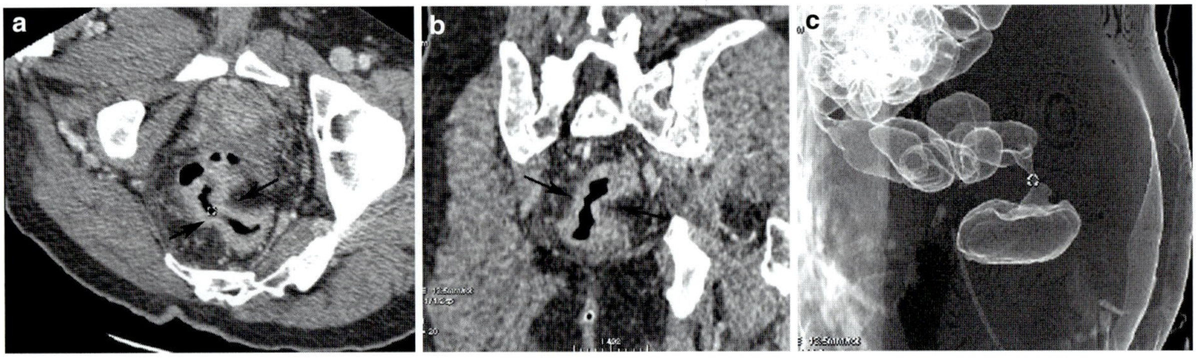

Fig. 17.39. Scirrhous cancer demonstrates luminal constriction, irregularity, and wall thickening in the mid-rectum on 2D MPR images (**a**, **b**), with the luminal constriction best highlighted on the virtual barium enema rendering (**c**).

and distal shouldering (Fig. 17.38). The intraluminal margins of the mass are irregular. Irregularity and extension of soft tissue into the pericolonic tissue signal invasion, as does regional lymphadenopathy or hepatic metastases. Annular cancers are best observed using 2D and 3D MPR images using soft-tissue window settings.

Scirrhous cancers are the most common type of cancer in our experience that are often missed by radiologists learning colonography (Fidler 2004). Scirrhous cancers are annular lesions that constrict the colonic lumen, and may be confused with luminal collapse or contraction, particularly when adjacent collapse obscures the shouldering of the carcinoma (Fig. 17.39). However, focal wall thickening of soft-tissue attenuation and irregular intraluminal margins clearly separate these lesions from collapse. Segmental regions of luminal narrowing observed in one position or in both positions should be considered as potential scirrhous cancers, until repositioning and reinflation can disprove their presence.

17.6 Conclusion

CT colonography interpretation requires radiologists to interactively view 2D and 3D images of the colonic lumen, use a variety of window and level settings, and compare the supine and prone 3D datasets. Colonic datasets are interrogated systematically to screen for potential colorectal lesions, employing well-established problem-solving techniques at the computer workstation to distinguish true neoplasms from benign and normal structures. A visual understanding of the normal appearance of colorectal structures, benign lesions, disease mimics, and colorectal neoplasia is necessary in utilizing the capabilities of modern CT colonography computer workstations to accurately diagnose the disease.

References

Chen SC, Lu DSK, Hecht JR et al (1999) CT colonography: value of scanning in both the supine and prone positions. AJR 172:595–599

Dachman AH, Kuniyoshi JK, Boyle CM et al (1998) CT colonography with three-dimensional problem solving for detection of colonic polyps. AJR 171:989–995

Fenlon HM, Nunes DP, Schroy PC et al (1999) A comparison of virtual and conventional colonoscopy for the detection of colorectal polyps. N Engl J Med 341(20):1496–1503

Fidler JL (2004) Understanding interpretive errors in radiologists learning computed tomography colonography. Acad Radiol 11:750–756

Fidler JL, Johnson CD, Maccarty RL et al (2002) Detection of flat lesions in the colon with CT colonography. Abdom Imaging 27(3):292–300

Fletcher JL, Johnson CD, Maccarty RL et al (1999) CT colonography: potential pitfalls and problem-solving techniques. AJR Am J Roentgenol 172(5):1271–1278

Fletcher JG, Johnson CD, Reed JE et al (2001) Feasibility of planar virtual pathology: a new paradigm in volume-rendered CT colonography. JCAT 25:864–869

Fletcher JG, Johnson CD, Welch TJ et al (2000) Optimization of CT colonography technique: a prospective trial in 180 patients. Radiology 216:704–711

Galdino GM, Yee J (2003) Carpet lesion on CT colonography: a potential pitfall. AJR Am J Roentgenol 180(5):1332–1334

Graser A, Stieber P, Nagel D et al (2008) Comparison of CT colonography, colonoscopy, sigmoidoscopy, and fecal occult blood tests for the detection of advanced adenoma in an average risk population. Gut 2009; 58:241–8.

Gryspeerdt SS, Herman MJ, Baekelandt MA et al (2004) Supine/left decubitus scanning: a valuable alternative to supine/prone scanning in CT colonography. Eur Radiol 14 (5):768–777

Halligan S, Altman DG, Taylor SA et al (2005) CT colonography in the detection of colorectal polyps and cancer: systematic review, meta-analysis, and proposed minimum data set for study level reporting. Radiology 237(3):893–904

Hara AK, Johnson CD, Reed JE (1997) Colorectal lesions: evaluation with CT colography. Radiographics 17(5):1157–1167; discussion 1167–1168

Hara AK, Johnson CD, MacCarty RL et al (2001) CT colonography: single- versus multi-detector row imaging. Radiology 219(2):461–465

Johnson CD, Chen MH, Toledano AY et al (2008) Accuracy of CT colonography for detection of large adenomas and cancers. N Engl J Med 359:1207–1217

Johnson CD, Fletcher JG, MacCarty RL et al (2007) Effect of slice thickness and primary 2D versus 3D virtual dissection on colorectal lesion detection at CT colonography in 452 asymptomatic adults. Am J Roentgenol 189(3): 672–680

Macari M, Bini E, Jacobs SL et al (2003) Filling defects at CT colonography: pseudo- and diminutive lesions (the good), polyps (the bad), flat lesions, masses, and carcinomas (the ugly). Radiographics 23(5):1073–1091

Macari M, Bini E, Jacobs SL et al (2004) Colorectal polyps and cancers in asymptomatic average-risk patients: evaluation with CT colonography. Radiology 230(3):629–636

Macari M, Megibow AJ (2001) Pitfalls of using three-dimensional CT colonography with two-dimensional imaging correlation. AJR 176:137–143

Macari M, Milano A, Lavelle M et al (2000) Comparison of time-efficient CT colonography with two- and three-dimensional colonic evaluation for detecting colorectal polyps. AJR Am J Roentgenol 174(6):1543–1549

Morrin MM, Farrell RJ, Kruskal JB et al (2000) Utility of intravenously administered contrast material at CT colonography. Radiology 217(3):765–771

O'Connor SD, Summers RM, Choi JR (2006) Oral contrast adherence to polyps on CT colonography. J Comput Assist Tomogr 30(1):51–57

Pickhartdt PJ (2003) Computed tomographic virtual colonoscopy to screen for colorectal neoplasia in asymptomatic adults. N Engl J Med 349:2191–2200

Pickhardt PJ, Kim DH, Taylor AJ (2008) Asymptomatic pneumatosis at CT colonography: a benign self-limited imaging finding distinct from perforation. AJR Am J Roentgenol 190(2): W112–W117

Silva AC, Beaty SD, Hara AK et al (2007) Spectrum of normal and abnormal CT appearances of the ileocecal valve and cecum with endoscopic and surgical correlation. Radiographics 27(4):1039–1054

Silva AC, Vens EA, Hara AK et al (2006) Evaluation of benign and malignant rectal lesions with CT colonography and endoscopic correlation. Radiographics 26(4): 1085–1099

Yee J, Akerkar GA, Hung RK et al (2001) Colorectal neoplasia: performance characteristics of CT colonography for detection in 300 patients. Radiology 219:685–692

Yee J (2003) Comparison of supine and prone scanning separately and in combination at CT colonography. Radiology 226(3):653–661

Subject Index

A

B

C

D

E

F

Q

R

S

T

U

V

W

Z

List of Contributors

Yasuaki Arai, MD
Diagnostic RadiologyDivision
National Cancer Center Hospital
1-1 Tsukiji 5-chome
Chuo-ku, Tokyo
Japan

Didier Bielen, MD
UZ Gasthuisberg
Herestraat
3000 Leuven
Belgium
Email: didier.bielen@uz.kuleuven.ac.be

Fargol Booya, MD
Department of Radiology
Mayo Clinic Rochester
Mayo Building East 2-B
200 First Street SW
Rochester, MN 55905
USA

David Burling, MD
Intestinal Imaging Unit
Level 4V, St Mark's Hospital
Watford Road, Harrow
Middlesex HA1 3UJ
UK
Email: burling@doctors.org.uk

Francesca Cerri, MD
Department of Oncology
Diagnostic and Interventional Radiology, Transplants, and Advanced Technologies in Medicine
University of Pisa
Via Roma 67
56100 Pisa
Italy

Abraham H. Dachman, MD, FACR
Department of Radiology
The University of Chicago
5841 South Maryland Avenue
Chicago, IL 60645
USA
Email: ahdachma@uchicago.edu

Ayso H. de Vries, MD
Department of Radiology
Academic Medical Center
University of Amsterdam
Meibergdreef 9
1105 AZ G1-226 Amsterdam
The Netherlands
Email: ayso.devries@amc.uva.nl

Helen Fenlon, MD
Department of Radiology
Mater Misericordiae University Hospital
Eccles Street, Dublin 7
Ireland
Email: helen.fenlon@nbsp.ie

Joel G. Fletcher, MD
Department of Radiology
Mayo Clinic Rochester
Mayo Building East 2-B
200 First Street SW
Rochester, MN 55905
USA
Email: Fletcher.Joel@mayo.edu

Stefaan Gryspeerdt, MD
Department of Radiology
Stedelijk Ziekenhuis
Bruggesteenweg 90
8800 Roeselare
Belgium
Email: stefaan.gryspeerdt@szr.be

Luis S. Guimaraes, MD
Department of Radiology
Hospital de São Teotónio
Avenida Rei D. Duarte
3504-509 Viseu
Portugal

Steve Halligan, MD
Department of Imaging
University College Hospital
2F Podium, 235 Euston Road
London NW1 2BU
UK

Email: s.Halligan@imperial.ac.uk

Gen Iinuma, MD, PhD
Diagnostic Radiology Division
National Cancer Center Hospital
1-1 Tsukiji 5-chome
Chuo-ku, 104-0045
Japan

Email: giinuma@ncc.go.jp

Andrea Laghi, MD
Department of Radiological Sciences
University of Rome "La Sapienza"
ICOT Hospital
Latina
Italy

Email: andlaghi@gmail.com

Philippe Lefere, MD
Department of Radiology, Stedelijk Ziekenhuis
Bruggesteenweg 90
8800 Roeselare
Belgium

Email: radiologie@skynet.be

A. Maier, MD
Department of Radiology
Medical University of Vienna
Waehringer Guertel 18-20
1090 Vienna
Austria

Thomas Mang, MD
Department of Radiology
Medical University of Vienna
Waehringer Guertel 18-20
1090 Vienna
Austria

Email: thomas.mang@meduniwien.ac.at

Beth G. McFarland, MD
Center for Diagnostic Imaging
Chesterfield, MO 63017
USA

Email: mcfarlandb123@gmail.com

Richard Mendelson, MD
Department of Diagnostic & Interventional Radiology
Royal Perth Hospital, Wellington Street, Perth
West Australia

Email: Richard.Mendelson@health.wa.gov.au

Mototaka Miyake, MD
Diagnostic RadiologyDivision
National Cancer Center Hospital
1-1 Tsukiji 5-chome
Chuo-ku, Tokyo
Japan

Noriyuki Moriyama, MD
Cancer Screening Division
Research Center for Cancer Prevention and Screening
1-1 Tsukiji 5-chome
Chuo-ku, Tokyo
Japan

Koenraad J. Mortelé, MD
Department of Radiology
Brigham and Women's Hospital
Harvard Medical School
75 Francis Street
Boston, MA 02115
USA

Email: kmortele@partners.org

Yukio Muramatsu, MD
Cancer Screening Division
Research Center for Cancer Prevention and Screening
1-1 Tsukiji 5-chome
Chuo-ku, Tokyo
Japan

Darra Murphy, MD
Department of Radiology
Mater Misericordiae University Hospital
Eccles Street
Dublin 7
Ireland

Email: darramurphy@me.com

Emanuele Neri, MD
Department of Oncology
Diagnostic and Interventional Radiology, Transplants, and Advanced Technologies in Medicine
University of Pisa
Via Roma 67
56126 Pisa
Italy
Email: neri@med.unipi.it

Piotr R. Obara, MD
Department of Radiology
The University of Chicago
5841 South Maryland Avenue
Chicago, IL 60645
USA

Ayodale S. Odulate, MD
Department of Radiology
Brigham and Women's Hospital
Harvard Medical School
75 Francis Street
Boston, MA 02115
USA
Email: ajohnson16@partners.org

Alan O'Hare
Department of Radiology
Mater Misericordiae University Hospital
Eccles Street
Dublin, 7
Ireland

M. Raquel Oliva, MD, PhD
Abdominal Imaging and Intervention Section
Brigham and Women's Hospital
Harvard Medical School
75 Francis Street
Boston, MA 02115
USA
Email: moliva@partners.org

P. Pokieser, MD
Department of Radiology
Medical University of Vienna
Waehringer Guertel 18-20
1090 Vienna
Austria

W Schima, MD
Department of Radiology
Medical University of Vienna
Waehringer Guertel 18-20
1090 Vienna
Austria

Jaap Stoker, MD, PhD
Department of Radiology
Academic Medical Center
University of Amsterdam
Meibergdreef 9
1105 AZ Amsterdam
The Netherlands
Email: j.stoker@amc.uva.nl

Stuart A. Taylor, MD, MRCP, FRCR
Department of Imaging
University College Hospital
2F Podium, 235 Euston Road
London NW1 2BU
UK
Email: csytaylor@yahoo.co.uk

Francesca Turini, MD
Department of Oncology
Diagnostic and Interventional Radiology,
Transplants, and Advanced Technologies in Medicine
University of Pisa
Via Roma 67
56100 Pisa
Italy

Kaori Uchida, MD
Diagnostic RadiologyDivision
National Cancer Center Hospital
1-1 Tsukiji 5-chome
Chuo-ku, Tokyo
Japan

Judy Yee, MD
University of California San Francisco
San Francisco VA Medical Center
4150 Clement Street
San Francisco, CA 94121
USA
Email: Judy.Yee@med.va.gov

Hiroyuki Yoshida, PhD
Department of Radiology
Massachusetts General Hospital
75 Blossom Court
Boston, MA 02114
USA
Harvard Medical School, Boston, MA 02114, USA

Email: yoshida@uchicago.edu

Michael E. Zalis, MD
Department of Radiology
Massachusetts General Hospital
55 Fruit Street
Boston, MA 02114
USA

Email: mzalis@partners.org

Medical Radiology Diagnostic Imaging and Radiation Oncology

Titles in the series already published

Diagnostic Imaging

Radiological Imaging of Sports Injuries
Edited by C. Masciocchi

Modern Imaging of the Alimentary Tube
Edited by A. R. Margulis

Diagnosis and Therapy of Spinal Tumors
Edited by P. R. Algra, J. Valk and J. J. Heimans

Interventional Magnetic Resonance Imaging
Edited by J. F. Debatin and G. Adam

Abdominal and Pelvic MRI
Edited by A. Heuck and M. Reiser

Orthopedic Imaging
Techniques and Applications
Edited by A. M. Davies and H. Pettersson

Radiology of the Female Pelvic Organs
Edited by E. K. Lang

Magnetic Resonance of the Heart and Great Vessels
Clinical Applications
Edited by J. Bogaert, A. J. Duerinckx, and F. E. Rademakers

Modern Head and Neck Imaging
Edited by S. K. Mukherji and J. A. Castelijns

Radiological Imaging of Endocrine Diseases
Edited by J. N. Bruneton in collaboration with B. Padovani and M.-Y. Mourou

Radiology of the Pancreas
2nd Revised Edition
Edited by A. L. Baert. Co-edited by G. Delorme and L. Van Hoe

Trends in Contrast Media
Edited by H. S. Thomsen, R. N. Muller, and R. F. Mattrey

Functional MRI
Edited by C. T. W. Moonen and P. A. Bandettini

Emergency Pediatric Radiology
Edited by H. Carty

Liver Malignancies
Diagnostic and Interventional Radiology
Edited by C. Bartolozzi and R. Lencioni

Spiral CT of the Abdomen
Edited by F. Terrier, M. Grossholz, and C. D. Becker

Medical Imaging of the Spleen
Edited by A. M. De Schepper and F. Vanhoenacker

Radiology of Peripheral Vascular Diseases
Edited by E. Zeitler

Radiology of Blunt Trauma of the Chest
P. Schnyder and M. Wintermark

Portal Hypertension
Diagnostic Imaging and Imaging-Guided Therapy
Edited by P. Rossi.
Co-edited by P. Ricci and L. Broglia

Virtual Endoscopy and Related 3D Techniques
Edited by P. Rogalla, J. Terwisscha van Scheltinga and B. Hamm

Recent Advances in Diagnostic Neuroradiology
Edited by Ph. Demaerel

Transfontanellar Doppler Imaging in Neonates
A. Couture, C. Veyrac

Radiology of AIDS
A Practical Approach
Edited by J. W. A. J. Reeders and P. C. Goodman

CT of the Peritoneum
A. Rossi, G. Rossi

Magnetic Resonance Angiography
2nd Revised Edition
Edited by I. P. Arlart, G. M. Bongartz, and G. Marchal

Applications of Sonography in Head and Neck Pathology
Edited by J. N. Bruneton in collaboration with C. Raffaelli, O. Dassonville

3D Image Processing
Techniques and Clinical Applications
Edited by D. Caramella and C. Bartolozzi

Imaging of the Larynx
Edited by R. Hermans

Pediatric ENT Radiology
Edited by S. J. King and A. E. Boothroyd

Imaging of Orbital and Visual Pathway Pathology
Edited by W. S. Müller-Forell

Radiological Imaging of the Small Intestine
Edited by N. C. Gourtsoyiannis

Imaging of the Knee
Techniques and Applications
Edited by A. M. Davies and V. N. Cassar-Pullicino

Perinatal Imaging
From Ultrasound to MR Imaging
Edited by F. E. Avni

Diagnostic and Interventional Radiology in Liver Transplantation
Edited by E. Bücheler, V. Nicolas, C. E. Broelsch, X. Rogiers and G. Krupski

Imaging of the Pancreas
Cystic and Rare Tumors
Edited by C. Procacci and A. J. Megibow

Imaging of the Foot & Ankle
Techniques and Applications
Edited by A. M. Davies, R. W. Whitehouse and J. P. R. Jenkins

Radiological Imaging of the Ureter
Edited by F. Joffre, Ph. Otal and M. Soulie

Radiology of the Petrous Bone
Edited by M. Lemmerling and S. S. Kollias

Imaging of the Shoulder
Techniques and Applications
Edited by A. M. Davies and J. Hodler

Interventional Radiology in Cancer
Edited by A. Adam, R. F. Dondelinger, and P. R. Mueller

Imaging and Intervention in Abdominal Trauma
Edited by R. F. Dondelinger

Radiology of the Pharynx and the Esophagus
Edited by O. Ekberg

Radiological Imaging in Hematological Malignancies
Edited by A. Guermazi

Functional Imaging of the Chest
Edited by H.-U. Kauczor

Duplex and Color Doppler Imaging of the Venous System
Edited by G. H. Mostbeck

Multidetector-Row CT of the Thorax
Edited by U. J. Schoepf

Radiology and Imaging of the Colon
Edited by A. H. Chapman

Multidetector-Row CT Angiography
Edited by C. Catalano and R. Passariello

Focal Liver Lesions
Detection, Characterization, Ablation
Edited by R. Lencioni, D. Cioni, and C. Bartolozzi

Imaging in Treatment Planning for Sinonasal Diseases
Edited by R. Maroldi and P. Nicolai

Clinical Cardiac MRI
With Interactive CD-ROM
Edited by J. Bogaert, S. Dymarkowski, and A. M. Taylor

Dynamic Contrast-Enhanced Magnetic Resonance Imaging in Oncology
Edited by A. Jackson, D. L. Buckley, and G. J. M. Parker

Contrast Media in Ultrasonography
Basic Principles and Clinical Applications
Edited by E. Quaia

Paediatric Musculoskeletal Disease
With an Emphasis on Ultrasound
Edited by D. Wilson

MR Imaging in White Matter Diseases of the Brain and Spinal Cord
Edited by M. Filippi, N. De Stefano, V. Dousset, and J. C. McGowan

Imaging of the Hip & Bony Pelvis
Techniques and Applications
Edited by A. M. Davies, K. Johnson, and R. W. Whitehouse

Imaging of Kidney Cancer
Edited by A. Guermazi

Magnetic Resonance Imaging in Ischemic Stroke
Edited by R. von Kummer and T. Back

Diagnostic Nuclear Medicine
2nd Revised Edition
Edited by C. Schiepers

Imaging of Occupational and Environmental Disorders of the Chest
Edited by P. A. Gevenois and P. De Vuyst

Virtual Colonoscopy
A Practical Guide
Edited by P. Lefere and S. Gryspeerdt

Contrast Media
Safety Issues and ESUR Guidelines
Edited by H. S. Thomsen

Head and Neck Cancer Imaging
Edited by R. Hermans

Vascular Embolotherapy
A Comprehensive Approach
Volume 1: *General Principles, Chest, Abdomen, and Great Vessels*
Edited by J. Golzarian. Co-edited by S. Sun and M. J. Sharafuddin

Vascular Embolotherapy
A Comprehensive Approach
Volume 2: *Oncology, Trauma, Gene Therapy, Vascular Malformations, and Neck*
Edited by J. Golzarian.
Co-edited by S. Sun and M. J. Sharafuddin

Vascular Interventional Radiology
Current Evidence in Endovascular Surgery
Edited by M. G. Cowling

Ultrasound of the Gastrointestinal Tract
Edited by G. Maconi and G. Bianchi Porro

Parallel Imaging in Clinical MR Applications
Edited by S. O. Schoenberg, O. Dietrich, and M. F. Reiser

MRI and CT of the Female Pelvis
Edited by B. Hamm and R. Forstner

Imaging of Orthopedic Sports Injuries
Edited by F. M. Vanhoenacker, M. Maas and J. L. Gielen

Ultrasound of the Musculoskeletal System
S. Bianchi and C. Martinoli

Clinical Functional MRI
Presurgical Functional Neuroimaging
Edited by C. Stippich

Radiation Dose from Adult and Pediatric Multidetector Computed Tomography
Edited by D. Tack and P. A. Gevenois

Spinal Imaging
Diagnostic Imaging of the Spine and Spinal Cord
Edited by J. Van Goethem, L. van den Hauwe and P. M. Parizel

Computed Tomography of the Lung
A Pattern Approach
J. A. Verschakelen and W. De Wever

Imaging in Transplantation
Edited by A. Bankier

Radiological Imaging of the Neonatal Chest
2nd Revised Edition
Edited by V. Donoghue

Radiological Imaging of the Digestive Tract in Infants and Children
Edited by A. S. Devos and J. G. Blickman

Pediatric Chest Imaging
Chest Imaging in Infants and Children
2nd Revised Edition
Edited by J. Lucaya and J. L. Strife

Color Doppler US of the Penis
Edited by M. Bertolotto

Radiology of the Stomach and Duodenum
Edited by A. H. Freeman and E. Sala

Imaging in Pediatric Skeletal Trauma
Techniques and Applications
Edited by K. J. Johnson and E. Bache

Image Processing in Radiology
Current Applications
Edited by E. Neri, D. Caramella, C. Bartolozzi

Screening and Preventive Diagnosis with Radiological Imaging
Edited by M. F. Reiser, G. van Kaick, C. Fink, S. O. Schoenberg

Percutaneous Tumor Ablation in Medical Radiology
Edited by T. J. Vogl, T. K. Helmberger, M. G. Mack, M. F. Reiser

Liver Radioembolization with ^{90}Y Microspheres
Edited by J. I. Bilbao, M. F. Reiser

Pediatric Uroradiology
2nd Revised Edition
Edited by R. Fotter

Radiology of Osteoporosis
2nd Revised Edition
Edited by S. Grampp

Gastrointestinal Tract Sonography in Fetuses and Children
A. Couture, C. Baud, J. L. Ferran, M. Saguintaah and C. Veyrac

Intracranial Vascular Malformations and Aneurysms
2nd Revised Edition
Edited by M. Forsting and I. Wanke

High-Resolution Sonography of the Peripheral Nervous System
2nd Revised Edition
Edited by S. Peer and G. Bodner

Imaging Pelvic Floor Disorders
2nd Revised Edition
Edited by J. Stoker, S. A. Taylor, andJ. O. L. DeLancey

Coronary Radiology
2nd Revised Edition
Edited by M. Oudkerk and M. F. Reiser

Integrated Cardiothoracic Imaging with MDCT
Edited by M. Rémy-Jardin and J. Rémy

Multislice CT
3rd Revised Edition
Edited by M. F. Reiser, C. R. Becker, K. Nikolaou, G. Glazer

MRI of the Lung
Edited by H.-U. Kauczor

Imaging in Percutaneous Musculoskeletal Interventions
Edited by A. Gangi, S. Guth, and A. Guermazi

Contrast Media. Safety Issues and ESUR Guidelines
2nd Revised Edition
Edited by H. Thomsen, J.A.W. Webb

Inflammatory Diseases of the Brain
Edited by S. Hähnel

Imaging of Bone Tumors and Tumor-Like Lesions - Techniques and Applications
Edited by A.M. Davies, M. Sundaram, and S.J. James

MR Angiography of the body
Technique and Clinical Applications
Edited by E. Neri, M. Cosottini and D. Caramella

Virtual Colonoscopy
A Practical Guide
Edited by P. Lefere and S. Gryspeerdt

Diffusion-Weighted MR Imaging
Applications in the Body
Edited by D.-M. Koh and H.C. Thoeny

MRI of the Gastroinestinal Tract
Edited by J. Stoker

Digital Mammography
Edited by U. Bick and F. Diekmann

Springer

MEDICAL RADIOLOGY Diagnostic Imaging and Radiation Oncology

Titles in the series already published

RADIATION ONCOLOGY

Lung Cancer
Edited by C. W. Scarantino

Innovations in Radiation Oncology
Edited by H. R. Withers and L. J. Peters

Radiation Therapy of Head and Neck Cancer
Edited by G. E. Laramore

Gastrointestinal Cancer – Radiation Therapy
Edited by R. R. Dobelbower, Jr.

Radiation Exposure and Occupational Risks
Edited by E. Scherer, C. Streffer, and K.-R. Trott

Interventional Radiation
Therapy Techniques – Brachytherapy
Edited by R. Sauer

Radiopathology of Organs and Tissues
Edited by E. Scherer, C. Streffer, and K.-R. Trott

Concomitant Continuous Infusion
Chemotherapy and Radiation
Edited by M. Rotman and C. J. Rosenthal

Intraoperative Radiotherapy – Clinical Experiences and Results
Edited by F. A. Calvo, M. Santos, and L. W. Brady

Interstitial and Intracavitary Thermoradiotherapy
Edited by M. H. Seegenschmiedt and R. Sauer

Non-Disseminated Breast Cancer
Controversial Issues in Management
Edited by G. H. Fletcher and S. H. Levitt

Current Topics in Clinical Radiobiology of Tumors
Edited by H.-P. Beck-Bornholdt

Practical Approaches to Cancer Invasion and Metastases
A Compendium of Radiation Oncologists' Responses to 40 Histories
Edited by A. R. Kagan with the Assistance of R. J. Steckel

Radiation Therapy in Pediatric Oncology
Edited by J. R. Cassady

Radiation Therapy Physics
Edited by A. R. Smith

Late Sequelae in Oncology
Edited by J. Dunst, R. Sauer

Mediastinal Tumors. Update 1995
Edited by D. E. Wood, C. R. Thomas, Jr.

Thermoradiotherapy and Thermochemotherapy
Volume 1: *Biology, Physiology, and Physics*

Volume 2: *Clinical Applications*
Edited by M. H. Seegenschmiedt, P. Fessenden and C. C. Vernon

Carcinoma of the Prostate
Innovations in Management
Edited by Z. Petrovich, L. Baert, and L. W. Brady

Radiation Oncology of Gynecological Cancers
Edited by H. W. Vahrson

Carcinoma of the Bladder
Innovations in Management
Edited by Z. Petrovich, L. Baert, and L. W. Brady

Blood Perfusion and Microenvironment of Human Tumors
Implications for Clinical Radiooncology
Edited by M. Molls and P. Vaupel

Radiation Therapy of Benign Diseases
A Clinical Guide
2nd Revised Edition
S. E. Order and S. S. Donaldson

Carcinoma of the Kidney and Testis, and Rare Urologic Malignancies
Innovations in Management
Edited by Z. Petrovich, L. Baert, and L. W. Brady

Progress and Perspectives in the Treatment of Lung Cancer
Edited by P. Van Houtte, J. Klastersky, and P. Rocmans

Combined Modality Therapy of Central Nervous System Tumors
Edited by Z. Petrovich, L. W. Brady, M. L. Apuzzo, and M. Bamberg

Age-Related Macular Degeneration
Current Treatment Concepts
Edited by W. E. Alberti, G. Richard, and R. H. Sagerman

Radiotherapy of Intraocular and Orbital Tumors
2nd Revised Edition
Edited by R. H. Sagerman and W. E. Alberti

Modification of Radiation Response
Cytokines, Growth Factors, and Other Biolgical Targets
Edited by C. Nieder, L. Milas and K. K. Ang

Radiation Oncology for Cure and Palliation
R. G. Parker, N. A. Janjan and M. T. Selch

Clinical Target Volumes in Conformal and Intensity Modulated Radiation Therapy
A Clinical Guide to Cancer Treatment
Edited by V. Grégoire, P. Scalliet, and K. K. Ang

Advances in Radiation Oncology in Lung Cancer
Edited by B. Jeremi´c

New Technologies in Radiation Oncology
Edited by W. Schlegel, T. Bortfeld, and A.-L. Grosu

Multimodal Concepts for Integration of Cytotoxic Drugs and Radiation Therapy
Edited by J. M. Brown, M. P. Mehta, and C. Nieder

Technical Basis of Radiation Therapy
Practical Clinical Applications
4th Revised Edition
Edited by S. H. Levitt, J. A. Purdy, C. A. Perez, and S. Vijayakumar

CURED I • LENT
Late Effects of Cancer Treatment on Normal Tissues
Edited by P. Rubin, L. S. Constine, L. B. Marks, and P. Okunieff

Radiotherapy for Non-Malignant Disorders
Contemporary Concepts and Clinical Results
Edited by M. H. Seegenschmiedt, H.-B. Makoski, K.-R. Trott, and L. W. Brady

CURED II • LENT
Cancer Survivorship Research and Education
Late Effects on Normal Tissues
Edited by P. Rubin, L. S. Constine, L. B. Marks, and P. Okunieff

Radiation Oncology
An Evidence-Based Approach
Edited by J. J. Lu and L. W. Brady

Primary Optic Nerve Sheath Meningioma
Edited by B. Jeremi´c, and S. Pitz

Function Preservation and Quality Life in Head and Neck Radiotherapy
Edited by P.M. Harari, N.P. Connor, and C. Grau

Nasopharyngeal Cancer
Edited by J.J. Lu, J.S. Cooper and A.W.M. Lee

Springer

Printing and Binding: Stürtz GmbH, Würzburg